Senotherapeutics

This book provides a comprehensive overview of the emerging field of senotherapeutics and its potential applications in various diseases. The initial chapter elucidates the central role of cellular senescence and the senescence-associated secretory phenotype (SASP) in the intricate balance between health and disease. The subsequent chapter examines the origin of senotherapeutics, introducing the concepts of senolytics and senomorphics for combating senescence and its associated disorders. The book also focuses on the potential of senotherapeutics in managing neurological disorders and neurodegenerative diseases. Furthermore, it investigates the intersection of senotherapeutics with cancer therapy, shedding light on innovative treatments and their role against cancer. It also discusses the broader role of senotherapeutics in aging and its associated disorders such as osteoporosis and osteoarthritis, offering insights into their implications for geriatric medicine. The book reviews the novel application of senotherapeutics in skincare and dermatological diseases, as well as metabolic disorders. This book is intended for researchers in the fields of biomedicine, pharmacology, and gerontology, as well as healthcare professionals.

Key Features

- Offers a comprehensive exploration of senotherapeutics, spanning various diseases and conditions, providing a holistic understanding of its potential applications.
- Provides a conceptual framework for cellular senescence and the senescence-associated secretory phenotype (SASP) and their relevance to health and disease.
- Examines the potential of senotherapeutics in addressing neurological disorders, neurodegenerative diseases, and cancer therapy.
- Explores the broader role of senotherapeutics in the context of aging and associated disorders such as osteoarthritis and osteoporosis.
- Reviews the application of senotherapeutics in skincare and dermatological concerns, as well as metabolic disorders.

Senotherapeutics

From Cellular Senescence to Disease Management

Edited by
Razia Khanam and Divya Vohora

CRC Press
Taylor & Francis Group
Boca Raton London New York

CRC Press is an imprint of the
Taylor & Francis Group, an **informa** business

Designed cover image: Razia Khanam

First edition published 2026
by CRC Press
2385 NW Executive Center Drive, Suite 320, Boca Raton FL 33431

and by CRC Press
4 Park Square, Milton Park, Abingdon, Oxon, OX14 4RN

CRC Press is an imprint of Taylor & Francis Group, LLC

ISBN: 978-1-032-79808-0 (hbk)
ISBN: 978-1-032-79809-7 (pbk)
ISBN: 978-1-003-49396-9 (ebk)

DOI: 10.1201/9781003493969

Typeset in Times New Roman
by Apex CoVantage, LLC

Contents

Preface

The rapid advancements in the fascinating field of cellular senescence and senolytics, combined with its growing translational value in recent medicine, has urged me to initiate writing a book that could serve both as a foundation and a clinical reference. However, it was during a casual yet inspiring metro ride through Dubai with Dr. Divya Vohora that this long-cherished vision took shape. From our informal conversations to specific literature review, we finalized the idea of writing and editing a book that may bridge the gap between the basic principles and clinical applications of serotherapy.

Senotherapeutics: From Cellular Senescence to Disease Management is the result of our initiative and its implementation. As editors and contributors, we have worked collaboratively with a team of authors to create a resource that covers both basics and clinical relevance. The book includes basic principles of cellular senescence and its role in different diseases/disorders and presents updated clinical insights, and emerging prospects. Starting from the origin of senotherapeutics to their role in various diseases/disorders including aging and age-related disorders, bone disorders, cancer, diabetes, lung disorders, neurological and various skin conditions, as well as a discussion on challenges that lie ahead, this book is a comprehensive resource for researchers, students, and professionals interested to work on senotherapeutics as exciting possibilities for future treatments. In this rapidly evolving field, we sincerely hope that this book serves as a useful and inspirational resource for the journey ahead.

About the Editors

Razia Khanam holds both an M.Pharm. and a Ph.D. degree from Jamia Hamdard University, New Delhi, India. Currently positioned as a professor specializing in pharmacology at Gulf Medical University in Ajman, UAE, she boasts an extensive tenure of 23 years in the realms of teaching and research. Her scholarly contributions have garnered significant attention, amassing over 1110 citations. She also holds the distinction of being an esteemed member of the editorial boards of various renowned journals. Her accomplishments further encompass accolades such as the 1999 Gold Medal from Jamia Hamdard and the Career Award for Young Scientists conferred by the All-India Council for Technical Education (AICTE).

Divya Vohora holds the position of Professor of Pharmacology in the School of Pharmaceutical Education and Research (SPER) at Jamia Hamdard University, New Delhi. With over 25 years of teaching and research experience, she has served in various roles such as head of the Department for Pharmacology, assistant dean for student's welfare, director of the Department of Distance and Online Learning (DODL), and in-charge of Pharmaceutical Medicine (a collaborative doctoral program with Sun Pharmaceuticals). She has published more than 200 research articles in both national and international journals of high repute and has authored and edited five books. She has earned prestigious fellowships throughout her career. She is an Elected Fellow of the National Academy of Medical Sciences (FAMS) in India, a Fellow of the Indian Pharmacological Society (FIPS), a Fellow of the British Pharmacological Society (FBPhS), and a Fellow of the Royal Society of Biology in the UK (FRSB). She has received numerous awards in recognition of her outstanding work, including the Dr. B. K. Anand Oration Award, the Dr. Vinod Kumar Bhargava Award from the National Academy of Medical Sciences (NAMS), the Distinguished Woman Scientist Award from the ISCB, the Dr. D. N. Prasad Memorial Oration Award from ICMR, the Career Award for Young Teachers from AICTE, and the Fast Track Award for Young Scientists from DST, Government of India, among others. She also plays an active role on the international stage, serving as a member of the International Advisory Group of the

British Pharmacological Society in the UK and as an expert member evaluating research grants submitted to institutions like the National Science Centre in Poland and the La Caixa Foundation in Spain. Her primary areas of research interest are in neuropharmacology, with a particular focus on epilepsy, neurodegenerative diseases (including Alzheimer's disease), and their associated co-morbidities including bone diseases.

Contributors

Aftab Ahmad
Health Information Technology Department
The Applied College, King Abdulaziz University
Jeddah, Saudi Arabia
Pharmacovigilance and Medication Safety Unit, Center of Research Excellence for Drug Research and Pharmaceutical Industries
King Abdulaziz University
Jeddah, Saudi Arabia

Aleeta Maria Jolly
Department of Pharmacology, Amrita School of Pharmacy
Amrita Vishwa Vidyapeetham
Ponekkara, 682041, Kochi, India

Anjana Krishna
Department of Pharmacology, Amrita School of Pharmacy
Amrita Vishwa Vidyapeetham
Ponekkara, 682041, Kochi, India

Anwar A. Alghamdi
Health Information Technology Department
The Applied College, King Abdulaziz University
Jeddah, Saudi Arabia
Pharmacovigilance and Medication Safety Unit, Center of Research Excellence for Drug Research and Pharmaceutical Industries
King Abdulaziz University
Jeddah, Saudi Arabia

Asif Husain
Department of Pharmaceutical Chemistry
School of Pharmaceutical Education and Research
Jamia Hamdard
New Delhi, India

Divya Vohora
Department of Pharmacology
School of Pharmaceutical Education and Research (SPER)
Jamia Hamdard
New Delhi, India

Faraha Ahmed
Department of Pharmacology
School of Pharmaceutical Education and Research
Jamia Hamdard
New Delhi, India

Gurpreet Kaur
Department of Pharmaceutics
School of Pharmaceutical Sciences

Delhi Pharmaceutical Sciences and Research University
New Delhi, India

Ishita Kakkar
Department of Pharmacy Practice
SGT College of Pharmacy
SGT University
Gurugram, Haryana, India

Jaya Thomas
Department of Pharmacology
Amrita School of Pharmacy
Amrita Vishwa Vidyapeetham
Ponekkara, Kochi, India

Mansha Jain
Department of Pharmaceutics
Adina Institute of Pharmaceutical Sciences
Sagar, Madhya Pradesh, India

Mintu Mathew
Department of Pharmacology
Amrita School of Pharmacy
Amrita Vishwa Vidyapeetham
Ponekkara, Kochi, India

Mohammad Jaffar Sadiq Mantargi
Department of Pharmaceutical Sciences
Pharmacy Program, Batterjee Medical College
Jeddah, Saudi Arabia

Mohit Agarwal
Department of Pharmacology
Amrita School of Pharmacy
Amrita Vishwa Vidyapeetham
Ponekkara, Kochi, India

Muhammad Afzal
Department of Pharmaceutical Sciences
Pharmacy Program
Batterjee Medical College
Jeddah, Saudi Arabia

Neha Sharma
Neurobehavioral Pharmacology Laboratory
Department of Pharmacology
School of Pharmaceutical Education and Research
Jamia Hamdard, New Delhi, India

Razia Khanam
Prof. Razia Khanam
Department of Biomedical Sciences
College of Medicine
Gulf Medical University
Ajman, United Arab Emirates

Saima Zameer
Department of Neurodegenerative Science
Van Andel Institute
Grand Rapids, MI
United States of America

Saurabh Mittal
Centre of Pharmaceutics
Amity Institute of Pharmacy
Amity University
Noida, Uttar Pradesh, India

Shah Alam Khan
Department of Pharmaceutical Chemistry
College of Pharmacy
National University of Science and Technology
Bousher, Muscat, Oman

Shreshta Jain
Neurobehavioral Pharmacology Laboratory
Department of Pharmacology
School of Pharmaceutical Education and Research
Jamia Hamdard, New Delhi, India

Sonal Setya
Department of Pharmacy Practice
SGT College of Pharmacy

SGT University
Gurugram, Haryana, India

Sushama Talegaonkar
Department of Pharmaceutics
School of Pharmaceutical Sciences
Delhi Pharmaceutical Sciences and Research University
New Delhi, India

Syed Sufian Ahmad
Department of Pharmacology
School Pharmaceutical Education and Research
Jamia Hamdard, New Delhi, India

Vaishali Yadav
Department of Pharmacology
Adina Institute of Pharmaceutical Sciences
Sagar, Madhya Pradesh, India

Vivek Jain
Department of Pharmaceutics
Adina Institute of Pharmaceutical Sciences
Sagar, Madhya Pradesh, India

Yashasvi Sharma
Centre of Pharmaceutics
Amity Institute of Pharmacy
Amity University
Noida, Uttar Pradesh, India

Chapter 1

Origin of Senotherapeutics

Senolytics and Senomorphics

Vaishali Yadav, Mansha Jain, Vivek Jain, and Divya Vohora

Abbreviations

AD: Alzheimer's disease; Aβ: amyloid beta; BBB: blood-brain barrier; CDK: cyclin-dependent kinase; GM-CSF: granulocyte-macrophage colony-stimulating factor; HDACs: histone deacetylases; HIF-1: hypoxia-inducible factor; HNSCC: head and neck squamous cell carcinoma; IL-6: interleukin 6; IL-8: interleukin 8; IL-1α: interleukin 1-alpha; IL-1R: interleukin-1 receptor; MMPs: metalloproteinases; mTOR: mammalian target of rapamycin; NF-κB: nuclear factor-κB; NFTs: neurofibrillary tangles; p38 MAPK: p38 mitogen-activated protein kinase; PD: Parkinson's disease; RB: retinoblastoma protein; ROS: reactive oxygen species; SA-β-gal: senescence-associated β-galactosidase; SASP: senescence-associated secretory phenotype; SCAP: senescent cell anti-apoptotic pathway; SenCells: senescent cells; SenHCPAPCells: senescent human cultured primary adipocyte progenitor cells; SenHUVECell: senescent cultured human umbilical vein endothelial cells; TGN: translational geroscience network.

1.1 INTRODUCTION

Senescent cells (SenCells) gradually proliferate in many tissues as people age. The process of cellular senescence seems diverse and influenced by environmental, genetic, and epigenetic variables. Numerous factors, including diminution of telomeric length, radiation-induced genome injury, oncogene induction, and mitochondrial malfunction along with endoplasmic reticulum stress, can cause senescence. Broadly, two types of senescence are addressed in relevance to physiology: stress-associated preterm senescence and replicative senescence (Toussaint et al. 2002). The Hayflick limit, sometimes referred to as replicative senescence, was initially discovered in human primary fibroblasts, which cease to divide after several divisions. Telomeric DNA shortening is a result of this kind of cellular senescence. Numerous internal and external causes, including oxidative stress, ionizing radiation, genotoxic stress, neoplastic transformation, and different infections, can lead to stress-associated preterm senescence

DOI: 10.1201/9781003493969-1

(Campisi 1997; Debacq-Chainiaux et al. 2016). The aging process can affect nearby cells in a positive or negative way. On one hand, the process of senescence is essential for preventing unchecked cell division. For instance, senescent cell buildup in aging plays a crucial role in the anti-oncogene system, an aberrant cell cycle state which inhibits malignant cell growth and oncogenic formation. However, numerous recent reports have also revealed cellular decline may trigger a number of harmful processes, including organismal aging, immunological surveillance, and chronic inflammation. SenCells create a senescence-associated secretory phenotype (SASP) which includes cytokines that promote inflammation, biologically active lipids, and other elements which process the autocrine and paracrine action of SenCells, despite growth suppression. Furthermore, age-related illnesses and chronic inflammation can be brought on by these variables. These stimuli raise senescence-associated β-galactosidase (SA-β-gal) activity, cause cell cycle arrest, activate senescence-associated signalling pathways, and have a paracrine effect on nearby young cells. SenCells have reduced reactivity towards exogenous cues, including aberrant morphology, growth hormones, and dysfunctional mitochondria. SenCells are flattened, metabolically active, and vacuolate. Moreover, accumulating lipofuscin and the absence of lamin A/B have been connected to SenCells (Childs et al. 2015; de Magalhães et al. 2018; Warner 1999; Van Deursen 2014).

Targeting the negative effects of cellular senescence therapeutically has been the focus of a lot of recent studies. Neurodegenerative disease, ocular degenerative disease, coronary artery disease, cartilage degeneration, eye diseases, carcinogenesis, hypertrophy of the heart, impaired renal function, lipodystrophy, and sarcopenia have all been demonstrated to be improved by senolysis in animal models of disease. In addition to extending health span, senolysis further improves average rodent longevity. Such senescence-associated diseases have been found to improve when senotherapeutics, a class of pharmaceutical interventions, target SenCells. Three development methodologies can be applied to senotherapeutics:

1. Senolytics remove SenCells on a selective basis.
2. Senomorphics slow down the transition of young cells into SenCells or cause SenCells to adopt the shape and activities of youthful cells.
3. The abolition of SenCells is mediated through immunotherapeutics that target SenCells (Zhang et al. 2023; Niedernhofer and Robbins 2018; Raffaele and Vinciguerra 2022).

In this chapter, we will explore the origins of senotherapeutics, tracing the journey from initial scientific observations to the development of targeted therapies. We will delve into the key discoveries that highlight the development of the first senolytic, examining the pioneering research that paved the way for therapeutic interventions, and will discuss the evolving strategies aimed at selectively eliminating or modulating SenCells. By understanding the origin and development of senotherapeutics, we can appreciate the potential of these innovative treatments to transform healthcare and improve the quality of life for aging populations. This chapter will provide a comprehensive overview of the scientific breakthroughs, disputes, and foresight in the field of senotherapeutics, setting a stage for a deeper understanding of this promising area of medical research.

1.2 FOUNDATION OF SENESCENCE

Weismann's 1881 essay "The Duration of Life" presented a groundbreaking idea for its time, suggesting that aging and death are tied to the finite capacity of cells to divide and renew themselves. He proposed that as tissues wear out and cells reach their limit of division, organisms inevitably age and eventually die (Joshi 2023). This concept lay dormant until 1961, when Leonard Hayflick's research provided empirical evidence supporting the notion of a restricted extent for cellular proliferation in mammalian cells. Hayflick's experiments demonstrated that normal mammalian cells are capable of splitting a certain number of times before ceasing division and entering a state known as cellular senescence. This situation, known as the "Hayflick limit", marked a pivotal moment in understanding the cellular basis of aging. It confirmed Weismann's earlier theoretical assertion that aging is linked to cellular processes and limitations. Today, the concept of the Hayflick limit remains a cornerstone in the study of aging and has significant implications in understanding age-linked ailments and potential avenues for extending healthy lifespan (Rattan 2016).

This concept of Weismann and Hayflick derives a common conclusion that the decline of the non-dividing cells' capacity to support tissue repair is a hallmark of aging tissue. Further, the discovery of a different class of non-dividing cells, known today as SenCells, caused by cellular stress posed a threat for distinct reasons. SenCells impair regular tissue performance through producing substances that draw in inflamed cells, alter the extracellular matrix, induce unintended cell destruction, create fibrosis, and prevent stem cell activity, in addition to their incapacity to proliferate and assist in tissue repair. These SenCells are intimately associated with the signs of natural aging as they expand gradually and harm the cellular system they dwell in (Kameda et al. 2021).

1.3 SCREENING AND RECOGNITION OF SENCELLS

Hayflick and Moorehead illustrated in 1961 that mammalian cell culture has a restricted capacity for replication. Most cultured cells eventually lose their ability to divide, but they nonetheless stay viable and engaged in metabolism after about 50 divisions. It was believed that the decrease in tissue repair and cell replacement that comes with aging was caused by this limited proliferative potential, which is now known as replicative senescence.

The identification of SenCells in experimental animals was initially facilitated through identifying enzymatic activity that was enriched in SenCells. Specifically, β-galactosidase exhibits a peak enzymatic action at around pH 6 in SenCells, while more commonly found β-galactosidase isoforms peak around pH 4. Such β-galactosidase action is now known as SA-β-gal. This realisation made it possible to create a straightforward colorimetric assay that is currently widely used for senescent cell labelling and detection (Faragher 2021; Gasek et al. 2021).

Furthermore, intracellular lipofuscin accumulation, $p16^{Ink4a}$ (a CDK blocker that works as a key controller of cell cycle halt in SenCells) and p19ARF-associated regulation of the transcription factor p53 were recognised as attributes for SenCells, contributing a crucial in vivo indicator of SenCells (Kamal et al. 2020).

1.3.1 Significant Traits of SenCells

SenCells possesses the following characteristics:

1. *Engagement in a permanent cell cycle arrest*: CDK2, CDK4, and CDK6 are inhibited by the activation of the p53-p21 and $p16^{Ink4a}$ cell cycle stall circuits in the aftermath of pro-senescence stressors such as ROS formation, genome injury, and others. Thus, the under-phosphorylated form of RB inhibits the production of S-phase transcripts by adhering to and retaining the transcription factors E2F, DP1, and DP2, and additionally attracting HDACs which communicate with heterochromatin (Kumari and Parmjit 2021).
2. *Resistance to cell death signalling*: SenCells refrain from mitochondria-associated programmed cell death (PCD) via upregulating B cell lymphoma 2 components; these components adhere as well as tether BAX and BCL-2 related agonist of cell death. Such tethering prevents BAX and BCL-2 related agonist of cell death from forming pores, which prevents the expulsion of pro-apoptotic cytochrome c, second mitochondria-derived activator of caspase, as well as mitochondrial outer membrane permeabilization. SenCells further inhibit extrinsic apoptosis via over-expressing decoy receptor 2; they seem to silence FAS ligand encoded on cytotoxic immune cells (Di Micco et al. 2021; Hu et al. 2022).
3. *Secretion of a biologically activated secretome, referred to as SASP*: SenCells produce dynamic and bioactive secretome. SASP formation begins and is carried on through chronic DNA damage response (DDR) referred to as "DNA-SCARS" (DNA segments with chromatin alterations reinforcing senescence). Notch signalling regulates TGF-β secretion (can be referred to as "early SASP"), which works through a cell-autonomous process to instigate cell cycle halt. A further decrement in the Notch pathway stimulates a transfer to a DDR-dependent "transitional SASP", which is amplified by mTOR, where cell surface–mediated IL-1α integrates with IL-1R. Subsequently, IL-1α signal or p38 MAPK action travels via NF-κB, leading to production of a "late SASP" that encompasses MMPs, IL-6, and IL-8 apart

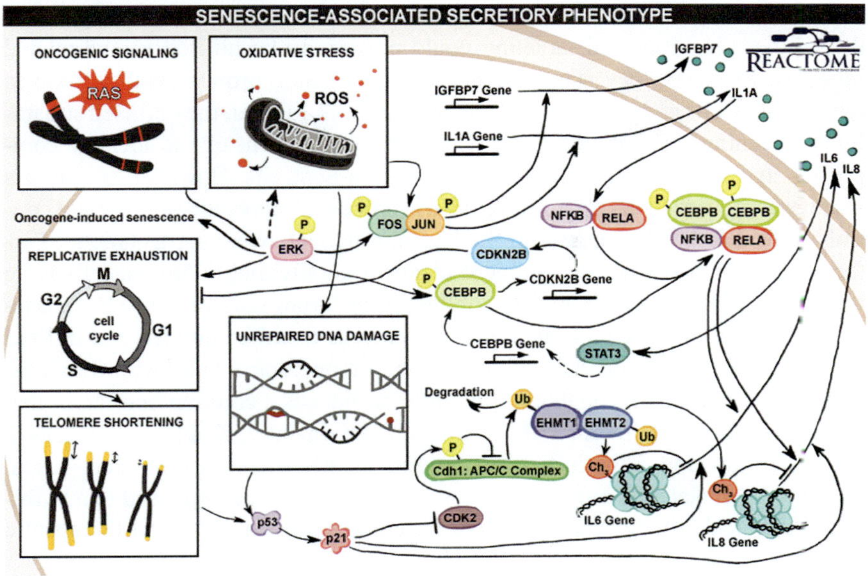

Figure 1.1 Senescence-associated secretory phenotype (SASP) pathway and related signalling molecules. SenCells secrete various proteins, forming the SASP, which is also referred as the senescence messaging secretome (SMS). SASP elements include inflammatory cytokines (e.g., IL-6 and IL-8), growth factors (e.g., IGFBPs), shed cell surface molecules (e.g., TNF receptors), and survival factors. SASP is consistent across different senescence triggers and cell types. Persistent DNA damage is a key SASP initiator. SASP components function both autocrine, reinforcing senescence, and paracrine, potentially promoting epithelial-to-mesenchymal transition (EMT) and neoplasm in neighbours (Ohtani 2022).

Source: The pathway is retrieved from "Senescence-Associated Secretory Phenotype (SASP)". Reactome, https://reactome.org/PathwayBrowser/#/R-HSA-2559582 (date of access: 10 January 2025).

from several other elements. Finally, IL-6 and IL-8 may further cause cell cycle halt (Ohtani 2022; Rodier 2013). Figure 1.1 shows SASP cascade and related signalling molecules.

1.4 JOURNEY OF SENOLYTICS

Krikland and Tchkonia initiated the search for therapies that eliminate SenCells in 2004 after reading an article from the Sharpless group. According to Krishnamurthy et al. (2004), Ames dwarf mice, having pituitary hormone deficits as well as a calorie-restricted murine system, have longer lifespans and improved health, exhibiting delayed senescent cell formation. They observed a delayed increase of p16^{Ink4a}, SA-β-gal–affirmative cells in this murine system, suggesting a simple concept that the population of SenCells and health span are inversely correlated.

This was a major factor in motivating Krikland and Tchkonia to investigate the theory that senescent cell targeting could potentially be utilised in age-related illnesses. By 2005, they started trying to create fusion proteins with a toxin to remove SenCells and a recognition site for SenCells. Further, they utilised streamlined screening for mammalian SenCells versus non-SenCells to identify compounds that will eliminate SenCells but not non-SenCells. However, no success was observed with such approaches, as the process of choosing appropriate controls proved to be challenging in the high-throughput screening technique. Furthermore, serum-starved or confluent identical nondividing, non-SenCells were required to inhibit replication. But confluence or serum starvation results in artefactual outcomes. As an alternative, non-SenCells could be divided and utilised like controls. The comparison of such proliferating control cells with SenCells, which are inherently incapable of dividing, introduces a confounding factor that makes it difficult to interpret the findings. Consequently, Krikland and Tchkonia (2020) developed the initial senolytic medicines by using a theorem-based, technique-associated therapeutic identification framework as opposed to an arbitrary large-scale therapeutics pool assessment or other conventional therapeutic identification techniques.

E. Wang in 1995 demonstrated that SenCells resist apoptosis, and this served as the foundation for Krikland and Tchkonia's proposal, who predicted the senolytic drug discovery on the following hypotheses. SenCells have two characteristics similar to cancerous cells that are incapable of multiplying: (1) such cells are resilient for cell death and exhibit metabolic changes; and (2) they can withstand apoptotic stimuli, suggesting enhanced persistence and downregulation of cell death mechanisms. They further postulated that protection of SenCells from downregulation of the cell death pathway network could shield SenCells from being removed. Furthermore, they discovered that such cells expressed SenCell downregulation of cell death strategies more highly than non-SenCells after searching through transcriptome and proteomic databases. They used RNA interference to probe the senescent cell anti-apoptotic pathway (SCAP) network and showed that pro-apoptotic SenCells do, in fact, rely on this network to avoid self-destruction (Wissler et al. 2020; Zhu et al., 2015). According to them, the specific senescent cell type would determine which small interfering RNAs (siRNAs) were successful in selectively reducing senescent cell viability by targeting anti-apoptotic regulators. For instance, as demonstrated by others, they discovered that siRNAs that reduce B-cell lymphoma extra-large was successful in specifically inducing cell death of SenCells versus non-senescent human umbilical vein endothelial primary cells. The identical siRNAs, however, were unable to distinguish between senescent and non-senescent human primary adipocyte progenitor cells in order to preferentially induce apoptosis. Furthermore, killing specific kind of SenCells required targeting multitudinous SCAPs, suggesting SenCell defences in opposed to apoptosis are sometimes unnecessary (Yosef et al. 2016; Zhu et al. 2016). Table 1.1 captures the progression from the discovery of SenCells to the expansion and clinical application of senolytic therapeutics.

Table 1.1 Timeline of Senolytic Research

Year	*Progress in Senolytic Research*
1961	Senescent cells (SenCells) discovered in vitro: *senescence at anatomical levels* was a phrase used to describe the restricted ability of primary mammalian cells in vitro to replicate
1965	Hypothesized that cellular senescence causes organismal aging by depleting the body's ability to heal damaged tissue
1980	SenCells escalates upon age as determined in human skin
1990	SenCells escalates upon age as determined in rat fat tissue
1995	SenCells resist apoptosis and identification of senescence-associated β-galactosidase (SA-β-gal) as a trait for SenCells
1996	Discovery of CDK suppressor $p16^{Ink4a}$; crucial modulator of the senescence cell cycle halt
2002	SenCells found in endothelium of mammalian atherogenic plaques
2004	Observations towards SenCells aged humans and murine cellular system by exploring SA-β-gal and $p16^{Ink4a}$ traits
2005	Age corresponding enhancement in SenCells retarded by exposing with therapies that enhance health span
2006	Preadipocytes with restricted replicative potential from old rats produce TNF-α
2008	Inflammatory, protein degrading, and growth factor–rich biologically active secretome (consequently leading to SASP) identified in multiple types of SenCells
2011	Prototype model illustrating SenCells elimination ameliorates precursor phenotypes in Bub1b-mutant mice
2013	Hypothesis-driven discovery of senolytics and senolytic targets, including BCL-XL
2015	Term *senolytic* first published along with dasatinib and quercetin as first senolytics
	Navitoclax, which targets BCL-xL, was reported as senolytic
2016	Senescent cell killing extends health span in normal-aged rodents
	Senescent cell removal via drug exposure/bioengineering suppresses atherosclerosis
	Dasatinib + quercetin alleviates age and high-fat diet–stimulated vasomotor dysfunction and vascular calcification
2017	Identification of senolytic traits in BCL-2 suppressors
	Osteoarthritis demonstrated to benefit medically from senolysis
	Dasatinib + quercetin alleviates bleomycin-induced pulmonary fibrosis
	Fisetin, A1331852, A1155463 are senolytic
	Dasatinib + quercetin alleviates hepatic steatosis
	Nutlin alleviates osteoarthritis
	FOX04-related peptide is senolytic
	Dasatinib + quercetin alleviates age-related osteoporosis

(Continued)

Table 1.1 (Continued) Timeline of Senolytic Research

Year	*Progress in Senolytic Research*
2018	HSP90 inhibitors are senolytic and alleviate progeria-related frailty
	Senolytic high-throughput screen
	A1331852 alleviates liver cirrhosis
	Dasatinib + quercetin alleviates frailty, lifespan, and health span in mice
	Dasatinib + quercetin clears SenCells from human fat explants
	Dasatinib + quercetin prevents clotting of dialysis fistulae
	Dasatinib + quercetin alleviates dementia in mice
	Fisetin alleviates frailty and improves lifespan and health span in mice
	Fisetin clears SenCells from human fat explants
2019	First investigation regarding senolytics in patients: dasatinib + quercetin
	Alleviates physical dysfunction in idiopathic pulmonary fibrosis
	In individuals, dasatinib + quercetin reduces the burden of SenCells

1.4.1 Discovery of First Senolytic

Bioinformatic techniques played a major role in developing senolytic agents. Krikland and Tchkonia screened specific agents with action towards SCAP network nodes, as they are crucial to defence against SenCells from apoptosis. Several such potential SCAPs like ephrins/dependence receptors; PI3Kδ/Akt/metabolic; Bcl-xl)/Bcl-w; p53/FOXO4a/p21/serpine [PAI-1&2]; and HIF-1α and HSP-90 pathway were identified. They discovered 46 substances that may act as senolytic where quercetin and dasatinib were on the top of the hit targets and were also evaluated in the cell line system (Hickson et al. 2019; Kirkland and Tchkonia 2020). Quercetin is found in ecology, one of the particularly prominent used bioflavonoids for management of metabolic and inflammatory disorders. One more senolytic flavonoid that occurs naturally is fisetin. Senolytic flavonoids function in part by suppressing hypoxia-inducible factor-1, extra SCAP elements, and components from the bcl2 chain, composing bcl-xL. On the other hand, dasatinib is a fabricated compact drug suppressor of Src-chain protein tyrosine kinases that is orally accessible. It has been licensed for clinical use in the United States since 2006 and binds to these kinases to suppress their growth-promoting properties. Further, dasatinib elevates cell death associated with dependence receptors, encompassing ephrins, and also by suppressing Src kinase (Zhu et al. 2017; Blagosklonny 2021; Yousefzadeh et al. 2018). In the same line of drug development, more tyrosine kinase blockers, encompassing imatinib, did not present any affinity towards SCAP network nodes. The chemicals that Krikland and Tchkonia initially concentrated on drug repurposing, where they emphasised medications and compounds in ecology previously utilised for various human applications, many of them as anti-cancer medicines, to speed translation into clinical application (Kirkland and Tchkonia 2020).

It is further anticipated that dasatinib could aim for Sen-HCPAPCells and quercetin could aim for Sen-HUVECells based on their known targets. These forecasts turned out to be accurate. Sen-HUVECell and Sen-HCPAPCells underwent apoptosis when exposed to the combination of dasatinib and quercetin; neither non-senescent adipocyte progenitor cells nor HUVECs underwent this process. Additionally, in certain cell types, such as rodent embryonic fibroblasts, neither dasatinib nor quercetin alone is senolytic; rather, the combination of dasatinib + quercetin is senolytic, most likely due to the redundancy of SCAP pathways (Nieto et al. 2024; Fan et al. 2022).

The effect of dasatinib + quercetin and of fisetin is also studied in a mouse model, where it has been demonstrated that they do not kill non-SenCells while decreasing the mass of SenCells in vivo. Following the abdominal intervention graft of radiation-triggered syngeneic Sen adipocyte precursor into middle-aged mice, which were identified by constitutive spleen focus–forming virus-promoter–driven luciferase expression, oral dasatinib + quercetin treatment for 3 days caused a substantial reduction of luminescence 2 days following the last drug administration. Neither the luminosity of rodent transplanted with non-senescent luciferase-expressing cells nor that of mice treated with dasatinib + quercetin or vehicle showed any discernible decrease after treating mice with senescent cell transplants. Progeroid Ercc-/Δ mice that expressed luciferase-associated $p16^{Ink4a}$ regulatory domain showed reduced luminosity when given fisetin orally, although vehicle administration did not affect such mice. This illustrates that dasatinib + quercetin and fisetin are senolytic in mice, removing 30%–70% of indigenous or transplanted SenCells, correspondingly (Park and Dong 2022; Bousset and Jesús 2022).

The effect of dasatinib + quercetin was further investigated in human tissues, where abdominal subcutaneous adipose tissue fragments, newly detached over surgical treatment from individuals who are overweight with diabetes, with substantial adipose tissue SenCells gathered, were promptly put in culture dishes and subjected to dasatinib + quercetin. The quantity of SenCells was reduced by 70% in 48 hours. Further, amplification in caspase-3 paralleled the process revealing apoptosis as source for the drop. In addition, conditioned media from the culture dishes subjected to dasatinib + quercetin showed a substantial decrement in SASP elements, IL-6, IL-8, MCP-1, PAI-1, and GM-CSF, when compared to vehicle. Fisetin was also found to decrease the number of SenCells in organ cultures made of adipose tissue. As a result, within 2 days, dasatinib + quercetin and fisetin induce apoptosis in human tissue, reducing the quantity of SenCells (Hickson et al. 2019).

Bioinformatics findings of Krikland and Tchkonia further illustrated that SenCells are the intended targets for senolytics; they are not specific to any one receptor, enzyme, or metabolic pathway. In comparison to substances that operate on one molecular structure, such as a receptor or an enzyme, the search for senolytics involves identifying compounds that respond on multiple SCAP network nodes, which significantly improves accuracy towards SenCells, minimizes off-target impacts over non-SenCells, and probably narrows side-effect profiles (Kirkland

and Tchkonia 2020). This assumption is supported by the fact that candidates that do operate on singular or restricted targets, like navitoclax/nutlin3a, might possess significant off-target PCD impacts over immune and platelet cells, which may render them panolytic (Zhu et al. 2016).

Furthermore, nutlins themselves have the ability to induce senescence, and medications such as navitoclax, which target SCAP signalling elements, eradicate certain subset of SenCells. Navitoclax and drugs belonging to a similar category, for instance, A1331852 or A1155463, do not exhibit removal of SenCells in precursor cells of mammalian adipocyte, which are among prevalent SenCells found in older individuals, diabetic patients, and obese people. Therefore, compared to drugs or a blend of compounds that acts on numerous nodes throughout the SCAP matrix, agents which operate on one particular node or a restricted number of SCAP elements tend to be less precisely senolytic and more panolytic, contributing to PCD/malfunction of various cell types besides SenCells (Wyles et al. 2022).

Moreover, the development of senolytics has diverged from the traditional drug-development methodologies typically employed in other domains. Compared to the conventional one target, one drug, one illness approach, strategies to create senolytics are similar to those used to produce antibiotics. The pioneer generation senolytics were identified by leveraging bioinformatics techniques that temporarily disrupt the SCAP networks, allowing SenCells to live in venerable surroundings generated, which eliminate nearby non-SenCells. On the contrary, next-phase senolytic therapeutics are screened via conventional approaches, which include random high-throughput drug library screens, including one that solves the control cell problem by containing both SenCells and non-SenCells in similar wells. Dasatinib, quercetin, fisetin, piperlongumine, luteolin, navitoclax, curcumin, etc. are the first-generation senolytic agents which mainly came from the mechanism-associated target development approach, while second-generation senolytic agents such as KSL0608-Se utilized classic and associated target development technique such as high-throughput element library screens, toxin-loaded nanoparticles partially injured by SenCells, and utilisation of immune inflector (Dhokia et al. 2024).

1.5 ASSOCIATION OF CELLULAR SENESCENCE AND SENOTHERAPEUTICS IN AGE-RELATED DISEASES

In 2011, Baker and coworkers published the initial concrete proof of an immediate connection between Sen and age-associated ailments. SenCells were attempted to eliminate from rodents, a transgenic approach was used, utilising INK-ATTAC obtained from $p16^{Ink4a}$, an acknowledged indicator of cellular senescence, whereby SenCells seemed specifically eradicated by PCD on exposure to AP20187. The INK-ATTAC–expressing rodent was crossed over a $BubR1^{H/H}$-progeroid mouse to achieve $BubR1^{H/H}$-INK-ATTAC rodent. The scientists showed AP20187, given to mice either early (during weaning) or upon further (152 days) aging, illustrated a decrement of p16^{Ink4a}-positive SenCells and an interruption towards growth of p16^{Ink4a}-mediated age-linked phenotypes in muscle and adipose tissue (Baker et al. 2011). Some years later, Baker et al. published additional conclusive proof of the direct connection between age-related diseases and cellular senescence. In this experiment, they used male and female INK-ATTAC genetically engineered rodents having a mix of genetic pool (C57BL/6 and mixed) to show the impact of p16^{Ink4a}-positive senescent cell clearance. The administration of AP20187 medication for 18 months resulted in a 24% improvement in the period of existence of C57BL/6 and genetically pooled rodents. Additionally, the treatment extended the health span of C57BL/6 mice by 18% and that of mixed background mice by 25%. Furthermore, they showed that AP20187 prevented negative side effects to the kidney, heart, or adipose tissue while attenuating age-based depreciation of several organs. Age-based lipodystrophy, hepatic steatosis, age-based cardiac function and bone loss, and tau-associated brain diseases were all alleviated by the genetic ablation in SenCells utilising the INK-ATTAC genetically engineered rodent. Research conducted on a different p16^{Ink4a} genetically modified rodent, called the p16^{Ink4a}-trimodality reporter (p16–3MR) rodent, demonstrated that the elimination of senescent macrophages decremental growth in atherosclerotic plaque along with osteoarthritis in LDLR−/− background mice. This was achieved by clearing p16^{Ink4a}-positive SenCells through ganciclovir treatment. Mice that received senescent ear fibroblast transplants into the knee area developed osteoarthritis besides genetic eradication of SenCells. According to reports, it only took a relatively modest amount of senescent cell transplantation into young mice to induce physical impairment that persisted for a while and to propagate cellular senescence across the host tissues, which decreased lifespan (Baker et al. 2016; Prieto et al. 2020; González-Gualda et al. 2021; Di Micco et al. 2021). Thus, these proof-of-principle studies demonstrated the direct connection between cellular senescence and age-related diseases and further imply that therapeutic interventions aimed at eliminating SenCells or inhibiting their effects could constitute a unique approach to prolong life expectancy and prevent or treat age-related diseases in humans.

1.5.1 Implications of Senotherapeutics in Neurological Disorders

The prevalent vulnerability for neuronal-damaging illnesses relates to age. As people age, there is an increased likelihood of developing diseases like Alzheimer's disease (AD) and Parkinson's disease (PD), which are characterised by dementia, decline in neurons, and diminished connectivity between neurons. Axon, dendrite, and neuron destruction is a feature of inflammatory illnesses like multiple sclerosis, which are also associated with age. SenCells have been seen in neurological cells, such as microglia, astrocytes, oligodendrocytes, and neural stem cells. While neurons always exit the cell cycle, they may also build up damage to their DNA and develop other characteristics of senescence, such as activation of SASP. The pathophysiology of multiple sclerosis, frontotemporal dementia, PD, AD, and ischemia/stroke has been linked to these senescent cell types. Cellular senescence induces loss of regenerative characteristics, accelerates age-based decrease in the BBB and microvasculature, and stipulates deciding to the onset and/or development of neuronal degenerative disease (Martínez-Cué and Rueda 2020; Si et al. 2021; Sahu et al. 2022).

The hallmarks of SenCells have been identified in glial structure, and current experiments show senescence of astrocytes and microglia is associated with cerebral aging, specifically in AD and PD (Sikora et al. 2021). PD traits in rodents (p16–3MR) can be exacerbated through paraquat, which further exacerbates astrocytic senescence and SASP. Ganciclovir exposure allows for the specific eradication of SenCells in this revised mouse model, upgrades motor skills and reinstates adult neuronal generation (Chinta et al. 2018). The MAPTP301SPS19 mouse model, which represents tau-associated neuronal deterioration disease, assembles p16-positive senescent astrocytes and microglia. Clearing such cells in the INK-ATTAC genetically engineered rodent suppresses gliosis and hyperphosphorylation of both soluble and insoluble tau, thereby reimposing cognition. Pharmacological exposure with the senolytic ABT-263 illustrated effects to those achieved through bioengineering in PS19 mice (Bussian et al. 2018).

The dasatinib + quercetin combination is validated in several preclinical and clinical experiments. Ogrodnik et al. (2019) investigated senescence in obesity-accompanying neurological psychiatry dysfunction using the INK-ATTAC rodents, allowing for the elimination of $p16^{Ink4a}$-presenting SenCells. Obesity ushers accumulation of senescent glial cells near the lateral ventricle, an area involved in neuronal generation. By removing these SenCells from high-fat–fed or leptin receptor–deficient obese mice by exposing dasatinib and quercetin, they were able to restore neuronal generation and alleviate anxiety-like behaviour. They further demonstrated that SenCells are major contributors to obesity-induced anxiety and suggested senolytics could be a targeted approach for neurological psychiatry. In another study, Musi et al. (2018) established removal of senescent neurons, having neurofibrillary tangles (NFTs) in a rodent system of tauopathy, was neuroprotective, improving brain structure and cerebral blood flow by treatment with dasatinib and quercetin. This further supports the potential of senolytics in treating neurodegenerative conditions.

A senescent transcriptome signature was found in neuronal cells containing NFTs of agglomerated tau protein in a study employing micro-dissected post-mortem human AD. The expression of CDKN2A mRNA indicates a senescent phenotype in NFT-accumulating neurons across various AD murine models. These SenCells can be killed with dasatinib + quercetin treatment, which lowers NFT density and reduces neuronal loss (Carreno et al. 2021). Furthermore, studies suggest that senescent oligodendrocyte precursors, a subgroup of brain glial cells, have been seen in the APP/PS1 AD rodent and human AD. In both species, these SenCells are linked to amyloid beta (Aβ) plaques, and the research implies that senescent oligodendrocyte precursor senescence is initiated by Aβ fibrils.

The selective elimination of aged oligodendrocytes from the plaque environment allowed for the desired outcome. Senescent glial cells may also impact the brain's neuropsychiatric processes, among other things. In animal experiments, the SenCells exhibit increased amounts of CDKN2A (encoding $p16^{Ink4a}$) mRNA, co-expression of senescent oligodendrocyte precursor markers along with $p16^{Ink4a}$ and $p21^{Cip1}$, and are positive for SA-β gal staining. Senescent oligodendrocyte precursors in Aβ plaques are specifically killed by acute oral exposure to a senolytic medication consisting of dasatinib and quercetin, which lowers IL-6 levels. The deliberate destruction of these aged cells not only lessens neuroinflammation but also lowers Aβ levels and improves the cognitive deficits associated with AD (Zhang et al. 2019; Ahmed and Khanam 2024; Richardson and Des 2024). Second-phase clinical studies started off in patients with AD utilising this senolytic amalgamation (Gonzales et al. 2022). In another investigation, Currais et al. (2018) demonstrated that fisetin enhanced cognitive function in SAMP8 mice, a model of sporadic AD and dementia that matures quickly.

When taken as a whole, these data point to a high correlation between neurodegeneration and SenCells in the cerebrum, corroborated by strategic research using mouse models. Approaches for treating AD that specifically eliminate SenCells could be revolutionary.

1.5.2 Implications of Senotherapeutics in Cancer

Senolysis is a newer approach to cancer treatment, especially when used in conjunction with more conventional anticancer therapies. The pan-Bcl-2 inhibitor ABT-263 (navitoclax) prevents senescence-related anti-apoptosis and causes SenCells to die off. Furthermore, ABT-263 was able to eradicate senescence-like mammary (MDA-MB-231) and ovarian (OV4453 and OV1946) tumour cells in xenografts and culture after they had been pretreated with the PARP inhibitor olaparib. Triple-negative breast cancer, which resembles senescence, overexpresses bromodomain and extraterminal (BET) protein BRD4, indicating a possible therapeutic target for BET inhibitors. In order to destroy these cells, obatoclax, another pan-BCL2 family inhibitor, shows synergistic benefits with the BET inhibitor (Zhu et al. 2016; Estepa-Fernández et al. 2023).

Similarly, in tumour-bearing SenCells, mammalian target of rapamycin (mTOR) inhibitors have demonstrated senolytic effects. mTOR is a crucial regulator of the SASP. In prostatic carcinoma (PC3) and mammary (MDA-MB-468) carcinogenic cells and transplanted model, both simultaneous and consecutive intervention of chemotherapeutic agent (specifically docetaxel) and inhibitor of mTOR, temsirolimus (CCI-779), demonstrated substantial curative impact. According to a recent publication, hepatic carcinoma cells with p53 mutations (Huh7 and MHCC97H) were selectively induced to undergo senescence by XL413, a suppressor of DNA-replication kinase CDC7. The suppressive effects of AZD8055, an mTOR inhibitor, were further enhanced by this treatment (Xu et al. 2022; Zhang et al. 2023).

It is further demonstrated that a histone deacetylase (HDAC) blocker, panobinostat, enhanced senolysis of HNSCC and NSCLC cultures treated with chemotherapy (A549, H460; UMSCC47, FaDu). In recent times, cardiac glycosides, specifically digoxin, have been identified as universal senolytics that possess the ability to eradicate many kinds of therapy-generated cancer-Sen cells under culture and in rodent experiments, including those caused by bleomycin, gemcitabine, doxorubicin, etoposide, and palbociclib. Senostasis (SASP) inhibition may also be sufficient to enhance the response to cancer treatments. When administered to animals receiving the chemotherapy drug, mitoxantrone and rapamycin significantly inhibit the growth of prostatic cancerous transplants. Rodents treated with both doxorubicin and SASP inhibitor, metformin, showed similar outcomes in breast cancer xenografts (Samaraweera et al. 2017; Zhang et al. 2023).

Senotherapies possess the ability to prolong cancer patients' lives in addition to intensifying the removal of malignant cells. ABT-263 notably postponed cancer spread and recurrence in rodents with MMTV-PyMT mammary gland cancer and removed doxorubicin-induced SenCells in a preclinical mouse model. In rodents, rapamycin and metformin also lengthened their healthy lives. Hence, the intervention of the SASP suppressor might lessen the non-tumorigenic detrimental action linked to chemotherapy that induces senescence (Sorrenti et al. 2022).

1.6 BENCH TO BEDSIDE: CLINICAL STORIES OF SENOTHERAPEUTICS

Clinical trials were contemplated for senolytic drugs due to the encouraging preclinical results demonstrating their effectiveness on multiple disease models. Senolytics were initially investigated in victims with severe illnesses like hyperglycaemia, idiopathic pulmonary fibrosis, and bone loss due to their unique nature and unclear risk/benefit ratio. Traditionally existing flavonoids like quercetin and fisetin are investigated towards a number of clinical phases, encompassing ones involving non-diseased older persons, due to their excellent safety profiles. Since its introduction into clinics in 2006, dasatinib has shown a non-detrimental record. The first therapeutic study employing fisetin and dasatinib + quercetin commenced with FDA approval, and many more are in the planning phases (Kirkland et al. 2017; Gerdes et al. 2021; Chaib et al. 2022).

Furthermore, the Translational Geroscience Network (TGN) is set to perform a simultaneous therapeutic study of therapies addressing intrinsic aging phenomena in response towards the demand for efficient exposure and sluggishness of preclinical and clinical trials. Figure 1.2 presents the active and planned clinical trials for various senotherapeutics under TGN trials. The Mayo Clinic, Harvard, Johns Hopkins, Wake Forest, the Universities of Minnesota, Michigan, and Connecticut, the University of Texas Health Sciences Centre at San Antonio, and other collaborators like the Steadman Clinic and St. Jude Children's Cancer Hospital are among the institutions that make up the TGN. The TGN has subgroups,

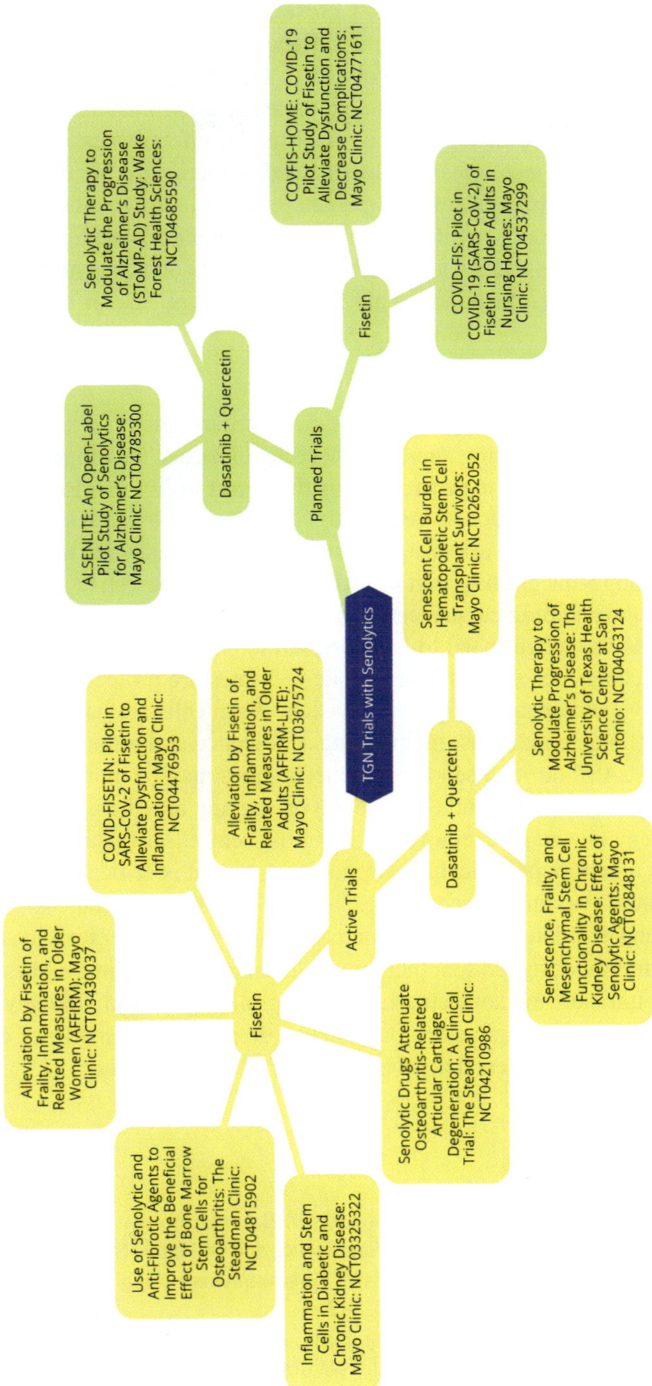

Figure 1.2 The active and planned clinical studies for various senotherapeutics under the Translational Geroscience Network.

specifically constituting the Facility for Geroscience Analysis (FGA). It also has a subcommittee for data management and statistical analysis. The FGA plays a key role in creating and synthesising novel assays for illness and aging markers. In rodent experiments and when conducted in patients, experiments are now utilised for evaluation of target engagement as well as the effectiveness of senolytics. Novel traits of aging techniques and associated ailments are being investigated by the FGA. By utilising a single infrastructure and pooling resources from several groups, the TGN could swiftly overcome challenges in starting and finishing experimental therapies that focus on elementary aging concepts, such as senolytics (Gonzales et al. 2021; Rolland et al. 2023; Wyles et al. 2022).

1.7 CONCLUSION

The probability of developing age-corresponding ailments, encompassing cancer, has grown along with life expectancy, thus the secret to living a longer life is to comprehend the aging process. SenCells proliferate in both human and mouse aging tissues, resulting in various age-corresponding ailments and tissue dysfunction. Eliminating SenCells has been shown in preclinical research to ameliorate and even reverse the pathological presentation of multiple illnesses in mice; nevertheless, numerous challenges need to be addressed to ensure a proper planned translation to the clinic. Senescence or apoptotic cell fates are protective mechanisms having positive and negative aspects that occur when cells are harmed and under stress. Under some conditions, maintaining senescence and reducing the harmful effects of the SASP through senomorphic techniques may be more interesting for tissue fitness; under other conditions, senolytic therapy may be a more beneficial clinical strategy towards the removal of SenCells. SenCells' resistance to apoptosis is caused by a variety of molecular mechanisms; thus it is critical to pinpoint the signalling pathways, unique secretomes, and factors that contribute to senescent arrest for each age-related disease. To increase efficacy and lower toxicity, rigorous picking of superior designed senotherapies is also necessary. Aging and associated ailments are intricate and sophisticated, and considering the individuality of each patient, future rejuvenating medical treatments are probably going to be designed to rely on unique biomarkers that offer a definite risk-benefit ratio.

REFERENCES

Ahmed, Faraha, and Razia Khanam. "Senolytics in Brain Disorders: A Novel Pharmacological Approach to Control Cellular Senescence and Oxidative Stress." In: Tulsawani and Vohora "Adaptation under Stressful Environments through Biological Adjustments and Interventions" (2024): 327–342.

Baker, Darren J., Bennett G. Childs, Matej Durik, Melinde E. Wijers, Cynthia J. Sieben, Jian Zhong, Rachel A. Saltness et al. "Naturally occurring p16Ink4a-positive cells shorten healthy lifespan." *Nature* 530, no. 7589 (2016): 184–189.

Baker, Darren J., Tobias Wijshake, Tamar Tchkonia, Nathan K. LeBrasseur, Bennett G. Childs, Bart Van De Sluis, James L. Kirkland, and Jan M. Van Deursen. "Clearance of p16Ink4a-positive senescent cells delays ageing-associated disorders." *Nature* 479, no. 7372 (2011): 232–236.

Blagosklonny, Mikhail V. "Anti-aging: Senolytics or gerostatics (unconventional view)." *Oncotarget* 12, no. 18 (2021): 1821.

Bousset, Laura, and Jesús Gil. "Targeting senescence as an anticancer therapy." *Molecular Oncology* 16, no. 21 (2022): 3855–3880.

Bussian, Tyler J., Asef Aziz, Charlton F. Meyer, Barbara L. Swenson, Jan M. van Deursen, and Darren J. Baker. "Clearance of senescent glial cells prevents tau-dependent pathology and cognitive decline." *Nature* 562, no. 7728 (2018): 578–582.

Campisi, Judith. "Aging and cancer: The double-edged sword of replicative senescence." *Journal of the American Geriatrics Society* 45, no. 4 (1997): 482–488.

Carreno, Gabriela, Romain Guiho, and Juan Pedro Martinez-Barbera. "Cell senescence in neuropathology: A focus on neurodegeneration and tumours." *Neuropathology and Applied Neurobiology* 47, no. 3 (2021): 359–378.

Chaib, Selim, Tamar Tchkonia, and James L. Kirkland. "Cellular senescence and senolytics: The path to the clinic." *Nature Medicine* 28, no. 8 (2022): 1556–1568.

Childs, Bennett G., Matej Durik, Darren J. Baker, and Jan M. Van Deursen. "Cellular senescence in aging and age-related disease: From mechanisms to therapy." *Nature Medicine* 21, no. 12 (2015): 1424–1435.

Chinta, Shankar J., Georgia Woods, Marco Demaria, Anand Rane, Ying Zou, Amanda McQuade, Subramanian Rajagopalan et al. "Cellular senescence is induced by the environmental neurotoxin paraquat and contributes to neuropathology linked to Parkinson's disease." *Cell Reports* 22, no. 4 (2018): 930–940.

Currais, Antonio, Catherine Farrokhi, Richard Dargusch, Aaron Armando, Oswald Quehenberger, David Schubert, and Pamela Maher. "Fisetin reduces the impact of aging on behavior and physiology in the rapidly aging SAMP8 mouse." *The Journals of Gerontology: Series A* 73, no. 3 (2018): 299–307.

de Magalhães, João Pedro, and João F. Passos. "Stress, cell senescence and organismal ageing." *Mechanisms of Ageing and Development* 170 (2018): 2–9.

Debacq-Chainiaux, F, R. Ben Ameur, E. Bauwens, E. Dumortier, M. Toutfaire, and O. Toussaint. "Stress-induced (premature) senescence." *Cellular Ageing and Replicative Senescence* (2016): 243–262.

Dhokia, Vinesh, Amal Albati, Hannah Smith, Gethin Thomas, and Salvador Macip. "A second generation of senotherapies: The development of targeted senolytics, senoblockers and senoreversers for healthy ageing." *Biochemical Society Transactions* (2024): BST20231066.

Di Micco, Raffaella, Valery Krizhanovsky, Darren Baker, and Fabrizio d'Adda di Fagagna. "Cellular senescence in ageing: From mechanisms to therapeutic opportunities." *Nature Reviews Molecular Cell Biology* 22, no. 2 (2021): 75–95.

Estepa-Fernández, Alejandra, Alba García-Fernández, Araceli Lérida-Viso, Juan F. Blandez, Irene Galiana, Félix Sancenon-Galarza, Mar Orzáez, and Ramón Martínez-Máñez. "Combination of palbociclib with navitoclax based-therapies enhances in vivo antitumoral activity in triple-negative breast cancer." *Pharmacological Research* 187 (2023): 106628.

Fan, Ting, Yi Du, Mingwan Zhang, Austin Rui Zhu, and Jianjun Zhang. "Senolytics cocktail dasatinib and quercetin alleviate human umbilical vein endothelial cell senescence via the TRAF6-MAPK-NF-κB axis in a YTHDF2-dependent manner." *Gerontology* 68, no. 8 (2022): 920–934.

Faragher, Richard GA. "Simple detection methods for senescent cells: Opportunities and challenges." *Frontiers in Aging* 2 (2021): 686382.

Gasek, Nathan S., George A. Kuchel, James L. Kirkland, and Ming Xu. "Strategies for targeting senescent cells in human disease." *Nature Aging* 1, no. 10 (2021): 870–879.

Gerdes, Erin O. Wissler, Avanish Misra, Jair Machado Espindola Netto, Tamar Tchkonia, and James L. Kirkland. "Strategies for late phase preclinical and early clinical trials of senolytics." *Mechanisms of Ageing and Development* 200 (2021): 111591.

Gonzales, Mitzi M., V. R. Garbarino, E. Marques Zilli, R. C. Petersen, J. L. Kirkland, T. Tchkonia, N. Musi, S. Seshadri, S. Craft, and Miranda E. Orr. "Senolytic therapy to modulate the progression of Alzheimer's disease (SToMP-AD): A pilot clinical trial." *The Journal of Prevention of Alzheimer's Disease* (2022): 1–8.

Gonzales, Mitzi M., Sudarshan Krishnamurthy, Valentina Garbarino, Ali S. Daeihagh, Gregory J. Gillispie, Gagan Deep, Suzanne Craft, and Miranda E. Orr. "A geroscience motivated approach to treat Alzheimer's disease: Senolytics move to clinical trials." *Mechanisms of Ageing and Development* 200 (2021): 111589.

González-Gualda, Estela, Andrew G. Baker, Ljiljana Fruk, and Daniel Muñoz-Espín. "A guide to assessing cellular senescence in vitro and in vivo." *The FEBS Journal* 288, no. 1 (2021): 56–80.

Hickson, LaTonya J., Larissa G. P. Langhi Prata, Shane A. Bobart, Tamara K. Evans, Nino Giorgadze, Shahrukh K. Hashmi, Sandra M. Herrmann et al. "Senolytics decrease senescent cells in humans: Preliminary report from a clinical trial of Dasatinib plus Quercetin in individuals with diabetic kidney disease." *EBioMedicine* 47 (2019): 446–456.

Hu, Li, Huiqin Li, Meiting Zi, Wen Li, Jing Liu, Yang Yang, Daohong Zhou, Qing-Peng Kong, Yunxia Zhang, and Yonghan He. "Why senescent cells are resistant to apoptosis: An insight for senolytic development." *Frontiers in Cell and Developmental Biology* 10 (2022): 822816.

Joshi, Amitabh. "August Weismann and the growth of biological understanding between Darwin and the rediscovery of Mendel." *Resonance* 28, no. 4 (2023): 513–525.

Kamal, Nor Shaheera Mohamad, Sabreena Safuan, Shaharum Shamsuddin, and Parisa Foroozandeh. "Aging of the cells: Insight into cellular senescence and detection Methods." *European Journal of Cell Biology* 99, no. 6 (2020): 151108.

Kameda, Masahiro, Takumi Mikawa, Masayuki Yokode, Nobuya Inagaki, and Hiroshi Kondoh. "Senescence research from historical theory to future clinical application." *Geriatrics & Gerontology International* 21, no. 2 (2021): 125–130.

Kirkland, James L., and Tamara Tchkonia. "Senolytic drugs: From discovery to translation." *Journal of Internal Medicine* 288, no. 5 (2020): 518–536.

Kirkland, James L., Tamara Tchkonia, Yi Zhu, Laura J. Niedernhofer, and Paul D. Robbins. "The clinical potential of senolytic drugs." *Journal of the American Geriatrics Society* 65, no. 10 (2017): 2297–2301.

Krishnamurthy, Janakiraman, Chad Torrice, Matthew R. Ramsey, Grigoriy I. Kovalev, Khalid Al-Regaiey, Lishan Su, and Norman E. Sharpless. "Ink4a/Arf expression is a biomarker of aging." *The Journal of Clinical Investigation* 114, no. 9 (2004): 1299–1307.

Kumari, Ruchi, and Parmjit Jat. "Mechanisms of cellular senescence: Cell cycle arrest and senescence associated secretory phenotype." *Frontiers in Cell and Developmental Biology* 9 (2021): 645593.

Martínez-Cué, Carmen, and Noemí Rueda. "Cellular senescence in neurodegenerative diseases." *Frontiers in Cellular Neuroscience* 14 (2020): 16.

Musi, Nicolas, Joseph M. Valentine, Kathryn R. Sickora, Eric Baeuerle, Cody S. Thompson, Qiang Shen, and Miranda E. Orr. "Tau protein aggregation is associated with cellular senescence in the brain." *Aging Cell* 17, no. 6 (2018): e12840.

Niedernhofer, Laura J., and Paul D. Robbins. "Senotherapeutics for healthy ageing." *Nature Reviews Drug Discovery* 17, no. 5 (2018): 377–377.

Nieto, Mario, Mina Konigsberg, and Alejandro Silva-Palacios. "Quercetin and dasatinib, two powerful senolytics in age-related cardiovascular disease." *Biogerontology* 25, no. 1 (2024): 71–82.

Ogrodnik, Mikolaj, Y. I. Zhu, Larissa G. P. Langhi, Tamar Tchkonia, Patrick Krüger, Edward Fielder, Stella Victorelli et al. "Obesity-induced cellular senescence drives anxiety and impairs neurogenesis." *Cell Metabolism* 29, no. 5 (2019): 1061–1077.

Ohtani, Naoko. "The roles and mechanisms of senescence-associated secretory phenotype (SASP): Can it be controlled by senolysis?" *Inflammation and Regeneration* 42, no. 1 (2022): 11.

Park, Jooho, and Dong Wook Shin. "Senotherapeutics and their molecular mechanism for improving aging." *Biomolecules & Therapeutics* 30, no. 6 (2022): 490.

Prieto, Luis I., Sara I. Graves, and Darren J. Baker. "Insights from in vivo studies of cellular senescence." *Cells* 9, no. 4 (2020): 954.

Raffaele, Marco, and Manlio Vinciguerra. "The costs and benefits of senotherapeutics for human health." *The Lancet Healthy Longevity* 3, no. 1 (2022): e67–e77.

Rattan, Suresh I. S. "Origins of the Hayflick system, the phenomenon and the limit." *Cellular Ageing and Replicative Senescence* (2016): 3–14.

Richardson, Miriam, and Des R. Richardson. "Pharmacological targeting of senescence with senolytics as a new therapeutic strategy for neurodegeneration." *Molecular Pharmacology* 105, no. 2 (2024): 64–74.

Rodier, Francis. "Detection of the senescence-associated secretory phenotype (SASP)." *Cell Senescence: Methods and Protocols* (2013): 165–173.

Rolland, Yves, Felipe Sierra, Luigi Ferrucci, Nir Barzilai, Rafael De Cabo, Joan Mannick, Anthony Oliva et al. "Challenges in developing Geroscience trials." *Nature Communications* 14, no. 1 (2023): 5038.

Sahu, Manas Ranjan, Linchi Rani, Rhea Subba, and Amal Chandra Mondal. "Cellular senescence in the aging brain: A promising target for neurodegenerative diseases." *Mechanisms of Ageing and Development* 204 (2022): 111675.

Samaraweera, Leleesha, Alfred Adomako, Alicia Rodriguez-Gabin, and Hayley M. McDaid. "A novel indication for panobinostat as a senolytic drug in NSCLC and HNSCC." *Scientific Reports* 7, no. 1 (2017): 1900.

Si, Zizhen, Linlin Sun, and Xidi Wang. "Evidence and perspectives of cell senescence in neurodegenerative diseases." *Biomedicine & Pharmacotherapy* 137 (2021): 111327.

Sikora, Ewa, Anna Bielak-Zmijewska, Magdalena Dudkowska, Adam Krzystyniak, Grazyna Mosieniak, Malgorzata Wesierska, and Jakub Wlodarczyk. "Cellular senescence in brain aging." *Frontiers in Aging Neuroscience* 13 (2021): 646924.

Sorrenti, Vincenzo, Francesca Benedetti, Alessandro Buriani, Stefano Fortinguerra, Giada Caudullo, Sergio Davinelli, Davide Zella, and Giovanni Scapagnini. "Immunomodulatory and antiaging mechanisms of resveratrol, rapamycin, and metformin: Focus on mTOR and AMPK signaling networks." *Pharmaceuticals* 15, no. 8 (2022): 912.

Toussaint, Olivier, Jose Remacle, Jean-François Dierick, Thierry Pascal, Christophe Frippiat, Stéphanie Zdanov, Joao Pedro Magalhaes, Véronique Royer, and Florence Chainiaux. "From the Hayflick mosaic to the mosaics of ageing: Role of stress-induced premature senescence in human ageing." *The International Journal of Biochemistry & Cell Biology* 34, no. 11 (2002): 1415–1429.

Van Deursen, Jan M. "The role of senescent cells in ageing." *Nature* 509, no. 7501 (2014): 439–446.

Warner, Huber R. "Apoptosis: A two-edged sword in aging." *Annals of the New York Academy of Sciences* 887, no. 1 (1999): 1–11.

Wissler Gerdes, Erin O., Yi Zhu, Tamar Tchkonia, and James L. Kirkland. "Discovery, development, and future application of senolytics: Theories and predictions." *The FEBS Journal* 287, no. 12 (2020): 2418–2427.

Wyles, Saranya P., Tamara Tchkonia, and James L. Kirkland. "Targeting cellular senescence for age-related diseases: Path to clinical translation." *Plastic and Reconstructive Surgery* 150 (2022): 20S–26S.

Xu, Weitong, Tingting Zhao, Honghan Chen, Ning Huang, Hui Gong, Jian Zhang, Yu Yang et al. "Pan-mTOR inhibitors sensitize the senolytic activity of navitoclax via mTORC2 inhibition-mediated apoptotic signaling." *Biochemical Pharmacology* 200 (2022): 115045.

Yosef, Reut, Noam Pilpel, Ronit Tokarsky-Amiel, Anat Biran, Yossi Ovadya, Snir Cohen, Ezra Vadai et al. "Directed elimination of senescent cells by inhibition of BCL-W and BCL-XL." *Nature Communications* 7, no. 1 (2016): 11190.

Yousefzadeh, Matthew J., Y. I. Zhu, Sara J. McGowan, Luise Angelini, Heike Fuhrmann-Stroissnigg, Ming Xu, Yuan Yuan Ling et al. "Fisetin is a senotherapeutic that extends health and lifespan." *EBioMedicine* 36 (2018): 18–28.

Zhang, Lei, Louise E. Pitcher, Vaishali Prahalad, Laura J. Niedernhofer, and Paul D. Robbins. "Targeting cellular senescence with senotherapeutics: Senolytics and senomorphics." *The FEBS Journal* 290, no. 5 (2023): 1362–1383.

Zhang, Peisu, Yuki Kishimoto, Ioannis Grammatikakis, Kamalvishnu Gottimukkala, Roy G. Cutler, Shiliang Zhang, Kotb Abdelmohsen et al. "Senolytic therapy alleviates Aβ-associated oligodendrocyte progenitor cell senescence and cognitive deficits in an Alzheimer's disease model." *Nature Neuroscience* 22, no. 5 (2019): 719–728.

Zhu, Y. I., Tamara Tchkonia, Heike Fuhrmann-Stroissnigg, Haiming M. Dai, Yuanyuan Y. Ling, Michael B. Stout, Tamar Pirtskhalava, N. Giorgadze, K. O. Johnson, C. B. Giles, J. D. Wren. "Identification of a novel senolytic agent, navitoclax, targeting the Bcl-2 family of anti-apoptotic factors." *Aging Cell* 2016 June; 15, no. 3: 428–435.

Zhu, Y. I., Tamara Tchkonia, Tamar Pirtskhalava, Adam C. Gower, Husheng Ding, Nino Giorgadze, Allyson K. Palmer et al. "The Achilles' heel of senescent cells: From transcriptome to senolytic drugs." *Aging Cell* 14, no. 4 (2015): 644–658.

Zhu, Yi, Ewald J. Doornebal, Tamar Pirtskhalava, Nino Giorgadze, Mark Wentworth, Heike Fuhrmann-Stroissnigg, Laura J. Niedernhofer, Paul D. Robbins, Tamara Tchkonia, and James L. Kirkland. "New agents that target senescent cells: The flavone, fisetin, and the BCL-XL inhibitors, A1331852 and A1155463." *Aging (Albany NY)* 9, no. 3 (2017): 955.

Chapter 2

Senotherapeutics in Neurological Disorders

Faraha Ahmed and Razia Khanam

Abbreviations

AD: Alzheimer's disease; ALS: amyotrophic lateral sclerosis; AMPK; AMP-activated protein kinase; Aβ: amyloid β; BACE-1: β-secretase 1; CDKN: cyclin-dependent kinase inhibitor; cGAS: cGMP-AMP synthase; CHIT1: chitinase 1; CNS: central nervous system; CRIPT: CXXC repeat containing interactor of PDZ3 domain; DNA: deoxyribonucleic acid; ERK: extracellular signal-regulated kinase; GATA4: GATA binding protein 4; HD: Huntington's disease; HIF-1α: hypoxia-inducible factor-1α; HSP-90: heat shock protein 90; IκKB: inhibitor of nuclear factor-κB kinase; IL-1A: interleukin-1A; M-CSF: macrophage colony-stimulating factor; MPTP 1: methyl 4 phenyl piperidinium MS: multiple sclerosis; mTOR: mammalian target of rapamycin; NF-κB: nuclear factor kappa B; Nrf-2: nuclear factor erythroid 2-related factor 2; p38MAPK: p38 mitogen-activated protein kinases; PAI-1: plasminogen activator factor-1; PD: Parkinson's disease; PON2: paraoxonase 2; PTH: parathyroid hormone; RB: retinoblastoma; RCT: randomized clinical trial; RNA: ribonucleic acid; SA-β gal^{+}: senescence-associated β-galactosidase; SCAPs: senescent cell anti-apoptotic pathways; SIRT3: sirtuins; SOD-1: superoxide dismutase-1; STING: stimulator of interferon genes; TRAF3IP: tumour necrosis factor-associated factor interacting protein 3; TNF-R: tumour necrosis factor; VSMC: vascular smooth muscle cell.

2.1 INTRODUCTION

Neurological disorders are mostly associated with age-related neurodegeneration caused by cellular senescence (Voisin et al. 2020). Senescence in cells takes place as an outcome of the inability of DNA to comprehensively replicate during its synthesis. Modification in the blood brain barrier (BBB), chronic inflammation, cerebral hypoperfusion, attenuated regenerative brain capacity or inconsistent post-mitotic neuronal activity significantly cause cellular senescence causing neurodegeneration (Kritsilis et al. 2018). The buildup of senescent cells accelerates

DOI: 10.1201/9781003493969-2

the aging progression. An aging brain exhibits inflamed astrocytes characterized by upregulated glial fibrillary acidic protein. Cellular senescence also decreases astrocyte activity implicating neurodegenerative disorders (Siracusa, Fusco, and Cuzzocrea 2019). Senescent cells can arise from mitotic or post-mitotic cells of the brain including endothelial cells, neurons, microglia, astrocytes and progenitor cells from oligodendrocytes (Russo and Riessland 2022). Protein modifications, stress, metabolic dysfunction, inflammation, oncogenes, telomere damage, nucleotide damage or microbial damage also cause senescence (Calcinotto et al. 2019; Ogrodnik 2021). The primary function of cellular senescence is to protect the body from tumorigenesis by inhibiting the replication of damaged DNA cells (Choi et al. 2022). But accumulation of senescent cells modifies the immune system and causes functional abnormalities in stem and progenitor cells. This subsequently gives rise to liver disorders, osteoarthritis, pulmonary fibrosis, atherosclerosis and neurodegenerative disorders, to name a few (Ogrodnik et al. 2019; Wissler Gerdes et al. 2020).

The natural human defence system of the body employs helper T cells to recognise the senescent cells, which are then subsequently eliminated by lymphocytes, macrophages and natural killer cells (Kowald, Passos, and Kirkwood 2020). Arrest of the cell cycle in cells undergoing senescence leads to suppression of malignancy and secretes senescence-associated secretory phenotype (SASP) that includes proliferative, immunomodulatory and extracellular matrix repairing factors (Triana-Martínez et al. 2019). There is stimulation of SASP-led cell senescence through the NF-κB signalling pathway. Nucleotides, growth factors, pro-inflammatory chemokines, interleukins, proteases, pro-coagulant factors, microvesicles and miRNAs are components of SASP (Xu et al. 2018; Martel et al. 2020). Biomarkers of cellular senescence include transcription factors like (p21) CDKN1A/p53, (p16) CDKN2A/RB, p27, $p16^{INK4a}$, $p21^{CIP1}$, $p19^{ARF}$, PAI-1 and Nrf-2 (Calcinotto and Alimonti 2017; Calcinotto et al. 2019; Casella et al. 2019; Hernandez-Segura, Nehme, and Demaria 2018; Shao et al. 2021). Upregulation of cyclin-dependent kinase inhibitor (CDKN) and elevated expression of CDKs p16 and p21 (Stein et al. 1999) in addition to an increase in SA-β-gal^{+} (senescence-associated β-galactosidase) functions are observed during senescence (Casella et al. 2019; Hernandez-Segura, Nehme, and Demaria 2018). The GATA-4 gene (zinc finger transcription factor) also regulates cellular senescence. It stimulates the NF-κB signalling mechanism via TRAF3IP and IL-1A, and therefore causes inflammation through DNA damage and autophagy (Kang et al. 2015). Mitochondrial dysfunction is observed with deficiency of PON2 (paraoxonase 2), a protein expressed in several regions of the brain (Costa et al. 2014). Downregulation of lamin B1 triggers methylation of chromatin to develop complete senescence and thus effects neurogenesis (Bedrosian et al. 2021).

Senescence initiates due to upregulation of p21 and p53. Activity of $p16^{INK4A}$ and p53-p21-RB which is mediated by CDK4/6 that hypo phosphorylates the RB protein to the arrest cell cycle at the S phase. NOTCH signalling, cGMP-AMP synthase, stimulator of interferon genes (STING), p38 mitogen-activated protein kinases (p38MAPK), mammalian target of rapamycin (mTOR) pathways, increased reactive oxygen species (ROS), and accumulation of lipofuscin also regulate cell senescence (Watanabe et al. 2017; Kritsilis et al. 2018; González-Gualda et al. 2021; Russo and Riessland 2022). Upregulation of the JAK/STAT signalling pathway suppresses the mitochondrial function that drives cells into senescence (C. Liu et al. 2019). Furthermore, oxidative stress, exposure to ionizing radiations, and drugs like etoposide and doxorubicin also cause senescence in cells (L. Zhang et al. 2021). Figure 2.1 illustrates factors causing cellular senescence.

Senotherapeutic agents do not have any intrinsic biochemical function but concretely target senescent cells to induce apoptosis (L. Zhang et al. 2021). Pathways that inhibit senescent cell death are called senescent cell anti-apoptotic pathways (SCAPs) and involve p53/FOXO4a/p21/serpine, Bcl-2/B-cell, ephrin receptors, PI3Kδ/Akt, HSP-90 and HIF-1α signalling (Wissler Gerdes et al. 2020). A few compounds demonstrate senotherapeutic effect. Drugs that selectively attack senescent cells by targeting SCAPs and other signalling mechanisms to induce senolysis by drugs are known as *senolytics*. Certain agents that weaken the SASP through senostasis are known as *senomorphics*. Senolytics target anti-apoptotic pathways like Bcl-2, AKT, p21, p53, P13K and FOXO4, whereas senomorphics attenuate SASP with pathways like p38MAPK, mTOR, NF-κB and IL-1α (L. Zhang et al. 2023; Papadopoulos et al. 2020).

Senescent cell death induced by senolytics can be achieved by intermittent dosing (Zhu et al. 2015). Senolytics such as quercetin and dasatinib cause kinase inhibition. The compounds of natural origin including piperlongumine, fisetin, curcumin, ouabain and others were identified as senolytics. These include Bcl-2

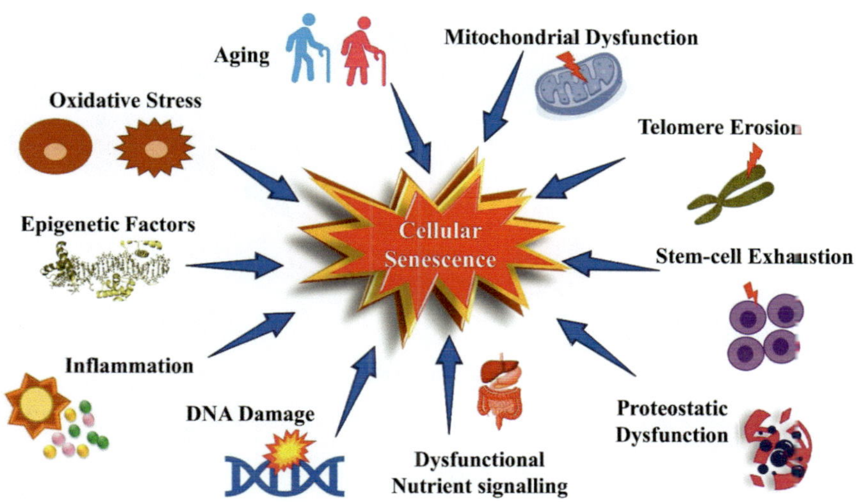

Figure 2.1 Pathological triggers underlying cellular senescence.

homology 3 mimetics or Bcl-2 blockers like navitoclax, A1155463, ABT-737, etc., MDM2/p53 blockers like P5091 and UBX0101, p53 suppressor FOXO4-DRI, histone deacetylase antagonist panobinostat and Hsp90 modulators like tanespimycin (Lagoumtzi and Chondrogianni 2021; Ahmed and Khanam 2023).

We summarise the mechanistic insights for development of cellular senescence in various neurodegenerative disorders. Further, the advancements in senotherapeutic actions in alleviating the disease conditions to improve the healthy lifespan are also explored.

2.2 MOLECULAR MECHANISMS OF SENESCENCE

The mechanisms of neurodegenerative disorders in discrete pathologies overlap, but still the different disorders display several contributors and factors involved in their pathogenesis as shown in Figure 2.2.

2.2.1 Alzheimer's Disease

Alzheimer's disease (AD) is characterized as an age-associated progressive neurological illness that causes dementia, cognitive dysfunction, and altered behaviour and personality in older people (Hou et al. 2019). With progressing age, lysosomal dysfunctions, abnormal autophagy and cellular senescence cause neurodegeneration (Saez-Atienzar and Masliah 2020). AD presents neuropathological hallmarks like β-amyloid (Aβ) crystals, senile plaques, neurofibrillary and hyperphosphorylated tau protein accumulations (R.-M. Liu 2022). Hippocampal

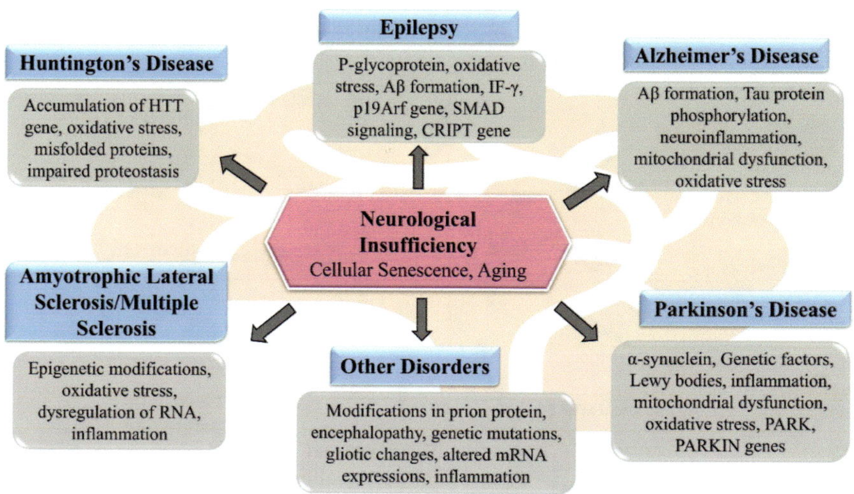

Figure 2.2 Shared and distinct mechanisms of neurodegenerative disorders.

regions of AD patients manifested elevated expressions of CDKN p53, $p21^{CIP1}$, p38MAPK, TNF-α, γH2AX IL-6/1β and transforming growth factor-β (TGF-β) (Kritsilis et al. 2018). Aβ is a primary player in the development of AD. Tau fibrillopathy and related neuronal decline are triggered by Aβ, which is formed by the successive degradation of the amyloid precursor protein (APP) by β/γ-secretases (Suelves et al. 2023). miR-101, miR106 and miR-124 generate Aβ by targeting APP and activating BACE1 (Aβ cleaving enzyme) (M. Fang et al. 2012). Attenuation of miR-9/29/29b/137/181c targets serine palmitoyl transferase enzyme, dislocates BACE1 in lipid rafts and increased conversion of APP to Aβ (Schonrock et al. 2012). Further, disturbed activity of calcium-dependent cysteine proteases known as calpains also cause pathological changes in AD (NIXON et al. 1994). Several mechanisms cause cellular senescence–associated AD.

2.2.2 Epilepsy

A neurological state that involves circuit reorganization, seizures, neuronal degeneration and other brain abnormalities is collectively known as epilepsy. It subsequently causes altered cognition, impaired memory and learning disability (Vrinda et al. 2019). In the pathophysiology of epilepsy, mitochondrial dynamics and oxidative stress are critically involved. The changes in functioning of mitochondria limit the production of ROS and energy. There is altered function of ion channels that stimulates the release of glutamate. This affects neuronal excitability affecting the calcium synaptic transmission causing excitotoxicity. The epigenetic changes include DNA methylation, histone modifications and modifications in expression of RNA (W. Xie et al. 2024). Epilepsy is triggered by cellular senescence and apoptosis that is marked by aging, neuronal incapacity, loss of tumour suppressor genes, changes in Aβ levels, shrinking of telomeres and epigenetic stress (Si, Sun, and Wang 2021; Innes et al. 2018). Integrity of genes is essentially maintained by telomeres that monitors cellular aging and related stress (Miranda et al. 2020). The miRNAs and IF-γ (interferon) signalling are involved in the development of post-traumatic epilepsy (Zhao et al. 2022).

Epileptic seizures elevate the P-glycoprotein (P-gp) expressions, which are efflux transporters of the BBB (Hartz et al. 2017). In mutant mice with decreased Ft1 genes (similar to AKTIP in humans), DNA damage, telomere changes and senescence were observed. Accelerated aging and skeletal abnormalities in addition to lipodystrophy were seen that triggered seizures. The Ft1 gene deletions caused elevated expression of inflammatory markers like TGF-β and IL−6. This association suggested the instrumental role of aging, DNA damage and epilepsy (Burla et al. 2018). Defect in neurogenesis forms malformed tissues and increases cellular senescence in epithelial cells in the brain. Rhinn et al. identified p19Arf as a powerful mediator of neuronal cell senescence (Rhinn et al. 2022). Sun et al. reported that mammalian chitinase, CHIT1, is associated with senescence when present in higher levels. The senescence is triggered due to activation of SMAD signalling causing toxicity to microglial cells (Sun et al. 2023). CRIPT, a protein coding gene, causes epilepsy and delay in neurodevelopmental and increases senescence of neuronal cells (Averdunk et al. 2023).

2.2.3 Amyotrophic Lateral Sclerosis and Multiple Sclerosis

Aging is identified as a critical contributor for development of amyotrophic lateral sclerosis (ALS) as both share several overlapping pathologies. In human tissues and animal models, senescence of glial cells is observed with ALS (Trias et al. 2019; Sivasubramanian et al. 2020). DNA repair is known to be facilitated by a number of proteins that are crucial in ALS such as valosin-containing protein-1 (VCP-1), Nek-1 c90rf72, c21orf2, TDP-43, FUS and SOD (superoxide dismutase), and senataxin (Konopka and Atkin 2022). The disease also exhibits disrupted neuromuscular junction, decreased SIRT1 expression, telomere shortening/dysfunction and retrograde axonal degeneration (Pandya and Patani 2020). ALS is also linked to the accumulation of SOD (Bhatia et al. 2020). There is degeneration of cortical and spinal motoneurons that progressively causes muscular paralysis, breathing difficulties and subsequently death within 2–5 years. The regular genetic cause of ALS include inadequate trafficking deficient lysosomal and mitochondrial function in iPSC (induced pluripotent stem cell)-generated spinal motor neurons in individuals with ALS who carry mutant TDP43 and fused sarcoma, and most common is the repeated expansion of intronic hexanucleotide in c90rf72 gene (Pal et al. 2021). ALS mice models Q331K and G93A carry TDP-43 function and exhibited elevated p16 and p21 mRNA, presence of glial protein and upregulated SA-β-gal activity indicating senescence. Moreover, SASP was indicated with elevated IL-1A/6 expression kindred with upregulated the protein M-CSF and TNF-R (Torres et al. 2022). The degeneration of motor neurons typically starts randomly in upper and lower motor neurons and then extends to the other areas of the motor area and spinal cord. In comparison to wild-type cells of the same age, the cultured astrocytes of ALS spinal cords exhibit a higher number of SA-β-gal and lower cell death. Further, a decreased expression of Ki-67 proliferation markers is also found to be involved in cellular senescence (Maximova, Werry, and Kassiou 2021). A decrease in NUP50 nucleoporin is also a risk for ALS. Nuclear architecture and protein import are also affected by mutated decrease in never-in-mitosis A-related kinase-1 in motor neurons produced by iPSC. There is currently wealth of evidence linking DNA damage to the ALS pathogenesis. Patients with ALS experience hyper-methylation of histone H3 and H4 near the promoter CpG-island (Jagaraj et al. 2024).

Multiple sclerosis (MS) is a demyelinating condition associated with immune dysfunction. The pathology of MS involves chronic demyelination leading to axonal degeneration causing neuronal deterioration. Progressing age limits the efficiency of remyelination, therefore MS is also affected by aging (Koutsoudaki et al. 2020). Primarily, oxidative stress-induced lipid peroxidation is involved in pathogenesis of MS, which is a systemic inflammatory condition. Cellular senescence is caused by capped chromosomal ends, telomere shortening with every cycle of cell division (J.-Z. Guan et al. 2015). The signs of aging contributing for MS include cellular decline, telomere loss, epigenetic alterations, mitochondrial impairment, suppression of proteostasis, genetic aberration, imbalance in cell signalling, altered nutrient sensing and fatigued stem cells (Oost et al. 2018). There is increased risk of developing MS with HLA gene variants including DQA1, DRB5 and DRB1. There is suppressed immunity and premature immunosenescence. Increased oxidative stress and shortened telomeres are responsible for brain atrophy and disability (Dema et al. 2021). Different molecules have been investigated for decreasing the senescent load in ALS and MS. Most studies showed a positive role of senotherapeutics for disease management.

2.2.4 Parkinson's Disease

Parkinson's disease (PD) is also an aging disorder that affects brain activity. It is identified with loss of DA (dopaminergic) neurons in the midbrain, specifically the substantia nigra pars compacta region indicated by motor dysfunctions. Senescence of cells is crucially involved in the dysfunction of neurons causing PD (Lee et al. 2021). PD displays features such as the accumulation of ubiquitinated protein α-synuclein; neuronal damage in the midbrain, specifically the substantia nigra; and there is existence of Lewy bodies and Lewy neuritis in cytoplasm (Kritsilis et al. 2018; Yoon et al. 2022). Brain tissue of PD patients exhibited cellular senescence markers, with elevated expression of $p16^{INK4a}$ mRNA, cell cycle genes and higher levels of SASP elements like IL-α/6/8 (Chinta et al. 2018). Lysosomal dysfunction along with iPSC are also responsible for development of PD (Wallings et al. 2019). PD patients also showed altered iron metabolism and elevated reactive oxygen intermediates leading to oxidative stress and neuron loss. Further, mutations in PD specific genes like *PARK2*, *PINK-1, LRRK2*, *SNCA* and *DJ-1* led to mitochondrial dysfunction causing apoptosis and cell death (Trist, Hare, and Double 2019). An ICICLE- PD study on PD patients demonstrated elevated inflammatory markers like TNF-α and IL-10, decreased p21 expression and short telomere length (Martin-Ruiz et al. 2020). Endothelial cells present at the BBB impair the integrity of this barrier along with SASP responsible for recruitment of T-cells at the midbrain. Moreover, senescence-vulnerable cells like astrocytes, DA neurons and microglia in the midbrain of PD patients may also augment senescence to other cells through SASP, attract more T cells and impair BBB permeability to attenuate DA neurons. These events cause inflammation and recruit immune cells to kill the senescence in DA neurons (Russo and Riessland 2022).

2.2.5 Huntington's Disease

Neuronal degeneration also causes Huntington's disease (HD), which exhibits similar aging hallmarks like DNA damage, telomere shortening, cellular senescence, altered signalling mechanisms, mitochondrial dysfunction, epigenetic changes, dysfunctional nutrient sensing through altered IGF-1, and dysregulated amino acid metabolism (Machiela and Southwell 2020). HD demonstrates an increase in glutathione reductase and activities of glucose metabolizing enzymes including hexokinase, glucose-6-phosphate dehydrogenase and pyruvate kinase. In addition, there are low levels of reduced glutathione in red cells (Zanella et al. 1980). HD is an autosomal dominant disorder that occurs due to repeated CAG code. Altered telomere length of leucocytes is an indicator for HD onset clinically (Scarabino et al. 2019). Cellular senescence is developed when FOXO3-ETS2-p16^{INK4a} is affected with neuronal differentiation (Voisin et al. 2020). Polymorphic sequence of glutamines modulate the function of the protein Huntingtin (HTT) that encodes HD (Clabough and Zeitlin 2006). Mitochondrial dysfunction takes place when there is an accumulation of mutant HTT that engages more IRS-2 that subsequently stimulates FOXO1 through the PI3K/Akt/FOXO1 signalling pathway (L. Li et al. 2021). Increased expressions of FOXO1 protein participate in protein maturation and processing linked to the pathology of HD. This alters the apoptosis of cells and autophagy of aggregated misfolded proteins developed due to ER stress. FOXO1 protein activation interferes with mitochondrial function including oxidation and phosphorylation that in turn causes ATP deficiency and affects metabolic homeostasis (Liyang Liu et al. 2022).

2.2.6 Others

A neurodegenerative fatal disease known as "prion's disease" occurs to conformational changes in cellular prion proteins (PrP^C). PrP^C is ubiquitously present in brain and other cells. The features of disease include spongiform degeneration and encephalopathy, glial cell activation, neuronal insufficiency, and deposition of amyloid-like plaques (PrP^{Sc}). In prion's disease, PrP^C are transformed into PrP^{Sc}. Additionally autophagy is also observed with increased expressions of p62 and LC3 and mutation is specific PRNP gene causing cellular senescence (Sigurdson, Bartz, and Glatzel 2019; Hao and Wang 2020; Baiardi et al. 2023).

Another progressive neurologic disorder, multiple system atrophy (MSA), is an uncommon condition caused due to gliotic changes and neuronal deficiency. The gliosis is found in several regions of the central nervous system such as structures with central autonomic functions, the olivopontocerebellar region and the striatonigral regions. Accumulation of protein α-synuclein and misfolded protein in oligodendroglial cytoplasmic cells is a classic hallmark of MSA (Poewe et al. 2022). Furiya et al. reported α-1-antichymotrypsin genotypic variation as a determinant of MSA (Furiya et al. 2005). In MSA patients, neuroinflammation was found to be triggered by abnormal expression of several miR-19a-3p/27b-3p/124-3p/29c-3p in the striatum region (Kim, Valera, and Desplats 2019). There is altered permeability of BBB that increases chances of injury to cells and increased excitability of neurons. The brain samples of MSA patients have presented elevated microglia class II^+ antigens, increased T cells ($CD3^+$, $CD4^+$ and $CD8^+$) and enhanced responses of cytokines that promote inflammation like IL-1A/1B/8/2/3 and

TNF-α, suggesting immune activation. Further, increased expression of STING genes and TANK-binding kinase-1 was found in astrocytes that also contribute in inflammation. The function of immune system is also modified by TREM-2 (triggering receptor expressed on myeloid cells-2) and NOD-2 (nucleotide-binding oligomerization domain containing-2) (Leńska-Mieciek et al. 2023).

The group of neurological disorders referred to as motor neuron disease is also induced by cellular senescence. In the hSOD1-G93A motor neuron disease model of transgenic mice, higher expressions of mRNA proteins p16 and p21 were found in glial cells indicating mitotic arrest in the absence of canonical upregulation and SA-β-gal function. Along with SASP, an elevated expression of M-CSF, IL-1A/6 and TNF-R were identified. Moreover, a DNA-binding protein TAR transcribed by gene *Tardbp* was compromised in association with *Adipor2* levels causing cell senescence (Torres et al. 2022). Recently, Guan et al. revealed that in neural stem cells, oxidized human SOD1 is identified as an underlying cause for senescent-associated changes. Elevated levels of these antioxidants and stimulation of p53, SA-β-gal and dislocation of extracellular HMGB1 genes directs towards cellular senescence in motor neuron disease (T. Guan et al. 2024).

2.3 ROLE OF SENOTHERAPEUTICS (SENOLYTICS/SENOMORPHICS)

Senotherapeutics as a drug target for cellular senescence has made significant advancements in several neurodegenerative disorders. Several studies have investigated the role of senolytics and senomorphics to alleviate degenerative neurological diseases. In this section we discuss the therapeutic capacity of this class in neurodegenerative disorders.

2.3.1 Alzheimer's Disease

Dementia in the aging population due to AD is a disturbing issue. More than a decade ago, Dong and team identified the in vitro neuroprotective capacity of tanshinone IIA (herb) in Aβ-induced cytotoxicity in PC-12 cell lines (pheochromocytoma cells). Tanshinone IIA after 24-hour treatment exhibited neuroprotection by decreasing apoptosis and enhanced cell viability by targeting activation of P13/AKT signalling and phosphorylation of activation and GSK3β signal transduction (Dong et al. 2012).

Intervention with 25 mg/kg fisetin orally in bigenic APPswe/PS1dE9 AD rodents (3–12 months) decreased oxidative stress. Reduction in carbonylation of protein and increased phosphorylation of signal-regulated kinase (ERK) in cytoplasm was also observed. The brain samples of mice demonstrated lower expressions of p25 responsible for degeneration and inflammation of neurons. Improved memory and learning with fisetin treatment in vivo exhibited ameliorative effects in AD (Currais et al. 2014). In 2017, Ahmad and team also investigated the neuron-sparing function of fisetin in learning, and memory preclinically in an AD $A\beta_{1-42}$ mice model. An $A\beta_{1-42}$ (3 μL) injection given intra-cerebroventricular for 5 minutes to animals caused memory loss, neuroinflammation and neurodegeneration. Fisetin administered after 24 hours demonstrated significant decline in Aβ accumulation, decreased tau protein and reduced phosphorylation. Morris water maze assessment showed improvement in memory as a reversal of $A\beta_{1-42}$-induced increased pre- and post-synaptic proteins like SNAP-23/25, SYN, phospho-GLuR1, phospho-CREB (p-CREB), post-synaptic density protein-95, and phospho-calcium/calmodulin-stimulated protein kinase II was observed. Further, decreased neurodegeneration and neuroinflammation was evidenced with elevated expressions of p-GSK3β, p-PI3K an p-Akt and in animals (Ahmad et al. 2017).

In APP/PSI mice model efficacy of quercetin and dasatinib (50 and 12 mg/kg, respectively) were evaluated after 9 days of treatment. The quantification of accumulated amyloid and OPC (oligodendrocyte progenitor cells) in brains of AD mice showed senescence in the cells that was linked to lysosomal dysfunction, neuronal degeneration and neuronal inflammation. Senolytic treatment downregulation of p16 and OPC and suppressed the activation of microglial cells and proinflammatory cytokines in animals. Moreover, improved learning and memory in the mice was also observed, suggesting the ability of quercetin and dasatinib to alter cellular senescence (P. Zhang et al. 2019). The effect of fisetin (100 mg/kg) alone or combined effect of quercetin with dasatinib (50 mg/kg + 5 mg/kg) was assessed for their capacity to ameliorate cellular senescence in AD preclinically. $APP^{NL-F/NL-F}$ mice of both genders were subjected to the combined treatment monthly. Results revealed that quercetin and dasatinib increased the energy expenditure and consumption of oxygen in $APP^{NL-F/NL-F}$ mice that led to decrease in body weight. Further, an improved spatial memory was identified due to hippocampal decrease in SA-β-gal activity, $A\beta_{42,}$ senescence markers and SASP. These changes attenuated the risk of dementia (Y. Fang et al. 2023).

Senotherapeutic effect of navitoclax (ABT-263) was studied in cognitive dysfunction in p16–3MR transgenic mice. Navitoclax reversed the cellular senescence induced with 5-Gy irradiation–influenced aging, modified the neurovascular coupling in astrocytes and induced cognition defects (Yabluchanskiy et al. 2020). Another study reported beneficial effects of navitoclax in a pre-clinical rodent model. The treatment given to middle-aged mice for a month induced attrition of hippocampal senescent cells and elevated the expression of hippocampal neural cells. After the therapy for a year, the drug exhibited 3-fold increase in subgranular SA-β-gal-positive cells. Along with this, the spatial navigation test called Morris test revealed enhanced cognition in mice (Fatt et al. 2022). In a preclinical study with 5XFAD Aβ-based mice model, efficacy of PTH_{1-34} (50 μg/kg) for 5 days/week was assessed in 2-month-old mice for 3 months in bone and AD. PTH_{1-34} showed a senolytic effect in mice as treatment exhibited improvement in bone health as well as in AD pathology. A decrease in dystrophic neurons, inflammatory cytokines, Aβ deposits and glial cell activation was observed in mice along with enhanced cognitive functions (Chen et al. 2023).

An unblinded pilot phase-1 trial was performed in five elderly nascent AD patients for 12 weeks. The drugs quercetin and dasatinib were orally administered to determine their viability, penetration, efficacy and safety in the CNS. The senolytic drugs were well tolerated and were detected in the blood and cerebrospinal fluid of participants. A decrease in senescence-related chemokines and cytokines was observed, suggesting the safety of the drugs as well (Gonzales et al. 2023).

The tyrosine-kinase inhibitor masitinib regulates the function of mast cells by inhibiting their migration and survival. In a preclinical study, the effect of the drug was investigated in APPswe/PSEN1dE9 transgenic mice as they express genes APP and PS1 that carry AD mutations. Treatment for 2.5 months at dose of 75 mg/kg restored the special learning. It also restored the mast cells and improved impaired synaptic activity in mice (T. Li et al. 2020). A decade ago, Piette et al. performed phase 2 random placebo-controlled trial with masitinib on 26 AD patients. Administration of masitinib (3–6 mg/kg) for 24 weeks significantly lowered the cognitive subscale-AD assessment scale and improved the AD pathology (Piette et al. 2011).

Senotherapeutics like fisetin, dasatinib and quercetin have been investigated preclinically for alleviating AD by targeting cellular senescence, though to further establish the activity for clinical purpose, investigations through clinical trials are needed.

2.3.2 Epilepsy

Effective therapeutic measures for epilepsy have been developed through modification of oxidative stress, apoptosis, neuronal inflammation or mTOR signalling. Transplantation of stem cells provides potential benefits in attenuating frequency and intensity of seizures for neurological benefits (Alayli et al. 2023).

Metformin, an antidiabetic drug, has been reported to mitigate neuronal loss in epilepsy via multiple mechanisms including suppression of inflammation, oxidative stress and activating the AMPK pathway (Yimer et al. 2019; H S, Paudel, and K L 2019). In several studies, quercetin has been explored extensively to demonstrate its potency as a therapeutic alternative for epilepsy (Akyuz et al. 2021). In a drug-induced epileptic mice model, quercetin (in combination with rutin) exhibited weak, short-term but safe therapy for psychomotor seizures (Nieoczym et al. 2014). Pentylenetetrazol (PTZ)-induced seizures are a promising model for evaluation of antiepileptic efficacy of drugs. Several preclinical studies were performed employing this model. Nanoparticles of quercetin at doses of 25 and 50 mg/kg fabricated with Fe_3O_4-β-cyclodextrin significantly reduced the activation of astrocytes, seizures and neuronal loss in PTZ-induced seizures in rodents (Hashemian et al. 2019). In the similar model, Ahmed et al. reported that 100 mg/kg quercetin effectively decreased the number of seizures and delayed the seizure onset time. In addition, a notable behavioural improvement was observed via dark and light behavioural model, elevated plus maze and rotarod test (H. Ahmed et al. 2021). A novel compound Q808 also exhibited efficacy through this model. The compound targeted several genes and pathways that would cause cellular senescence leading to epilepsy. A decrease in apoptosis of cells and morphological change in neurons was also observed (X. Li et al. 2024). Quercetin exhibited remarkable neuron protection from seizure led neuronal death both discrete models. It showed favourable effects in cognitive function impairment by targeting SIRT1/Nrf2/SLC7A11/GPX4 signal (R. Xie et al. 2022). Given a dosage of 25 mg/kg quercetin lowered the proinflammatory cytokines and decreased the absence seizures in WAG/Rij rodents implanted with triode electrodes. A decrease in NO, TNF-α and IL-6 was identified in rat brains in addition to the decrease in spike-wave discharge suggesting its efficacy in absence seizures (Kızılaslan et al. 2023). Effect of quercetin (10 μL or 100 mg/kg) was also explored in discrete model of epilepsy. Interestingly, a neurotoxin, kainic acid (KA) was employed to induce seizures in BALB/c mice. The study revealed that quercetin significantly suppressed the KA-induced seizures frequency. It also downregulated NF-κB signalling, TNF-α and IL-1β, contributing to anti-seizure benefits (Wu et al. 2020).

Quercetin with dasatinib together have proven efficacy against cellular senescence in several pathologies including neurodegeneration. A few studies reported the role of this combination against epilepsy as well. Recent study in a unique dysplasia type II (FCDII) in vivo rodent model role of senolytic therapy was promising. The therapy with dasatinib and quercetin remarkably attenuated the senescent cell load and reduced the frequency of seizures associated with $Mtor^{S2215F}$ mutations. Further, the treatment also altered the presence of senescent markers like p53/p16, SASP and SA-β-gal activity in animals (Ribierre et al. 2024). In addition to treatment benefits a recent study reported the prophylactic potential of this combination of drugs in aged mouse. The treatment to C57BL/6J mice demonstrated a significant decline in mortality and intensity of seizures. Furthermore, the senolytic intervention suppressed the SA-β-gal activity p16 function that aided in age-related deterioration (Khan et al. 2024). The studies regarding senolytic management of epilepsy is limited to quercetin as most research have focussed on this flavonoid.

2.3.3 Amyotrophic Lateral Sclerosis and Multiple Sclerosis

ALS is a fatal disease that progressively damages the nervous system. The progress can be slowed down by targeting motor neurons. Therapeutic approaches that may target increased senescent cells may serve as promising therapeutic approaches for the treatment. Oxidative stress is a key player that leads to disease progression (Maximova, Werry, and Kassiou 2021).

Katsumata et al. used motor neuron cells of mice to identify the causative gene for ALS. They discovered the mutation of Cu/Zn SOD accentuated the c-Abl gene that subsequently increased activity of the caspase-3 enzyme in the G93A-SOD1 transgenic mice model of ALS. Oral administration of dasatinib reduced the phosphorylation of c-Abl, inactivated enzyme caspase-3 and augmented the innervations of neuromuscular junction suggesting neuroprotection and amelioration of ALS (Katsumata et al. 2012). In an RCT, curcumin (600 mg/day) oral supplementation was found to decrease the disease progression in ALS patients. Six months of treatment with the supplementation decreased oxidative stress, oxidative protein products and improved the aerobic metabolism affecting the pathology of ALS (Chico et al. 2018).

Wang and team assessed the effect of fisetin in different hSOD1 ALS models considering the fact that oxidative stress leads to significant advancement in disease pathology. Transgenic mice and drosophila with mutant $hSOD1^{G93A}$, $hSOD1^{G85}$ NSC34 cells were employed. An increase in survival rate, reduced motor impairment and decreased free radical damage was observed after fisetin treatment. The probable mechanism involved was found to be raised in phosphorylated ERK levels and enhanced antioxidants. Further, fisetin also decreased the hSOD1 expression in various models. These fisetin-led alterations provide insight for the capacity of fisetin for ALS therapy (T. H. Wang et al. 2018).

In MS there is continuous demyelination that causes neurodegeneration. The cumulative axonal and neuronal loss leads to disability. Therefore, re-myelination and myelin repair with senotherapeutic compounds that can help to preserve the axons from damage may serve as an effective therapy for preventing or delaying the disease progression (Koutsoudaki et al. 2020).

An adaptive and innate immune-mediated preclinical autoimmune encephalomyelitis rodent model for MS was employed by Azizi et al. to investigate the effect of dasatinib. This is an inflammation-based model that causes demyelination and axonal impairment. C57BL/6 mice were used for the study model, which was established using myelin oligodendrocyte glycoprotein emulsion. Dasatinib treatment reduced the damage and delayed the onset of MS in just 21 days. It also decreased the oxidative stress and elevated TNF-α, NO in vivo. Further in vitro assessment of dasatinib activity in C6 astrocytoma cells demonstrated a decrease in MMP-2 activity and inhibited cell growth. These observations showed the effect of potential of dasatinib to alleviate MS (Azizi et al. 2015).

Recently, the role of curcumin was also investigated in MS model. In vitro evaluation in lipopolysaccharide (LPS)-stimulated CD-D18 cells showed curcumin (10 μM) altered the cytokines Th1/Th2/Th17. Additionally, curcumin (100 mg/kg) attenuated the neurological symptoms in an autoimmune encephalomyelitis model and regulated the CD3 and CD4 expressions in lymphocytes. These results suggest the therapeutic capacity of curcumin to alter MS pathology, decrease demyelination and restore motor and behavioural impairment through its properties including antioxidant capacity and anti-inflammatory effects (ELBini-Dhouib et al. 2022). Ahmadi and team investigated the immunomodulatory effects of quercetin in vitro in peripheral blood mononuclear cells to study its potential role in modifying MS. The compound modulated the TH17 cells and decreased the IL-17 gene and thus attenuated the mechanism of neuroinflammation, indicating its efficacy for treatment of MS (Ahmadi et al. 2023).

A multicentre, randomized clinical trial with 35 patients of MS assessed the effect of masitinib. The drug administered orally (3–6 mg/kg) for a year showed a decline in the progression of MS and also affected relapse-free secondary progressive MS. This was evidence with improved scores of multiple sclerosis functional composite (Vermersch et al. 2012).

Senotherapy combined with regenerative therapies including haematopoietic stem cells oligodendrocyte precursors, microglia, monocytes, thymus and immune cells can attenuate immune senescence and offer therapeutic benefits in MS (Dema et al. 2021).

2.3.4 Parkinson's Disease

Oxidative damage or inflammation of neurons induced by senescent cells and are major players for causing progression of PD. The pathology of disease displays accumulation of neurotic plaques (Kakoty et al. 2023). Removal of senescent astrocytes reversed the elevated SASP factors, caused a decline in neuronal cell death and ameliorated the paraquat-triggered PD in vitro (Chinta et al. 2018). Mitochondrial overactivity is also observed during the initiation of PD. In view of this, it was found that antidiabetic drug metformin was found to modulate mitochondrial respiration and improve neuronal viability and motor function. These effects indicate metformin is a promising agent for PD therapy (Mor et al. 2020).

Effect of fisetin was assessed in vitro in MPTP/MPP^+-triggered cytotoxicity in PC12 cells. MPTP caused apoptosis and inflammation in cells which was evidenced with upregulated pro-inflammatory cytokines, mediators of apoptosis and transcription factors. Pre-treatment of cells with fisetin suppressed the inflammatory mediators, apoptosis and expression of α-synuclein. These changes by fisetin ameliorated PD development (Patel et al. 2012). PD developed through rotenone is a well-established model. The effects of fisetin (10 and 20 mg/kg) in this model were investigated in animals after 25 days of oral treatment. Analysis of rat brains showed enhanced motor activity in a cylinder test. Moreover, the treatment also reversed the altered mitochondrial activity, dopamine levels in striatum and antioxidant enzyme levels and prevented PD (Alikatte et al. 2021).

The flavonoid quercetin also covalently binds with α-synuclein and has the capacity to alter PD pathology (Singh et al. 2020). The influence of quercetin in PD was identified in 6-hydroxydomaine–induced neuronal damage in primary cultured rat cortical cells and rodent models (Haleagrahara et al. 2011; Bakoyiannis et al. 2019). Quercetin modifies cellular senescence by stimulation of SIRT1 genes and autophagy, alteration of Nrf2 pathway, suppression of SASP and induces PON2 (Kida and Goligorsky 2016; Shao et al. 2021; Acıkara et al. 2022). The neuroprotective effect of this drug was explored in the 6-hydroxydopamine (6-OHDA)-stimulated damage in the PD rodent model and in vitro in 6-OHDA-exposed PC12 cells. Quercetin administration in PD rats reversed the 6-OHDA-induced changes like neuronal death, mitochondrial damage and motor symptoms. Further, in vitro treatment of PC12 cells with quercetin (20 μM) decreased α-synuclein, attenuated the oxidative stress, improved mitochondrial function, and also increased the expressions of *PINK1* and *PARKIN* genes. These results suggested neuroprotective effects against PD (W.-W. Wang et al. 2021).

Oral supplementation with 50 mg/kg quercetin in PD caused by rotenone in rats modified the motor functions, cognitive behaviour and depression-like symptoms in rats. Brain samples raised the levels of neurotransmitters and increased the levels of antioxidants and cognition. These improvements were observed after intervention with quercetin (Madiha et al. 2021). In another preclinical study, intervention with 30 mg/kg quercetin for 2 months ameliorated PD in rotenone-induced neurotoxicity in a rat model. Quercetin altered the rotenone-induced changes like increased inflammatory markers, downregulation of striatal dopaminergic fibres and increased astrocyte function in the hippocampus and substantia nigra. Further, quercetin also improved the memory function identified via T- and Y-maze recognition tests, increased time for immobility in the forced swim test and also altered the compromised muscle strength of animals. These results exhibited that quercetin has the potential to attenuate neuroinflammation and enhanced cognitive functions and memory (Jain et al. 2022). In the same year, Josiah et al. also investigated the effect of quercetin in neurotoxic PD rat model induced by rotenone. Diseased animals exhibited inflammation-altered NF-κB, TNF-α, IκKB and IL-1β. Further modulation of the p53 gene was also identified. Quercetin 20 mg/kg attenuated the expressions of IκKB and NF-κB. Further, it also demonstrated reduction in oxidative stress, regulated dopamine metabolism, decreased inflammatory activity and apoptosis in animal models, exhibiting its potential for PD therapy (Josiah et al. 2022).

Metal contamination is also correlated with health risk in humans, specifically neurodegenerative diseases. Copper is an essential co-factor for some enzymes including cytochrome oxidase. The effect of quercetin was investigated in copper-induced toxicity in neuroblastoma SH-SY5Y human cells. Results suggested that quercetin reversed the copper-induced changes like increased oxidative stress, altered mitochondrial function and apoptosis. Anti-apoptotic effects were attributed to upregulated microtubules linked protein light chain–3. Quercetin also modified the response of endoplasmic reticulum–mediated homeostasis in cell organelles. The modifications after quercetin treatment shed light on its effective therapeutic behaviour for PD (Joyeeta Chakraborty et al. 2022).

Overall, the senotherapeutic approach for PD therapy mostly relies on its antioxidant and anti-inflammatory behaviour along with the impact on α-synuclein which might help to delay the disease progression.

2.3.5 Huntington's Disease

HD is an autosomal genetic disorder that influences cognition, psychological and motor behaviour. The therapies available only provide some level of symptomatic relief. The target therapy using senotherapeutics may offer delay in development of disease.

The effects and mechanism of fisetin were studied in various HD models like PC12 cells that express the mutant *Httex* gene, drosophila that also express mutant *Httex* and R6/2 mice model. Fisetin treatment attenuated the effect of mutant HTT in all the models and was found to activate Ras-extracellular signal regulating the cascade mechanism that involves MAPK (Maher et al. 2011). The fisetin derivative CMS121 was investigated for its effects on HD mice models R6/2 and YAC128. CMS121 showed a decline in HD-induced changes in gene expression and oxidative phosphorylation. Further improved motor function was also restored that is associated with better health span (Ates, Taguchi, and Maher 2023).

In a preclinical study, a sub-chronic intra-peritoneum dose of 3-nitropropioic (3-NP) acid was employed for induction of HD in animals. Analysis of biochemical and neuro-behavioural parameters assured neurodegeneration. A quercetin supplement (25 mg/kg) for 21 days modulated the 3-NP–led changes in respiratory chain, swelling ATP levels and mitochondrial oxidative damage. Quercetin also restored the enzyme activities of catalase and superoxide dismutase. Neuro-behavioural assessment with footprint analysis and beam walk improved motor function. Further, histopathological analysis of the brain demonstrated decreased striatal astrogliosis and pyknotic nuclei. All these changes induced by quercetin exhibit its significant role in regulating mitochondrial activity for the therapy of HD (Sandhir and Mehrotra 2013). In the following year, another study was conducted on the similar model, and the effect of 4 days quercetin treatment was investigated. Assessment of biogenic amines present at the striatum and monoamine oxidase activity revealed potential of quercetin to alter the metabolism of serotonin. A significant decrease in gait despair, anxiety and motor incoordination was also observed with quercetin in 3-NP–exposed animals. Further, attenuation of astrocytes and microglial proliferation was also in neurons. These changes alleviated HD pathology by improving motor coordination and anxiety behaviour (Joy Chakraborty et al. 2014).

2.3.6 Others

The effect of quercetin was investigated on the progression of prion's disease (transmissible spongiform encephalopathies), which is a fatal neurodegenerative disorder. The treatment led to the formation of proteinase-sensitive aggregates and disaggregate mouse prion protein. Amyloid fibrils bound to quercetin disturbed the erythrocyte function, decreased oxidative stress, and cytotoxicity for neuroblastoma cells. These effects were different from typical anti-amyloidogenic agents but may help for therapy of the disease (Yu and Lee 2020). Quercetin and dasatinib decreased the expression of p16/21 in an hSOD1-G93A model. This ameliorated the motor neuron disease pathology (Torres et al. 2022).

Neuronal toxicity and apoptosis can be induced by aluminium chloride ($AlCl_3$) and cause discrete central nervous disorders. Neuroprotective effect of fisetin were explored in $AlCl_3$-induced neuronal degeneration in male Swiss albino mice. Aluminium caused increased oxidative stress, aggregation of Aβ and accelerated apoptosis. Cortical and hippocampal regions showed higher expressions of caspase 3/9, cytochrome 3, p53, p-JNK (c-Jun N-terminal kinase) and apoptosis-stimulating kinase (ASK-1) and altered Bax/Bcl-2 gene. These factors were altered by fisetin treatment (15 mg/kg) (Prakash and Sudhandiran 2015). In a similar model, quercetin (10 mg/kg) interfered with displacement of cytochrome-c, enhanced Bcl-2 gene, decreased caspase-3, p53 and Bax levels and also prevented DNA fragmentation. The treatment also suppressed cristae loss, mitochondrial swelling and chromosome condensation. These outcomes suggest neuroprotective potential of quercetin (Sharma et al. 2016).

Efficacy of senolytic fisetin was evaluated in Hutchinson-Gilford progeria syndrome (HGPS) model. For the accelerated aging model, WT and Zmpste24$^{-/-}$ (Z24$^{-/-}$) mice were used. Accelerated aging witness increased activity of fibro-adipogenic progenitors (FAPs) that integrate with progenitor muscle cells. Aged mice exhibited elevated a two-fold increase in FAPs and decrease in these cells. There was impaired myogenic proliferation of cells in animals. Fisetin treatment enhanced the apoptosis of Z24$^{-/-}$ mice, reduced senescent FAPs and increased the MPCs that improved the pathology of muscle. The outcome proposed fisetin treatment as a therapeutic target for muscle-related diseases like progeria (Lei Liu et al. 2022). The influence of metformin was also investigated on HGPS premature aging disease and on other aging disorders. The treatment was found to delay senescence, decrease oxidative stress, improve nuclear phenotypes and enhance phosphorylation of AMP-stimulated protein kinase in dermal HGPS fibroblast cells. Elevated antioxidant mRNA enzyme expression was observed. These results postulated metformin as a potential therapeutic agent for HGPS for life extension (Park and Shin 2017).

Metformin (a drug used in diabetes) has also been explored for its effects on cellular senescence. Metformin treatment decreased the mitochondrial dysfunction and oxidative stress in aged adipose-derived stromal cells. This enhanced the adipogenic capacity of cells (Le Pelletier et al. 2021). In intervertebral disc deterioration that involves senescence of nucleus pulposus cells, Ren et al. propounded that metformin suppress cellular senescence through inactivation of the cGAS-STING signalling pathway (Ren et al. 2022). Metformin decreased inflammation and enhanced autophagy. Aging-related disorders are also caused by senescence of vascular smooth muscle cells (VSMC). Metformin was found to decrease angiotensin-II (Ang-II)-dependent cellular senesce in elderly arteries. It modulated structure of arteries, decreased SASP and improved stiffness of arteries along and migration and proliferation of senescent VSMC. Autophagic flux decreased in Ang-II was restored by metformin at the autophagosome-lysosome fusion level (Tai et al. 2022). Sung and team also reported that metformin ameliorates senescence of VSMC by increasing AMPK-induced mitochondrial antioxidants dependent on SIRT3 levels (Sung et al. 2022). In a recent controlled two-arm trial on 20 participants of both sexes, pre-treatment with metformin was found to alter cellular senescence through FAPs and SASP. Metformin reduced FAPs and modified fibroblast cells, and decreased pro-inflammatory transcriptional factors (Petrocelli et al. 2023).

Aging exhibits an increased incidence of neurological symptoms associated with cerebral micro-haemorrhages. Senolytic intervention with drugs like navitoclax may arrest senescence and effectively delay the onset, decrease the incidence of disease and offer significant cerebro-microvascular protection in CMH (Faakye et al. 2023). In another study, in p16–3MR transgenic mice, navitoclax prevented the cell senescence in whole-brain irradiation-induced endothelial senescence along with improved capillarization in the cortex (Gulej et al. 2023) and reversed the chemotherapy-induced cognitive dysfunction as improved special memory, microvascular density and neovascular responses were observed (Ahire et al. 2023). Further, integrity of the BBB was restored, and cognition was improved in both studies.

In a recent study combined influence of quercetin and dasatinib was investigated for its neuroprotective potential in the aging female brain that encounters reduced hormonal levels. Female C57BL/6 mice were administered the drug till 14 months of age. The control aged animals exhibited inflammation and oxidative stress. These effects were reversed with the combined senolytic treatment as evidence with decrease in ROS and increased catalase activity. Additionally, the treatment prevented the declined activity of Na^+, K^+-ATPase. The study reported protective effect of the combined treatment in age-related neurochemical changes in the brain (Faria et al. 2024).

Senotherapeutics are being explored for several neurodegenerative disorders and the outcome from the studies suggests that the senotherapy may benefit several illnesses associated with age and neuronal damage. Table 2.1 briefly describes the clinical trials underway for assessment of senotherapeutic activity.

2.4 CONCLUSION

To improve health and longevity, senotherapeutics are being developed to ameliorate age-related neurodegeneration. This class of drugs was first identified in the year 2015, and since then several advancements have been reported preclinically. Clinically, around 35 clinical trials are ongoing to address several health issues related to age, diabetes, bone, cardiovascular system, central nervous system, etc. The science of senotherapeutics is anticipated to grow with investigations on drugs that may be optimally employed.

In specific regard to brain or neurological disorders, several clinical studies are being conducted to assess the potency in age-related ailments. The target of this class is to re-establish mitochondrial function, decrease inflammation, and modulate SA-β-gal activity and several SASP markers. Recent studies have identified specific biomarkers as therapeutic approaches to increase the specificity of drugs and reduce their adverse effects. This approach may help to establish the safety of senotherapeutics as drugs like navitoclax possess haematological toxicity. Tolerability, safety and efficacy need to be established with clinical trials. It is crucial to note that reported senotherapeutics have been investigated with single

Table 2.1 Clinical Trials Underway for Senotherapeutics

S.No	*Official Title*	*Registration Number*	*Drugs and Phase*
1	An Unblinded Pilot Study for AD	NCT04785300	Dasatinib with quercetin Phase 1 and Phase 2
2	Pilot Study to evaluate the safety and feasibility of Senotherapy to alter the Progression of AD (SToMP-AD)	NCT04063124	Dasatinib with quercetin Phase 1 and Phase 2
3	Phase 2 trial to assess the safety and feasibility of senotherapy in AD	NCT04685590	Dasatinib with quercetin Phase 2
4	Influence of combined treatment of curcumin and Resveratrol Liposomes with G04CB02 for improvement in ALS	NCT04654689	Curcumin Phase 2
5	Phase 2, prospective, multicenter, randomized, Double-blinded controlled study to evaluate the safety, tolerability, and Activity intravitreal injection of UBX1325 in Neovascular AMD	NCT05275205	UBX1325 Phase 2
6	A Pilot trial to assess the influence of senotherapy to alter the progression of AD (SToMP-AD)	NCT04063124	Dasatinib and quercetin
7	A lifestyle intervention protocol to identify changes in retinal amyloid in patients with cognitive impairment	NCT02741804	Fisetin and other interventions Phase NA

concentration. Moreover, their effectiveness relies on the measurement of senescent markers like p16^{INK4a} and p21^{CIP1} or SA-β-gal activity. In fact, senescence-like characteristics overlap with quiescent or proliferating cells that may require a discrete approach, or else it may lead to imprecise understanding of the mechanism. Therefore, in future, senotherapeutics must identify the characteristics of senescent cells to precisely employ the senescent markers and thereafter target them in several neurodegenerative disorders.

REFERENCES

Acıkara, Ozlem Bahadır, Gökçe Şeker Karatoprak, Çiğdem Yücel, Esra Küpeli Akkol, Eduardo Sobarzo-Sánchez, Maryam Khayatkashani, Mohammad Amjad Kamal, and Hamid Reza Khayat Kashani. 2022. "A Critical Analysis of Quercetin as the Attractive Target for the Treatment of Parkinson's Disease." *CNS & Neurological Disorders Drug Targets* 21 (9): 795–817. https://doi.org/10.2174/1871527320666211206122407.

Ahire, Chetan, Adam Nyul-Toth, Jordan DelFavero, Rafal Gulej, Janet A. Faakye, Stefano Tarantini, Tamas Kiss, et al. 2023. "Accelerated Cerebromicrovascular Senescence Contributes to Cognitive Decline in a Mouse Model of Paclitaxel (Taxol)-Induced Chemobrain." *Aging Cell* 22 (7). https://doi.org/10.1111/acel.13832.

Ahmad, Ashfaq, Tahir Ali, Hyun Young Park, Haroon Badshah, Shafiq Ur Rehman, and Myeong Ok Kim. 2017. "Neuroprotective Effect of Fisetin Against Amyloid-Beta-Induced Cognitive/Synaptic Dysfunction, Neuroinflammation, and Neurodegeneration in Adult Mice." *Molecular Neurobiology* 54 (3): 2269–2285. https://doi.org/10.1007/S12035-016-9795-4.

Ahmadi, Leila, Nahid Eskandari, Mustafa Ghanadian, Mahshid Rahmati, Neda Kasiri, Masoud Etamadifar, Mohadeseh Toghyani, and Fereshteh Alsahebfosoul. 2023. "The Immunomodulatory Aspect of Quercetin Penta Acetate on Th17 Cells Proliferation and Gene Expression in Multiple Sclerosis." *Cell Journal* 25 (2): 110–117. https://doi.org/10.22074/cellj.2022.557560.1073.

Ahmed, Hammad, Mahtab Ahmad Khan, Syed Awais Ali Zaidi, and Sajjad Muhammad. 2021. "In Silico and In Vivo: Evaluating the Therapeutic Potential of Kaempferol, Quercetin, and Catechin to Treat Chronic Epilepsy in a Rat Model." *Frontiers in Bioengineering and Biotechnology* 9 (November). https://doi.org/10.3389/fbioe.2021.754952.

Ahmed, Faraha, and Razia Khanam. 2023. "Senolytics in Brain Disorders: A Novel Pharmacological Approach to Control Cellular Senescence and Oxidative Stress." In *Adaptation under Stressful Environments through Biological Adjustments and Interventions*, 327–342. Singapore: Springer Nature Singapore. https://doi.org/10.1007/978-981-99-7652-2_20.

Akyuz, Enes, Yam Nath Paudel, Ayse Kristina Polat, Huseyin Emre Dundar, and Efthalia Angelopoulou. 2021. "Enlightening the Neuroprotective Effect of Quercetin in Epilepsy: From Mechanism to Therapeutic Opportunities." *Epilepsy & Behavior* 115 (February): 107701. https://doi.org/10.1016/j.yebeh.2020.107701.

Alayli, Adam, Gavin Lockard, Jonah Gordon, Jacob Connolly, Molly Monsour, Samantha Schimmel, Ike Dela Peña, and Cesar V. Borlongan. 2023. "Stem Cells: Recent Developments Redefining Epilepsy Therapy." *Cell Transplantation* 32 (January). https://doi.org/10.1177/09636897231158967.

Alikatte, Kanakalatha, Suresh Palle, Jadi Rajendra Kumar, and Naveen Pathakala. 2021. "Fisetin Improved Rotenone-Induced Behavioral Deficits, Oxidative Changes, and Mitochondrial Dysfunctions in Rat Model of Parkinson's Disease." *Journal of Dietary Supplements* 18 (1): 57–71. https://doi.org/10.1080/19390211.2019.1710646.

Ates, Gamze, Taketo Taguchi, and Pamela Maher. 2023. "CMS121 Partially Attenuates Disease Progression in Mouse Models of Huntington's Disease." *Molecular Neurobiology* (October). https://doi.org/10.1007/s12035-023-03711-2.

Averdunk, Luisa, Maxim A. Huetzen, Daniel Moreno-Andrés, Reinhard Kalb, Shane McKee, Tzung-Chien Hsieh, Annette Seibt, et al. 2023. "Biallelic Variants in CRIPT Cause a Rothmund-Thomson-like Syndrome with Increased Cellular Senescence." *Genetics in Medicine* 25 (7): 100836. https://doi.org/10.1016/j.gim.2023.100836.

Azizi, Gholamreza, Mahdi Goudarzvand, Sanaz Afraei, Reza Sedaghat, and Abbas Mirshafiey. 2015. "Therapeutic Effects of Dasatinib in Mouse Model of Multiple Sclerosis." *Immunopharmacology and Immunotoxicology* 37 (3): 287–294. https://doi.org/10.3109/08923973.2015.1028074.

Baiardi, Simone, Angela Mammana, Sabina Capellari, and Piero Parchi. 2023. "Human Prion Disease: Molecular Pathogenesis, and Possible Therapeutic Targets and Strategies."

Expert Opinion on Therapeutic Targets 27 (12): 1271–1284. https://doi.org/10.1080/14728222.2023.2199923.

Bakoyiannis, Ioannis, Afrodite Daskalopoulou, Vasilios Pergialiotis, and Despina Perrea. 2019. "Phytochemicals and Cognitive Health: Are Flavonoids Doing the Trick?" *Biomedicine & Pharmacotherapy = Biomedecine & Pharmacotherapie* 109 (January): 1488–1497. https://doi.org/10.1016/J.BIOPHA.2018.10.086.

Bedrosian, Tracy A., Judith Houtman, Juan Sebastian Eguiguren, Saeed Ghassemzadeh, Nicole Rund, Nicole M. Novaresi, Lauren Hu, et al. 2021. "Lamin B1 Decline Underlies Age-Related Loss of Adult Hippocampal Neurogenesis." *The EMBO Journal* 40 (3). https://doi.org/10.15252/embj.2020105819.

Bhatia, Nidhi K., Priya Modi, Shilpa Sharma, and Shashank Deep. 2020. "Quercetin and Baicalein Act as Potent Antiamyloidogenic and Fibril Destabilizing Agents for SOD1 Fibrils." *ACS Chemical Neuroscience* 11 (8): 1129–1138. https://doi.org/10 1021/acschemneuro.9b00677.

Burla, Romina, Mattia La Torre, Giorgia Zanetti, Alex Bastianelli, Chiara Merigliano, Simona Del Giudice, Alessandro Vercelli, et al. 2018. "P53-Sensitive Epileptic Behavior and Inflammation in Ft1 Hypomorphic Mice." *Frontiers in Genetics* 9 (November). https://doi.org/10.3389/fgene.2018.00581.

Calcinotto, Arianna, and Andrea Alimonti. 2017. "Aging Tumour Cells to Cure Cancer: 'Pro-Senescence' Therapy for Cancer." *Swiss Medical Weekly* 147 (January). https://doi.org/10.4414/SMW.2017.14367.

Calcinotto, Arianna, Jaskaren Kohli, Elena Zagato, Laura Pellegrini, Marco Demaria, and Andrea Alimonti. 2019. "Cellular Senescence: Aging, Cancer, and Injury." *Physiological Reviews* 99 (2): 1047–1078. https://doi.org/10.1152/PHYSREV.00020.2018.

Casella, Gabriel, Rachel Munk, Kyoung Mi Kim, Yulan Piao, Supriyo De, Kotb Abdelmohsen, and Myriam Gorospe. 2019. "Transcriptome Signature of Cellular Senescence." *Nucleic Acids Research* 47 (14): 7294–7305. https://doi.org/10.1093/NAR/GKZ555.

Chakraborty, Joy, Raghavendra Singh, Debashis Dutta, Amit Naskar, Usha Rajamma, and Kochupurackal P. Mohanakumar. 2014. "Quercetin Improves Behavioral Deficiencies, Restores Astrocytes and Microglia, and Reduces Serotonin Metabolism in 3-Nitropropionic Acid-Induced Rat Model of Huntington's Disease." *CNS Neuroscience & Therapeutics* 20 (1): 10–19. https://doi.org/10.1111/cns.12189.

Chakraborty, Joyeeta, Sourav Pakrashi, Arpita Sarbajna, Moumita Dutta, and Jaya Bandyopadhyay. 2022. "Quercetin Attenuates Copper-Induced Apoptotic Cell Death and Endoplasmic Reticulum Stress in SH-SY5Y Cells by Autophagic Modulation." *Biological Trace Element Research* 200 (12): 5022–5041. https://doi.org/10.1007/s12011-022-03093-x.

Chen, Li, Lei Xiong, Lingling Yao, Jinxiu Pan, Emily Arzola, Xiaojuan Zhu, Lin Mei, and Wen-Cheng Xiong. 2023. "Attenuation of Alzheimer's Brain Pathology in 5XFAD Mice by PTH1–34, a Peptide of Parathyroid Hormone." *Alzheimer's Research & Therapy* 15 (1): 53. https://doi.org/10.1186/s13195-023-01202-z.

Chico, Lucia, Elena Caldarazzo Ienco, Costanza Bisordi, Annalisa Lo Gerfo, Lucia Petrozzi, Antonio Petrucci, Michelangelo Mancuso, and Gabriele Siciliano. 2018. "Amyotrophic Lateral Sclerosis and Oxidative Stress: A Double-Blind Therapeutic Trial After Curcumin Supplementation." *CNS & Neurological Disorders Drug Targets* 17 (10): 767–779. https://doi.org/10.2174/1871527317666180720162029.

Chinta, Shankar J., Georgia Woods, Marco Demaria, Anand Rane, Ying Zou, Amanda McQuade, Subramanian Rajagopalan, et al. 2018. "Cellular Senescence Is Induced by the Environmental Neurotoxin Paraquat and Contributes to Neuropathology Linked to Parkinson's Disease." *Cell Reports* 22 (4): 930–940. https://doi.org/10.1016/J.CELREP.2017.12.092.

Choi, Ji Young, Samantha F. Yee, Tzvetelina Tchangalova, Guang Yang, and John P. Fisher. 2022. "Recent Advances in Senotherapeutics Delivery." *Tissue Engineering. Part B, Reviews* 28 (6): 1223–1234. https://doi.org/10.1089/ten.TEB.2021.0212.

Clabough, Erin B.D., and Scott O. Zeitlin. 2006. "Deletion of the Triplet Repeat Encoding Polyglutamine within the Mouse Huntington's Disease Gene Results in Subtle Behavioral/Motor Phenotypes in Vivo and Elevated Levels of ATP with Cellular Senescence in Vitro." *Human Molecular Genetics* 15 (4): 607–623. https://doi.org/10.1093/hmg/ddi477.

Costa, Lucio G., Rian De Laat, Khoi Dao, Claudia Pellacani, Toby B. Cole, and Clement E. Furlong. 2014. "Paraoxonase-2 (PON2) in Brain and Its Potential Role in Neuroprotection." *Neurotoxicology* 43: 3–9. https://doi.org/10.1016/J.NEURO.2013.08.011.

Currais, Antonio, Marguerite Prior, Richard Dargusch, Aaron Armando, Jennifer Ehren, David Schubert, Oswald Quehenberger, and Pamela Maher. 2014. "Modulation of P25 and Inflammatory Pathways by Fisetin Maintains Cognitive Function in Alzheimer's Disease Transgenic Mice." *Aging Cell* 13 (2): 379–390. https://doi.org/10.1111/ACEL.12185.

Dema, María, Herena Eixarch, Luisa M. Villar, Xavier Montalban, and Carmen Espejo. 2021. "Immunosenescence in Multiple Sclerosis: The Identification of New Therapeutic Targets." *Autoimmunity Reviews* 20 (9): 102893. https://doi.org/10.1016/j.autrev.2021.102893.

Dong, Huimin, Shanpin Mao, Jiajun Wei, Baohui Liu, Zhaohui Zhang, Qian Zhang, and Mingmin Yan. 2012. "Tanshinone IIA Protects PC12 Cells from β-Amyloid25–35-Induced Apoptosis via PI3K/Akt Signaling Pathway." *Molecular Biology Reports* 39 (6): 6495–6503. https://doi.org/10.1007/s11033-012-1477-3.

ELBini-Dhouib, Ines, Maroua Manai, Nour-Elhouda Neili, Soumaya Marzouki, Ghada Sahraoui, Warda Ben Achour, Sondes Zouaghi, Melika BenAhmed, Raoudha Doghri, and Najet Srairi-Abid. 2022. "Dual Mechanism of Action of Curcumin in Experimental Models of Multiple Sclerosis." *International Journal of Molecular Sciences* 23 (15). https://doi.org/10.3390/ijms23158658.

Faakye, Janet, Ádám Nyúl-Tóth, Mihaly Muranyi, Rafal Gulej, Boglarka Csik, Santny Shanmugarama, Stefano Tarantini, et al. 2023. "Preventing Spontaneous Cerebral Microhemorrhages in Aging Mice: A Novel Approach Targeting Cellular Senescence with ABT263/Navitoclax." *GeroScience* 46 (1): 21–37. https://doi.org/10.1007/s11357-023-01024-9.

Fang, Marong, Jing Wang, Xiaobing Zhang, Yu Geng, Zhiying Hu, John A. Rudd, Shucai Ling, Wei Chen, and Shu Han. 2012. "The MiR-124 Regulates the Expression of BACE1/β-Secretase Correlated with Cell Death in Alzheimer's Disease." *Toxicology Letters* 209 (1): 94–105. https://doi.org/10.1016/j.toxlet.2011.11.032.

Fang, Yimin, Mackenzie R. Peck, Kathleen Quinn, David Medina, Stephen Roy, Samuel A. McFadden, Andrzej Bartke, Kevin N. Hascup, and Erin R. Hascup. 2023. "Senolytic Intervention Improves Cognition, Metabolism, and Adiposity in Female APPNL-F/NL-F Mice." *BioRxiv: The Preprint Server for Biology* (December). https://doi.org/10.1101/2023.12.12.571277.

Faria, Olivia Wyse, Mayara Sandrielly Soares de Aguiar, Julia Eisenhardt de Mello, Fernando Lopez Alvez, Karina Pereira Luduvico, Driele Neske Garcia, Augusto Schneider, Michal M Masternak, Roselia Maria Spanevello, and Francieli Moro Stefanello.

2024. "Senolytics Prevent Age-Associated Changes in Female Mice Brain." *Neuroscience Letters* 826 (March): 137730. https://doi.org/10.1016/j.neulet.2024.137730.

Fatt, Michael P., Lina M. Tran, Gisella Vetere, Mekayla A. Storer, Jaclin V. Simonetta, Freda D. Miller, Paul W. Frankland, and David R. Kaplan. 2022. "Restoration of Hippocampal Neural Precursor Function by Ablation of Senescent Cells in the Aging Stem Cell Niche." *Stem Cell Reports* 17 (2). Elsevier: 259. https://doi.org/10.1016/J.STEMCR.2021.12.010.

Furiya, Yoshiko, Makito Hirano, Norio Kurumatani, Takuya Nakamuro, Ryusuke Matsumura, Naonobu Futamura, and Satoshi Ueno. 2005. "Alpha-1-Antichymotrypsin Gene Polymorphism and Susceptibility to Multiple System Atrophy (MSA)." *Brain Research. Molecular Brain Research* 138 (2): 178–181. https://doi.org/10.1016/j.molbrainres.2005.04.011.

Gonzales, Mitzi M., Valentina R. Garbarino, Tiffany F. Kautz, Juan Pablo Palavicini, Marisa Lopez-Cruzan, Shiva Kazempour Dehkordi, Julia J. Mathews, et al. 2023. "Senolytic Therapy in Mild Alzheimer's Disease: A Phase 1 Feasibility Trial." *Nature Medicine* 29 (10): 2481–2488. https://doi.org/10.1038/s41591-023-02543-w.

González-Gualda, Estela, Andrew G. Baker, Ljiljana Fruk, and Daniel Muñoz-Espín. 2021. "A Guide to Assessing Cellular Senescence In Vitro and In Vivo." *The FEBS Journal* 288 (1). FEBS J: 56–80. https://doi.org/10.1111/FEBS.15570.

Guan, Jing-Zhi, Wei-Ping Guan, Toyoki Maeda, Xie Guoqing, Wan GuangZhi, and Naoki Makino. 2015. "Patients with Multiple Sclerosis Show Increased Oxidative Stress Markers and Somatic Telomere Length Shortening." *Molecular and Cellular Biochemistry* 400 (1–2): 183–187. https://doi.org/10.1007/s11010-014-2274-1.

Guan, Teng, Ying Guo, Ting Zhou, Qiang Yu, Jingyi Sun, Baoliang Sun, Guohui Zhang, and Jiming Kong. 2024. "Oxidized SOD1 Accelerates Cellular Senescence in Neural Stem Cells." *Stem Cell Research & Therapy* 15 (1): 55. https://doi.org/10.1186/s13287-024-03669-5.

Gulej, Rafal, Ádám Nyúl-Tóth, Chetan Ahire, Jordan DelFavero, Priya Balasubramanian, Tamas Kiss, Stefano Tarantini, et al. 2023. "Elimination of Senescent Cells by Treatment with Navitoclax/ABT263 Reverses Whole Brain Irradiation-Induced Blood-Brain Barrier Disruption in the Mouse Brain." *GeroScience* 45 (5): 2983–3002. https://doi.org/10.1007/s11357-023-00870-x.

H S, Nandini, Yam Nath Paudel, and Krishna K L. 2019. "Envisioning the Neuroprotective Effect of Metformin in Experimental Epilepsy: A Portrait of Molecular Crosstalk." *Life Sciences* 233 (September). https://doi.org/10.1016/J.LFS.2019.116686.

Haleagrahara, Nagaraja, Cheng Jun Siew, Nilesh Kumar Mitra, and Mangala Kumari. 2011. "Neuroprotective Effect of Bioflavonoid Quercetin in 6-Hydroxydopamine-Induced Oxidative Stress Biomarkers in the Rat Striatum." *Neuroscience Letters* 500 (2): 139–143. https://doi.org/10.1016/J.NEULET.2011.06.021.

Hao, Zongbing, and Guanghui Wang. 2020. "Autophagy and Prion Disease." *Advances in Experimental Medicine and Biology* 1207: 75–85. https://doi.org/10.1007/978-981-15-4272-5_4.

Hartz, Anika M. S., Anton Pekcec, Emma L. B. Soldner, Yu Zhong, Juli Schlichtiger, and Bjoern Bauer. 2017. "P-Gp Protein Expression and Transport Activity in Rodent Seizure Models and Human Epilepsy." *Molecular Pharmaceutics* 14 (4): 999–1011. https://doi.org/10.1021/acs.molpharmaceut.6b00770.

Hashemian, Mona, Maryam Ghasemi-Kasman, Shahram Ghasemi, Atefeh Akbari, Monire Moalem-Banhangi, Leila Zare, and Seyed Raheleh Ahmadian. 2019. "Fabrication and Evaluation of Novel Quercetin-Conjugated Fe_3O_4–β-Cyclodextrin Nanoparticles for Potential Use in Epilepsy Disorder." *International Journal of Nanomedicine* 14 (August): 6481–6495. https://doi.org/10.2147/IJN.S218317.

Hernandez-Segura, Alejandra, Jamil Nehme, and Marco Demaria. 2018. "Hallmarks of Cellular Senescence." *Trends in Cell Biology* 28 (6): 436–453. https://doi.org/10.1016/J.TCB.2018.02.001.

Hou, Yujun, Xiuli Dan, Mansi Babbar, Yong Wei, Steen G. Hasselbalch, Deborah L. Croteau, and Vilhelm A. Bohr. 2019. "Ageing as a Risk Factor for Neurodegenerative Disease." *Nature Reviews. Neurology* 15 (10): 565–581. https://doi.org/10.1038/s41582-019-0244-7.

Innes, Kim E., Terry Kit Selfe, Kathleen Brundage, Caitlin Montgomery, Sijin Wen, Sahiti Kandati, Hannah Bowles, Dharma Singh Khalsa, and Zenzi Huysmans. 2018. "Effects of Meditation and Music-Listening on Blood Biomarkers of Cellular Aging and Alzheimer's Disease in Adults with Subjective Cognitive Decline: An Exploratory Randomized Clinical Trial." *Journal of Alzheimer's Disease: JAD* 66 (3): 947–970. https://doi.org/10.3233/JAD-180164.

Jagaraj, Cyril Jones, Sina Shadfar, Sara Assar Kashani, Sayanthooran Saravanabavan, Fabiha Farzana, and Julie D. Atkin. 2024. "Molecular Hallmarks of Ageing in Amyotrophic Lateral Sclerosis." *Cellular and Molecular Life Sciences: CMLS* 81 (1): 111. https://doi.org/10.1007/s00018-024-05164-9.

Jain, Juli, Whidul Hasan, Pronit Biswas, Rajesh S. Yadav, and Deepali Jat. 2022. "Neuroprotective Effect of Quercetin against Rotenone-Induced Neuroinflammation and Alterations in Mice Behavior." *Journal of Biochemical and Molecular Toxicology* 36 (10). https://doi.org/10.1002/jbt.23165.

Josiah, Sunday Solomon, Courage Dele Famusiwa, Olamide Olajusi Crown, Akeem O. Lawal, Mary Tolulope Olaleye, Afolabi Akintunde Akindahunsi, and Afolabi Clement Akinmoladun. 2022. "Neuroprotective Effects of Catechin and Quercetin in Experimental Parkinsonism through Modulation of Dopamine Metabolism and Expression of IL-1β, TNF-α, NF-KB, IκKB, and P53 Genes in Male Wistar Rats." *NeuroToxicology* 90 (May): 158–171. https://doi.org/10.1016/j.neuro.2022.03.004.

Kakoty, Violina, Sarathlal Kalarikkal Chandran, Monica Gulati, Bey Hing Goh, Kamal Dua, and Sachin Kumar Singh. 2023. "Senolytics: Opening Avenues in Drug Discovery to Find Novel Therapeutics for Parkinson's Disease." *Drug Discovery Today* 28 (6): 103582. https://doi.org/10.1016/j.drudis.2023.103582.

Kang, Chanhee, Qikai Xu, Timothy D. Martin, Mamie Z. Li, Marco Demaria, Liviu Aron, Tao Lu, Bruce A. Yankner, Judith Campisi, and Stephen J. Elledge. 2015. "The DNA Damage Response Induces Inflammation and Senescence by Inhibiting Autophagy of GATA4." *Science (New York, N.Y.)* 349 (6255). https://doi.org/10.1126/SCIENCE.AAA5612.

Katsumata, Ryu, Shinsuke Ishigaki, Masahisa Katsuno, Kaori Kawai, Jun Sone, Zhe Huang, Hiroaki Adachi, Fumiaki Tanaka, Fumihiko Urano, and Gen Sobue. 2012. "C-Abl Inhibition Delays Motor Neuron Degeneration in the G93A Mouse, an Animal Model of Amyotrophic Lateral Sclerosis." *PloS One* 7 (9): e46185. https://doi.org/10.1371/journal.pone.0046185.

Khan, Tahiyana, Abbas I. Hussain, Timothy P. Casilli, Logan Frayser, Michelle Cho, Gabrielle Williams, David McFall, and Patrick A. Forcelli. 2024. "Prophylactic Senolytic Treatment in Aged Mice Reduces Seizure Severity and Improves Survival from *Status Epilepticus*." *Aging Cell* 23 (9). https://doi.org/10.1111/acel.14239.

Kida, Yujiro, and Michael S. Goligorsky. 2016. "Sirtuins, Cell Senescence, and Vascular Aging." *Canadian Journal of Cardiology* 32 (5). Pulsus Group Inc.: 634–641. https://doi.org/10.1016/j.cjca.2015.11.022.

Kim, Taeyeon, Elvira Valera, and Paula Desplats. 2019. "Alterations in Striatal MicroRNA-MRNA Networks Contribute to Neuroinflammation in Multiple System Atrophy." *Molecular Neurobiology* 56 (10): 7003–7021. https://doi.org/10.1007/s12035-019-1577-3.

Kızılaslan, Nildem, Duygu Aydın, Orhan Sumbul, Reyhan Koroglu, and Hatice Aygun. 2023. "The Effect of Quercetin on Absence Epilepsy in WAG/Rij Rats." *Neurological Research* 45 (8): 701–707. https://doi.org/10.1080/01616412.2023.2194182.

Konopka, Anna, and Julie D. Atkin. 2022. "DNA Damage, Defective DNA Repair, and Neurodegeneration in Amyotrophic Lateral Sclerosis." *Frontiers in Aging Neuroscience* 14: 786420. https://doi.org/10.3389/fnagi.2022.786420.

Koutsoudaki, Paraskevi N., Dimitrios Papadopoulos, Panagiotis-Georgios Passias, Pinelopi Koutsoudaki, and Vassilis G. Gorgoulis. 2020. "Cellular Senescence and Failure of Myelin Repair in Multiple Sclerosis." *Mechanisms of Ageing and Development* 192 (December): 111366. https://doi.org/10.1016/j.mad.2020.111366.

Kowald, Axel, João F. Passos, and Thomas B.L. Kirkwood. 2020. "On the Evolution of Cellular Senescence." *Aging Cell* 19 (12). https://doi.org/10.1111/ACEL.13270.

Kritsilis, Marios, Sophia V. Rizou, Paraskevi N. Koutsoudaki, Konstantinos Evangelou, Vassilis G. Gorgoulis, and Dimitrios Papadopoulos. 2018. "Ageing, Cellular Senescence and Neurodegenerative Disease." *International Journal of Molecular Sciences* 19 (10). https://doi.org/10.3390/IJMS19102937.

Lagoumtzi, Sofia M., and Niki Chondrogianni. 2021. "Senolytics and Senomorphics: Natural and Synthetic Therapeutics in the Treatment of Aging and Chronic Diseases." *Free Radical Biology & Medicine* 171 (August): 169–190. https://doi.org/10.1016/J.FREERADBIOMED.2021.05.003.

Lee, Suckwon, Ellen Y. Wang, Alexandra B. Steinberg, Chaska C. Walton, Shankar J. Chinta, and Julie K. Andersen. 2021. "A Guide to Senolytic Intervention in Neurodegenerative Disease." *Mechanisms of Ageing and Development* 200 (December). https://doi.org/10.1016/J.MAD.2021.111585.

Leńska-Mieciek, Marta, Natalia Madetko-Alster, Piotr Alster, Leszek Królicki, Urszula Fiszer, and Dariusz Koziorowski. 2023. "Inflammation in Multiple System Atrophy." *Frontiers in Immunology* 14: 1214677. https://doi.org/10.3389/fimmu.2023.1214677.

Li, Li, Yun Sun, Yinong Zhang, Weixi Wang, and Cuifang Ye. 2021. "Mutant Huntingtin Impairs Pancreatic β-Cells by Recruiting IRS-2 and Disturbing the PI3K/AKT/FoxO1 Signaling Pathway in Huntington's Disease." *Journal of Molecular Neuroscience* 71 (12): 2646–2658. https://doi.org/10.1007/s12031-021-01869-9.

Li, Tengfei, Elodie Martin, Yah-Se Abada, Céline Boucher, Aurélia Cès, Ihsen Youssef, Grégory Fenaux, et al. 2020. "Effects of Chronic Masitinib Treatment in APPswe/PSEN1dE9 Transgenic Mice Modeling Alzheimer's Disease." *Journal of Alzheimer's Disease: JAD* 76 (4): 1339–1345. https://doi.org/10.3233/JAD-200466.

Li, Xiang, Ning Liu, Di Wu, Shu chang Li, Qing Wang, Dian-wen Zhang, Lian-lian Song, Min Huang, Xia Chen, and Wei Li. 2024. "Hippocampal Transcriptomic Analyses Reveal the Potential Antiapoptotic Mechanism of a Novel Anticonvulsant Agent Q808 on Pentylenetetrazol-Induced Epilepsy in Rats." *Biomedicine & Pharmacotherapy* 175 (June): 116746. https://doi.org/10.1016/j.biopha.2024.116746.

Liu, Chang, Rouven Arnold, Gonçalo Henriques, and Karima Djabali. 2019. "Inhibition of JAK-STAT Signaling with Baricitinib Reduces Inflammation and Improves

Cellular Homeostasis in Progeria Cells." *Cells* 8 (10). https://doi.org/10.3390/cells8101276.

Liu, Lei, Xianlin Yue, Zewei Sun, William S. Hambright, Jianming Wei, Ying Li, Polina Matre, et al. 2022. "Reduction of Senescent Fibro-Adipogenic Progenitors in Progeria-Aged Muscle by Senolytics Rescues the Function of Muscle Stem Cells." *Journal of Cachexia, Sarcopenia and Muscle* 13 (6): 3137–3148. https://doi.org/10.1002/jcsm.13101.

Liu, Liyang, Jun Bai, Fangxi Liu, Ying Xu, Mei Zhao, Chuansheng Zhao, and Zhike Zhou. 2022. "Cross-Talking Pathways of Forkhead Box O1 (FOXO1) Are Involved in the Pathogenesis of Alzheimer's Disease and Huntington's Disease." *Oxidative Medicine and Cellular Longevity* 2022 (February): 1–14. https://doi.org/10.1155/2022/7619255.

Liu, Rui-Ming. 2022. "Aging, Cellular Senescence, and Alzheimer's Disease." *International Journal of Molecular Sciences* 23 (4). https://doi.org/10.3390/ijms23041989.

Machiela, Emily, and Amber L. Southwell. 2020. "Biological Aging and the Cellular Pathogenesis of Huntington's Disease." *Journal of Huntington's Disease* 9 (2): 115–128. https://doi.org/10.3233/JHD-200395.

Madiha, Syeda, Zehra Batool, Saiqa Tabassum, Laraib Liaquat, Sadia Sadir, Sidrah Shahzad, Fizza Naqvi, et al. 2021. "Quercetin Exhibits Potent Antioxidant Activity, Restores Motor and Non-Motor Deficits Induced by Rotenone Toxicity." *PloS One* 16 (11): e0258928. https://doi.org/10.1371/journal.pone.0258928.

Maher, Pamela, Richard Dargusch, Laszlo Bodai, Paul E. Gerard, Judith M. Purcell, and J. Lawrence Marsh. 2011. "ERK Activation by the Polyphenols Fisetin and Resveratrol Provides Neuroprotection in Multiple Models of Huntington's Disease." *Human Molecular Genetics* 20 (2): 261–270. https://doi.org/10.1093/hmg/ddq460.

Martel, Jan, David M. Ojcius, Cheng Yeu Wu, Hsin Hsin Peng, Laurent Voisin, Jean Luc Perfettini, Yun Fei Ko, and John D. Young. 2020. "Emerging Use of Senolytics and Senomorphics against Aging and Chronic Diseases." *Medicinal Research Reviews* 40 (6): 2114–2131. https://doi.org/10.1002/MED.21702.

Martin-Ruiz, Carmen, Caroline H. Williams-Gray, Alison J. Yarnall, John J. Boucher, Rachael A. Lawson, Ruwani S. Wijeyekoon, Roger A. Barker, et al. 2020. "Senescence and Inflammatory Markers for Predicting Clinical Progression in Parkinson's Disease: The ICICLE-PD Study." *Journal of Parkinson's Disease* 10 (1): 193–206. https://doi.org/10.3233/JPD-191724.

Maximova, Alexandra, Eryn L. Werry, and Michael Kassiou. 2021. "Senolytics: A Novel Strategy for Neuroprotection in ALS?" *International Journal of Molecular Sciences* 22 (21). https://doi.org/10.3390/IJMS222112078.

Miranda, D. M., D. V. Rosa, B. S. Costa, N. F. Nicolau, L. A.V. Magno, J. J. de Paula, and M. A. Romano-Silva. 2020. "Telomere Shortening in Patients with Drug-Resistant Epilepsy." *Epilepsy Research* 166 (October). https://doi.org/10.1016/J.EPLEPSYRES.2020.106427.

Mor, Danielle E., Salman Sohrabi, Rachel Kaletsky, William Keyes, Alp Tartici, Vrinda Kalia, Gary W. Miller, and Coleen T. Murphy. 2020. "Metformin Rescues Parkinson's Disease Phenotypes Caused by Hyperactive Mitochondria." *Proceedings of the National Academy of Sciences of the United States of America* 117 (42): 26438–26447. https://doi.org/10.1073/PNAS.2009838117.

Nieoczym, Dorota, Katarzyna Socała, Grzegorz Raszewski, and Piotr Wlaź. 2014. "Effect of Quercetin and Rutin in Some Acute Seizure Models in Mice." *Progress in Neuro-Psychopharmacology and Biological Psychiatry* 54 (October): 50–58. https://doi.org/10.1016/j.pnpbp.2014.05.007.

Nixon, R. A., K.-I. Saito, F. Grynspan, W. R. Griffin, S. Katayama, T. Honda, P. S. Mohan, T. B. Shea, and M. Beermann. 1994. "Calcium-Activated Neutral Proteinase (Calpain) System in Aging and Alzheimer's Disease ^a^." *Annals of the New York Academy of Sciences* 747 (1): 77–91. https://doi.org/10.1111/j.1749-6632.1994.tb44402.x.

Ogrodnik, Mikolaj. 2021. "Cellular Aging beyond Cellular Senescence: Markers of Senescence Prior to Cell Cycle Arrest in Vitro and in Vivo." *Aging Cell* 20 (4). https://doi.org/10.1111/ACEL.13338.

Ogrodnik, Mikolaj, Yi Zhu, Larissa G. P. Langhi, Tamar Tchkonia, Patrick Krüger, Edward Fielder, Stella Victorelli, et al. 2019. "Obesity-Induced Cellular Senescence Drives Anxiety and Impairs Neurogenesis." *Cell Metabolism* 29 (5). Cell Press: 1233. https://doi.org/10.1016/j.cmet.2019.01.013.

Oost, Wendy, Nynke Talma, Jan F. Meilof, and Jon D. Laman. 2018. "Targeting Senescence to Delay Progression of Multiple Sclerosis." *Journal of Molecular Medicine (Berlin, Germany)* 96 (11): 1153–1166. https://doi.org/10.1007/s00109-018-1686-x.

Pal, Arun, Benedikt Kretner, Masin Abo-Rady, Hannes Glaβ, Banaja P. Dash, Marcel Naumann, Julia Japtok, et al. 2021. "Concomitant Gain and Loss of Function Pathomechanisms in C9ORF72 Amyotrophic Lateral Sclerosis." *Life Science Alliance* 4 (4). https://doi.org/10.26508/lsa.202000764.

Pandya, Virenkumar A., and Rickie Patani. 2020. "Decoding the Relationship between Ageing and Amyotrophic Lateral Sclerosis: A Cellular Perspective." *Brain: A Journal of Neurology* 143 (4): 1057–1072. https://doi.org/10.1093/brain/awz360.

Papadopoulos, Dimitrios, Roberta Magliozzi, Dimos D. Mitsikostas, Vassilis G. Gorgoulis, and Richard S. Nicholas. 2020. "Aging, Cellular Senescence, and Progressive Multiple Sclerosis." *Frontiers in Cellular Neuroscience* 14: 178. https://doi.org/10.3389/fncel.2020.00178.

Park, Seul-Ki, and Ok Sarah Shin. 2017. "Metformin Alleviates Ageing Cellular Phenotypes in Hutchinson–Gilford Progeria Syndrome Dermal Fibroblasts." *Experimental Dermatology* 26 (10): 889–895. https://doi.org/10.1111/exd.13323.

Patel, Mital Y., Hirenkumar V. Panchal, Othman Ghribi, and Kenza E. Benzeroual 2012. "The Neuroprotective Effect of Fisetin in the MPTP Model of Parkinson's Disease." *Journal of Parkinson's Disease* 2 (4): 287–302. https://doi.org/10.3233/JPD-012110.

Pelletier, Laura Le, Matthieu Mantecon, Jennifer Gorwood, Martine Auclair, Roberta Foresti, Roberto Motterlini, Mireille Laforge, et al. 2021. "Metformin Alleviates Stress-Induced Cellular Senescence of Aging Human Adipose Stromal Cells and the Ensuing Adipocyte Dysfunction." *ELife* 10 (September). https://doi.org/10.7554/eLife.62635.

Petrocelli, Jonathan J., Alec I. McKenzie, Naomi M. M. P. de Hart, Paul T. Reidy, Ziad S. Mahmassani, Alexander R. Keeble, Katie L. Kaput, et al. 2023. "Disuse-induced Muscle Fibrosis, Cellular Senescence, and Senescence-associated Secretory Phenotype in Older Adults Are Alleviated during Re-ambulation with Metformin Pre-Treatment." *Aging Cell* 22 (11). https://doi.org/10.1111/acel.13936.

Piette, François, Joël Belmin, Hélène Vincent, Nicolas Schmidt, Sylvie Pariel, Marc Verny, Caroline Marquis, et al. 2011. "Masitinib as an Adjunct Therapy for Mild-to-Moderate Alzheimer's Disease: A Randomised, Placebo-Controlled Phase 2 Trial." *Alzheimer's Research & Therapy* 3 (2): 16. https://doi.org/10.1186/alzrt75.

Poewe, Werner, Iva Stankovic, Glenda Halliday, Wassilios G. Meissner, Gregor K. Wenning, Maria Teresa Pellecchia, Klaus Seppi, Jose-Alberto Palma, and Horacio Kaufmann. 2022. "Multiple System Atrophy." *Nature Reviews. Disease Primers* 8 (1): 56. https://doi.org/10.1038/s41572-022-00382-6.

Prakash, Dharmalingam, and Ganapasam Sudhandiran. 2015. "Dietary Flavonoid Fisetin Regulates Aluminium Chloride-Induced Neuronal Apoptosis in Cortex and Hippocampus of Mice Brain." *The Journal of Nutritional Biochemistry* 26 (12): 1527–1539. https://doi.org/10.1016/j.jnutbio.2015.07.017.

Ren, Chenghao, Jie Jin, Chenchao Li, Jianwei Xiang, Yaosen Wu, Yifei Zhou, Liaojun Sun, Xiaolei Zhang, and Naifeng Tian. 2022. "Metformin Inactivates the CGAS-STING Pathway through Autophagy and Suppresses Senescence in Nucleus Pulposus Cells." *Journal of Cell Science* 135 (15). https://doi.org/10.1242/jcs.259738.

Rhinn, Muriel, Irene Zapata-Bodalo, Annabelle Klein, Jean-Luc Plassat, Tania Knauer-Meyer, and William M. Keyes. 2022. "Aberrant Induction of P19Arf-Mediated Cellular Senescence Contributes to Neurodevelopmental Defects." *PLOS Biology* 20 (6): e3001664. https://doi.org/10.1371/journal.pbio.3001664.

Ribierre, Théo, Alexandre Bacq, Florian Donneger, Marion Doladilhe, Marina Maletic, Delphine Roussel, Isabelle Le Roux, et al. 2024. "Targeting Pathological Cells with Senolytic Drugs Reduces Seizures in Neurodevelopmental MTOR-Related Epilepsy." *Nature Neuroscience* 27 (6): 1125–1136. https://doi.org/10.1038/s41593-024-01634-2.

Russo, Taylor, and Markus Riessland. 2022. "Age-Related Midbrain Inflammation and Senescence in Parkinson's Disease." *Frontiers in Aging Neuroscience* 14: 917797. https://doi.org/10.3389/fnagi.2022.917797.

Saez-Atienzar, Sara, and Eliezer Masliah. 2020. "Cellular Senescence and Alzheimer Disease: The Egg and the Chicken Scenario." *Nature Reviews. Neuroscience* 21 (8): 433–444. https://doi.org/10.1038/S41583-020-0325-Z.

Sandhir, Rajat, and Arpit Mehrotra. 2013. "Quercetin Supplementation Is Effective in Improving Mitochondrial Dysfunctions Induced by 3-Nitropropionic Acid: Implications in Huntington's Disease." *Biochimica et Biophysica Acta (BBA)—Molecular Basis of Disease* 1832 (3): 421–430. https://doi.org/10.1016/j.bbadis.2012.11.018.

Scarabino, Daniela, Liana Veneziano, Martina Peconi, Marina Frontali, Elide Mantuano, and Rosa Maria Corbo. 2019. "Leukocyte Telomere Shortening in Huntington's Disease." *Journal of the Neurological Sciences* 396 (January): 25–29. https://doi.org/10.1016/j.jns.2018.10.024.

Schonrock, Nicole, David T. Humphreys, Thomas Preiss, and Jürgen Götz. 2012. "Target Gene Repression Mediated by MiRNAs MiR-181c and MiR-9 Both of Which Are Down-Regulated by Amyloid-β." *Journal of Molecular Neuroscience* 46 (2): 324–335. https://doi.org/10.1007/s12031-011-9587-2.

Shao, Z., B. Wang, Y. Shi, C. Xie, C. Huang, B. Chen, H. Zhang, et al. 2021. "Senolytic Agent Quercetin Ameliorates Intervertebral Disc Degeneration via the Nrf2/NF-KB Axis." *Osteoarthritis and Cartilage* 29 (3): 413–422. https://doi.org/10.1016/J.JOCA.2020.11.006.

Sharma, D. R., W. Y. Wani, A. Sunkaria, R. J. Kandimalla, R. K. Sharma, D. Verma, A. Bal, and K. D. Gill. 2016. "Quercetin Attenuates Neuronal Death against Aluminum-Induced Neurodegeneration in the Rat Hippocampus." *Neuroscience* 324 (June): 163–176. https://doi.org/10.1016/j.neuroscience.2016.02.055.

Si, Zizhen, Linlin Sun, and Xidi Wang. 2021. "Evidence and Perspectives of Cell Senescence in Neurodegenerative Diseases." *Biomedicine & Pharmacotherapy = Biomedecine & Pharmacotherapie* 137 (May). https://doi.org/10.1016/J.BIOPHA.2021.111327.

Sigurdson, Christina J., Jason C. Bartz, and Markus Glatzel. 2019. "Cellular and Molecular Mechanisms of Prion Disease." *Annual Review of Pathology* 14 (January): 497–516. https://doi.org/10.1146/annurev-pathmechdis-012418-013109.

Singh, Ashish, Pratibha Tripathi, Arun Kumar Yadawa, and Sarika Singh. 2020. "Promising Polyphenols in Parkinson's Disease Therapeutics." *Neurochemical Research* 45 (8): 1731–1745. https://doi.org/10.1007/S11064-020-03058-3.

Siracusa, Rosalba, Roberta Fusco, and Salvatore Cuzzocrea. 2019. "Astrocytes: Role and Functions in Brain Pathologies." *Frontiers in Pharmacology* 10 (September). https://doi.org/10.3389/fphar.2019.01114.

Sivasubramanian, Mahesh Kumar, Raisa Monteiro, Priya Balasubramanian, and Madhan Subramanian. 2020. "Oxidative Stress-Induced Senescence Alters Glutamate Transporter Expression in Human Brainstem Astrocytes." *The FASEB Journal* 34 (S1). Wiley: 1–1. https://doi.org/10.1096/FASEBJ.2020.34.S1.06566.

Stein, Gretchen H., Linda F. Drullinger, Alexandre Soulard, and Vjekoslav Dulić. 1999. "Differential Roles for Cyclin-Dependent Kinase Inhibitors P21 and P16 in the Mechanisms of Senescence and Differentiation in Human Fibroblasts." *Molecular and Cellular Biology* 19 (3). American Society for Microbiology: 2109–2117. https://doi.org/10.1128/mcb.19.3.2109.

Suelves, Nuria, Shirine Saleki, Tasha Ibrahim, Debora Palomares, Sebastiaan Moonen, Marta J. Koper, Céline Vrancx, et al. 2023. "Senescence-Related Impairment of Autophagy Induces Toxic Intraneuronal Amyloid-β Accumulation in a Mouse Model of Amyloid Pathology." *Acta Neuropathologica Communications* 11 (1): 82. https://doi.org/10.1186/s40478-023-01578-x.

Sun, Shuhui, Jiaming Li, Si Wang, Jingyi Li, Jie Ren, Zhaoshi Bao, Le Sun, et al. 2023. "CHIT1-Positive Microglia Drive Motor Neuron Ageing in the Primate Spinal Cord." *Nature* 624 (7992): 611–620. https://doi.org/10.1038/s41586-023-06783-1.

Sung, Jin Young, Seul Gi Kim, Young Jin Kang, and Hyoung Chul Choi. 2022. "Metformin Mitigates Stress-Induced Premature Senescence by Upregulating AMPKα at Ser485 Phosphorylation Induced SIRT3 Expression and Inactivating Mitochondrial Oxidants." *Mechanisms of Ageing and Development* 206 (September): 111708. https://doi.org/10.1016/j.mad.2022.111708.

Tai, Shi, Jiaxing Sun, Yuying Zhou, Zhaowei Zhu, Yuhu He, Mingxian Chen, Hui Yang, et al. 2022. "Metformin Suppresses Vascular Smooth Muscle Cell Senescence by Promoting Autophagic Flux." *Journal of Advanced Research* 41 (November): 205–218. https://doi.org/10.1016/j.jare.2021.12.009.

Torres, Pascual, Carlos Anerillas, Omar Ramírez-Núñez, Anna Fernàndez, Mario Encinas, Mònica Povedano, Pol Andrés-Benito, et al. 2022. "A Motor Neuron Disease Mouse Model Reveals a Non-Canonical Profile of Senescence Biomarkers." *Disease Models & Mechanisms* 15 (8). https://doi.org/10.1242/dmm.049059.

Triana-Martínez, Francisco, Pilar Picallos-Rabina, Sabela Da Silva-Álvarez, Federico Pietrocola, Susana Llanos, Verónica Rodilla, Enrica Soprano, et al. 2019. "Identification and Characterization of Cardiac Glycosides as Senolytic Compounds." *Nature Communications* 10 (1): 4731. https://doi.org/10.1038/s41467-019-12888-x.

Trias, Emiliano, Pamela R. Beilby, Mariángeles Kovacs, Sofía Ibarburu, Valentina Varela, Romina Barreto-Núñez, Samuel C. Bradford, Joseph S. Beckman, and Luis Barbeito. 2019. "Emergence of Microglia Bearing Senescence Markers During Paralysis Progression in a Rat Model of Inherited ALS." *Frontiers in Aging Neuroscience* 11 (FEB). https://doi.org/10.3389/FNAGI.2019.00042.

Trist, Benjamin G., Dominic J. Hare, and Kay L. Double. 2019. "Oxidative Stress in the Aging Substantia Nigra and the Etiology of Parkinson's Disease." *Aging Cell* 18 (6): e13031. https://doi.org/10.1111/acel.13031.

Vermersch, Patrick, Rabah Benrabah, Nicolas Schmidt, Hélène Zéphir, Pierre Clavelou, Cyrille Vongsouthi, Patrice Dubreuil, Alain Moussy, and Olivier Hermine. 2012. "Masitinib Treatment in Patients with Progressive Multiple Sclerosis: A Randomized Pilot Study." *BMC Neurology* 12 (June): 36. https://doi.org/10.1186/1471-2377-12-36.

Voisin, Jessica, Francesca Farina, Swati Naphade, Morgane Fontaine, Kizito-Tshitoko Tshilenge, Carlos Galicia Aguirre, Alejandro Lopez-Ramirez, et al. 2020. "FOXO3 Targets Are Reprogrammed as Huntington's Disease Neural Cells and Striatal Neurons Face Senescence with P16 ^{INK4a} Increase." *Aging Cell* 19 (11). https://doi.org/10.1111/acel.13226.

Vrinda, M., S. Arun, B. N. Srikumar, Bindu M. Kutty, and B. S. Shankaranarayana Rao. 2019. "Temporal Lobe Epilepsy-Induced Neurodegeneration and Cognitive Deficits: Implications for Aging." *Journal of Chemical Neuroanatomy* 95 (January): 146–153. https://doi.org/10.1016/j.jchemneu.2018.02.005.

Wallings, Rebecca L., Stewart W. Humble, Michael E. Ward, and Richard Wade-Martins. 2019. "Lysosomal Dysfunction at the Centre of Parkinson's Disease and Frontotemporal Dementia/Amyotrophic Lateral Sclerosis." *Trends in Neurosciences* 42 (12): 899–912. https://doi.org/10.1016/j.tins.2019.10.002.

Wang, T. H., S. Y. Wang, X. D. Wang, H. Q. Jiang, Y. Q. Yang, Y. Wang, J. L. Cheng, C. T. Zhang, W. W. Liang, and H. L. Feng. 2018. "Fisetin Exerts Antioxidant and Neuroprotective Effects in Multiple Mutant HSOD1 Models of Amyotrophic Lateral Sclerosis by Activating ERK." *Neuroscience* 379 (May): 152–166. https://doi.org/10.1016/j.neuroscience.2018.03.008.

Wang, Wen-Wen, Ruiyu Han, Hai-Jun He, Jia Li, Si-Yan Chen, Yingying Gu, and Chenglong Xie. 2021. "Administration of Quercetin Improves Mitochondria Quality Control and Protects the Neurons in 6-OHDA-Lesioned Parkinson's Disease Models." *Aging* 13 (8): 11738–11751. https://doi.org/10.18632/aging.202868.

Watanabe, Sugiko, Shimpei Kawamoto, Naoko Ohtani, and Eiji Hara. 2017. "Impact of Senescence-Associated Secretory Phenotype and Its Potential as a Therapeutic Target for Senescence-Associated Diseases." *Cancer Science* 108 (4): 563–569. https://doi.org/10.1111/CAS.13184.

Wissler Gerdes, Erin O., Yi Zhu, Tamar Tchkonia, and James L. Kirkland. 2020. "Discovery, Development, and Future Application of Senolytics: Theories and Predictions." *The FEBS Journal* 287 (12): 2418–2427. https://doi.org/10.1111/FEBS.15264.

Wu, Dongmei, Zihui Zheng, Shaohua Fan, Xin Wen, Xinrui Han, Shan Wang, Yongjian Wang, et al. 2020. "Ameliorating Effect of Quercetin on Epilepsy by Inhibition of Inflammation in Glial Cells." *Experimental and Therapeutic Medicine* 20 (2): 854–859. https://doi.org/10.3892/ETM.2020.8742.

Xie, Ruijin, Wenjing Zhao, Scott Lowe, Rachel Bentley, Guoqin Hu, Huiya Mei, Xiaofan Jiang, Chenyu Sun, Yu Wu, and Yueying liu. 2022. "Quercetin Alleviates Kainic Acid-Induced Seizure by Inhibiting the Nrf2-Mediated Ferroptosis Pathway." *Free Radical Biology & Medicine* 191 (October): 212–226. https://doi.org/10.1016/J.FREERADBIOMED.2022.09.001.

Xie, Wen, Sushruta Koppula, Mayur B. Kale, Lashin S. Ali, Nitu L. Wankhede, Mohit D. Umare, Aman B. Upaganlawar, et al. 2024. "Unraveling the Nexus of Age, Epilepsy, and Mitochondria: Exploring the Dynamics of Cellular Energy and Excitability." *Frontiers in Pharmacology* 15 (September). https://doi.org/10.3389/fphar.2024.1469053.

Xu, Ming, Tamar Pirtskhalava, Joshua N. Farr, Bettina M. Weigand, Allyson K. Palmer, Megan M. Weivoda, Christina L. Inman, et al. 2018. "Senolytics Improve Physical

Function and Increase Lifespan in Old Age." *Nature Medicine* 24 (8): 1246–1256. https://doi.org/10.1038/S41591-018-0092-9.

Yabluchanskiy, Andriy, Stefano Tarantini, Priya Balasubramanian, Tamas Kiss, Tamas Csipo, Gábor A. Fülöp, Agnes Lipecz, et al. 2020. "Pharmacological or Genetic Depletion of Senescent Astrocytes Prevents Whole Brain Irradiation–Induced Impairment of Neurovascular Coupling Responses Protecting Cognitive Function in Mice." *GeroScience* 42 (2). Springer: 409. https://doi.org/10.1007/S11357-020-00154-8.

Yimer, Ebrahim M., Awol Surur, Dawit Zewdu Wondafrash, and Abadi Kahsu Gebre. 2019. "The Effect of Metformin in Experimentally Induced Animal Models of Epileptic Seizure." *Behavioural Neurology* 2019. https://doi.org/10.1155/2019/6234758.

Yoon, Ye-Seul, Jueng Soo You, Tae-Kyung Kim, Woo Jung Ahn, Myoung Jun Kim, Keun Hong Son, Diadem Ricarte, Darlene Ortiz, Seung-Jae Lee, and He-Jin Lee. 2022. "Senescence and Impaired DNA Damage Responses in Alpha-Synucleinopathy Models." *Experimental & Molecular Medicine* 54 (2): 115–128. https://doi.org/10.1038/s12276-022-00727-x.

Yu, Kun-Hua, and Cheng-I Lee. 2020. "Quercetin Disaggregates Prion Fibrils and Decreases Fibril-Induced Cytotoxicity and Oxidative Stress." *Pharmaceutics* 12 (11): 1081. https://doi.org/10.3390/pharmaceutics12111081.

Zanella, Alberto, Crescenzio Izzo, Giovanni Meola, Mariagabriella Mariani, Maria Teresa Colotti, Vincenzo Silani, Gabriella Pellegata, and Guglielmo Scarlato. 1980. "Metabolic Impairment and Membrane Abnormality in Red Cells from Huntington's Disease." *Journal of the Neurological Sciences* 47 (1): 93–103. https://doi.org/10.1016/0022-510X(80)90028-3.

Zhang, Lei, Louise E. Pitcher, Vaishali Prahalad, Laura J. Niedernhofer, and Paul D. Robbins. 2021. "Recent Advances in the Discovery of Senolytics." *Mechanisms of Ageing and Development* 200 (December). https://doi.org/10.1016/J.MAD.2021.111587.

Zhang, Lei, Louise E. Pitcher, Vaishali Prahalad, Laura J. Niedernhofer, and Paul D. Robbins. 2023. "Targeting Cellular Senescence with Senotherapeutics: Senolytics and Senomorphics." *The FEBS Journal* 290 (5): 1362–1383. https://doi.org/10.1111/febs.16350.

Zhang, Peisu, Yuki Kishimoto, Ioannis Grammatikakis, Kamalvishnu Gottimukkala, Roy G. Cutler, Shiliang Zhang, Kotb Abdelmohsen, et al. 2019. "Senolytic Therapy Alleviates Aβ-Associated Oligodendrocyte Progenitor Cell Senescence and Cognitive Deficits in an Alzheimer's Disease Model." *Nature Neuroscience* 22 (5): 719–728. https://doi.org/10.1038/S41593-019-0372-9.

Zhao, Gengshui, Yongqi Fu, Chao Yang, Xuehui Yang, and Xiaoxiao Hu. 2022. "Exploring the Pathogenesis Linking Traumatic Brain Injury and Epilepsy via Bioinformatic Analyses." *Frontiers in Aging Neuroscience* 14 (November). https://doi.org/10.3389/fnagi.2022.1047908.

Zhu, Yi, Tamara Tchkonia, Tamar Pirtskhalava, Adam C. Gower, Husheng Ding, Nino Giorgadze, Allyson K. Palmer, et al. 2015. "The Achilles' Heel of Senescent Cells: From Transcriptome to Senolytic Drugs." *Aging Cell* 14 (4): 644–658. https://doi.org/10.1111/ACEL.12344.

Chapter 3

Senolytics in Skin Care and Skin Diseases

Syed Sufian Ahmad and Faraha Ahmed

Abbreviations

AMPK: AMP-activated protein kinase; AP-1: activator protein-1; COX: cyclooxygenase; CREB: cAMP response element binding protein; DNA: deoxyribonucleic acid; ECM: extracellular matrix; ERK: extracellular signal-regulated kinase; FAK: focal adhesion kinase; GPx7: glutathione peroxidase 7; HDF: human dermal fibroblasts; HDMEC: human dermal microvascular endothelial cells; HMGB1: high-mobility group box-1; HO: heme oxygenase; IGF-1: insulin-like growth factor; Ikb: inhibitor of nuclear factor kappa B; IL: interleukin; iNOS: inducible nitric oxide synthase; JNK: Jun-N terminal kinase; MAPK: mitogen-activated protein kinase; MMPs: matrix metalloproteinases; NF-κB: nuclear factor kappa B; PGE2: prostaglandin E2; ROS: reactive oxygen species; SASP: senescence-associated secretory phenotypes; SA-β-gal: senescence-associated β-galactosidase; SCAPs: senescent cell–associated anti-apoptotic pathways; SDF-1: stromal cell–derived factor; TGF-β: transforming growth factor-β; TNF-α: tumor necrosis factor-α; UV: ultraviolet; VEGF: vascular endothelial growth factor.

3.1 INTRODUCTION

The human skin is intricate and is the largest dynamic organ having a unique structure. It is consistently subjected to internal and external factors that alter its morphology and functions. It is composed of three distinct layers: the epidermis (outermost), the dermis (middle) and the hypodermis (innermost). All these layers are individually required for functioning of the skin. The Langerhans cells of skin are immune cells that act as the first line of defense. The epidermis has four distinct layers: the stratum corneum, stratum granulosum, stratum spinosum and stratum basalis. These comprise discrete cells: keratinocytes, melanocytes, Langerhans cells and Merkel cells. The epidermis regulates body temperature, serves as a protective barrier to prevent loss of water from the body and the entry of outer substances inside the body. Under the epidermis lies the dermis, with nutrition and nerves for circulation. The dermis consists of macrophages, mast cells and dendritic cells. It has fibrous connective tissue and is

 DOI: 10.1201/9781003493969-3

formed from two different types of cells: elastin fibers and collagen. The elastin fibers allow flexibility and provide elasticity while collagen allows skin stability and tensile strength. Sweat glands, hair follicles and lymph vessels are also present in this layer. The border of the epidermis and dermis is the epidermal-dermal junction that forms the basement membrane with proteins. The innermost later hypodermis is primarily composed of adipocytes (fat cells), blood vessels and nerves. Aging, changes in weather, hot or cold temperatures, and other chronic skin ailments like psoriasis and eczema affect skin integrity (Payne 2020; Csekes and Račková 2021).

The skin serves as a defense and barrier against environmental toxins, harmful ultraviolet (UV) rays and also prevents water loss. The UV rays generate free radicals and damage skin due to inflammation. The continuous exposure causes degradation of proteins of the extracellular matrix such as collagen, elastin or fibronectin that causes skin to sag or wrinkle and consequently reduces its strength and resilience. The major structural protein of skin is collagen present in the dermis. The formation of collagen is regulated by factors including matrix metalloproteinases (MMPs), activator protein-1 (AP-1) and mitogen-activated protein kinase (MAPK) (Wu et al. 2017). Aging reduces the amount of collagen, papillary capillaries and fibroblasts. There is also a decline in stem cells that obstructs skin ulcers and wound healing and also causes frailty and atrophy of skin (Thompson et al. 2022).

The skin undergoes consistent damage due to environmental pollution, and therefore its ability to protect the internal structures decreases with time and age. Every layer of skin develops the changes that together reduce the functions of the skin. The epidermal later becomes thin and there is altered distribution of keratinocyte and melanocyte cells. The stratum corneum becomes stiffer with increased permeability that delays the recovery after an injury. Further, the flattening of epidermis and dermis junction reduces the resistance towards shearing forces (Branchet et al. 1990; Russell-Goldman and Murphy 2020).

Cellular senescence is a hallmark primarily associated with older skin. Several extrinsic and intrinsic factors lead to shortening of telomeres and increase in oxidative stress and cause a functional decline of skin by increasing the cellular senescence (Cristofalo et al. 2004; Passos et al. 2007). The telomers are very sensitive towards oxidative damage and result in the formation of components of DNA repair and accumulation of telomere-associated foci. Exposure to UV radiation and environmental pollution is critical for cellular senescence (J. Shin, Kim, and Kim 2012; Fitsiou et al. 2021). Genes like RAS and BRAF, which are responsible for skin cancer, also drive skin into aging due to senescence. Skin aging is contributed to by senescence of various skin cells like melanocytes, keratinocytes and fibroblasts (Lee et al. 2021; Pils et al. 2021).

Senotherapeutics are compounds designed to target and eliminate senescent cells. These agents mitigate the inflammation and restore the tissue healthy metabolism that increases the life span of skin. Senotherapeutics are classified as (1) senolytics and (2) senomorphics which selectively clear the senescent cells or decrease the activity of pathways that drive cells into senescence. These agents attenuate the upregulated senescent cell–associated anti-apoptotic pathways (SCAPs) and senescence-associated secretory phenotypes (SASP) to form pro-inflammatory secretomes. Several enzymes and pathways are targeted for senolysis like P13K, AKT, FOXO4, Bcl-2 family genes, p53 and p52, while senomorphics target interleukins, mTOR, p38 MAPK, NF-κB and other signaling cascades (Thompson et al. 2022).

Recent developments have improved the understanding of mechanisms involved in cellular senescence and the factors that inhibit cellular senescence. The novel approach that describes the removal of senescent cells is known as senotherapy. Researches showed that senotherapeutics improve the pathological age-related decline in health by preventing the hallmarks of senescence and significantly decreasing the number of senescent cells (Bulbiankova et al. 2023a).

3.2 CELLULAR SENESCENCE AND MECHANISMS OF SKIN AGING AND SKIN DISEASES

The natural process of cellular senescence was observed in cultured human cells in the 1960s by scientists Hayflick and Moorhead. They noted that human cells have limited capacity for cell division before entering permanent cell cycle arrest or senescence and termed this the "Hayflick limit" (Hayflick and Moorhead 1961). Causes of cellular senescence in skin include chronological aging, pollution and exposure to UV radiation. These factors cause DNA damage, increased skin pigmentation, reactive oxygen species (ROS) generation, inflammation and decreased immunosuppression response of skin, wrinkles, keratosis, dermatitis or acne (Chin et al. 2023). The mechanism of skin aging is depicted in Figure 3.1.

Cellular dysfunction alters protein expression causing replicative cell arrest to drive a cell into senescence, which causes stress and damages the cells. The quiescent cells undergo terminal differentiation while the senescent cells are arrested at

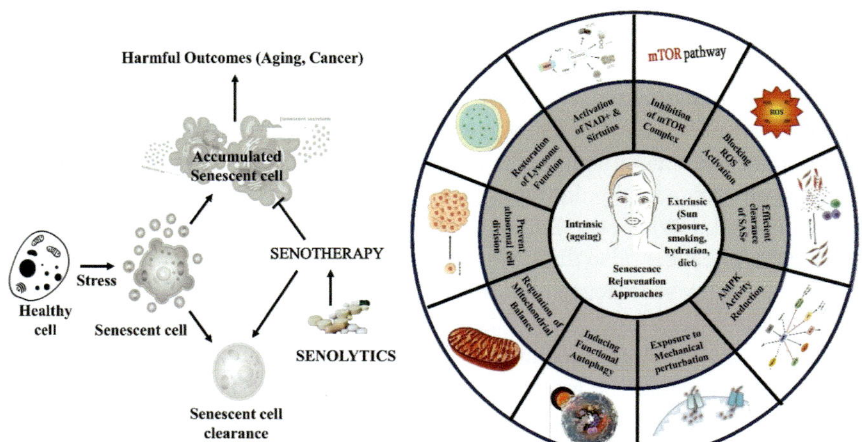

Figure 3.1 Mechanism of skin aging.

the mitotic phase and fail to proliferate. The nuclear structure of cells is altered by the protein lamin B1. The senescence in the cells is identified by several senescent markers. These include SASP, activity of senescence-associated β-galactosidase (SA-β-gal), cell cycle blockers like $p21^{CIP1}$ and $p16^{INK4A}$ (CDKN2A) along with the role of metalloproteinase, chemokines, growth factors and cytokines (A. S. Wang and Dreesen 2018; Shah et al. 2013; Ahmed and Khanam 2023). The persistent expression of $p16^{INK4A}$ in the epidermal cells of mice induced proliferation of keratinocytes, dysplasia and hyperplasia. It also induced epidermal papilloma and was identified as a strong component for senescence and cell cycle arrest (Azazmeh et al. 2020). Cytokines, proteases, growth factors and high-mobility box-1 (HMGB1) are the phenotypes of SASP exhibited by senescent cells. SASP tend to increase the inflammatory macrophage proteins and interleukins (IL-6/8/1α/1β). The SASP also generates senescence through TGF-β, vascular endothelial growth factor (VEGF) and activation of chemokines (Chin et al. 2023).

The epidermal keratinocytes regulate its homeostasis through continuous differentiation. This limits the impact on skin cells undergoing senescence. But exposure to UV irradiation, aging, and environmental pollution induce the senescence markers like MMPs, SASP, $p21^{CIP1}$, $p16^{INK4a}$, p53 and SA-β-gal activity and pro-inflammatory cytokines like TNF-α, IL-1α/1β/6 which increase the keratinocytes. The senescent cells increase the skin permeability by decreasing the cellular adhesion and extracellular matrix (Thompson et al. 2022). The density of fibroblasts present in dermis also decrease with aging. The senescent fibroblasts induce the apoptosis of adjacent cells. In addition, they increase the senescence phenotypes $p21^{CIP1}$, $p16^{INK4a}$ and p53 and upregulate SASP components like interleukins and MMPs. Aging-induced cellular senescence alters skin pigmentation by suppressing the expression of stromal cell–derived factor (SDF-1). Mitochondrial incapacity and oxidative damage in fibroblasts leads to a decrease in insulin-like growth factor (IGF-1) that in turn decreases the production of collagen and reduces the differentiation and proliferation of keratinocytes (Wlaschek et al. 2021). Aging also affects the density of melanocytes identified with reduced lamin B1 and elevated $p16^{INK4a}$ and telomere dysfunction in fibroblasts (Victorelli et al. 2019).

In pathological conditions like skin lesions, fibroblasts secrete platelet-derived growth factor for wound healing and repair of tissue. But during the process, myofibroblasts become senescent and lose their activity and are eliminated by the immune system. The stressor triggers the tumor suppressor genes $p16^{INK4A}$/pRB and p53/ $p21^{WAF1/CIP1}$ to initiate the cell cycle arrest. The $p16^{INK4A}$ is an inhibitor of CDK4/6 which inhibits the phosphorylation of RB that in turn causes arrest of the cell cycle at the G1 phase (Kanaki, Makrantonaki, and Zouboulis 2016; W. Y. Kim and Sharpless 2006). In addition to overexpression of $p16^{INK4a}$ gene some intrinsic factors like genetic predisposition, oxidative DNA damage and hormonal regulation also induce senescence in fibroblast cells (Reilly and Lozano 2021). Senescence also decreases vascularization and causes thinning of the epidermal dermal interface. This contributes to a decline in skin resilience and increased wrinkles (Puizina-Ivić 2008).

From recent developments it appears that the senotherapeutic class of drugs can improve age-related deterioration related to metabolic dysfunction, bones, vascular phenotypes and many more. These agents primarily target pro-apoptosis and pro-signaling pathways and inhibit them in the cells exposed to senescence (Bulbiankova et al. 2023b; Wyles et al. 2023).

Senescent can be initiated from developmental stages where p21 plays a crucial role to induce senescence in limbs. Huang et al. described the senescent pathways by various senescent inducers (Table 3.1).

3.3 SENOTHERAPEUTICS FOR SKIN CARE

Senotherapy is a newly discovered class for skin problems and as anti-aging agents. Though the removal of senescent cells improves skin conditions, there are no officially clinically approved drugs as a number of active clinical trials are being executed. Pre-clinical and clinical studies require a large time interval so that drugs may be attributed as a high standard for medical interventions.

Senotherapeutics are molecules categorized as senolytics, which are cytotoxic for senescent cells, while senomorphics are agents that attenuate and reverse the senescence phenotypes (E. C. Kim and Kim 2019). Many natural bioactive compounds, especially polyphenols (plant-derived metabolites) have effective senotherapeutic activity due to their potent antioxidant capacity. Flavonols are attracting considerable attention due to their multiple biological properties including cellular senescence. The bioactive compounds have drawn attention for skin therapy due to their safety index. Natural products show their cumulative effect in comparison to modern drugs and are speculated to work slower (Domaszewska-Szostek, Puzianowska-Kuźnicka, and Kuryłowicz 2021; Borchers and Pieler 2010; Dańczak-Pazdrowska et al. 2023). Various agents that have shown benefits in skin damage are described in Table 3.2.

Table 3.1 Pathways for Cellular Senescence

Senescence Inducer	*Pathway*
Epigenetic factors	Epigenetic histone modifications induce cellular senescence through p16-Rb signaling cascade
Replicative stress	Telomere shortening due to cell proliferation causes DNA damage
Mitochondrial dysfunction	It causes generations of reactive oxygen moieties that causes damage of DNA
Oncogene activation	Activation of oncogenes activates p38AMPK/p16 and MDM2/p53/p21 signaling
Decline of tumor suppressor genes	Reduced activity of tumor suppressor genes activates AKT/mTOR/p53 signaling to induce cellular senescence
Cytotoxic drugs and ionizing radiation	These agents cause cellular and DNA damage

Source: Huang et al. (2022).

Table 3.2 Compounds Exhibiting Senotherapeutic Benefits on Skin

S.No.	*Compound*	*Model*	*Mechanism*	*Reference*
1	Fisetin	UV-induced damage human fibroblast	↓ MAPK, JNK, ERK, p38, p65, NF-κB and IκB Targeting P13/AKT/CREB pathways	Chiang et al. (2015)
		Human HaCaT keratinocytes	↓ COX-2, iNOS, PGE2, IL-6/1β, NO, NF-κB, TNF-α, HO-1 mRNA and translocation of Nrf2 Targeting P13K/AKT	Seo and Jeong (2015)
		BALB/c hairless mice	↓ COX-2, MMPs, Nrf2	Seo and Jeong (2015)
2	Quercetin	C3H/HeN female mice	↓ TGF-β and skin fibrosis	Horton et al. (2013)
		Human dermal fibroblast cells	↓ p53, $p16^{INK4A}$, SOD, catalase and ↑ LPL and KCNE2 genes	Sohn et al. (2018)
		Human skin tissues	↓ COX-2, MMPs, AP-1 and NF-κB Targeting JAK2/PKCδ signaling	E. J. Shin et al. (2019)
		Human HaCaT keratinocytes	↓ IF-γ, TNF-α, IL-6/4, CC17, CC22 and lnc-C7orf30–2 gene	Hou et al. (2019)
		Human HaCaT keratinocytes	↓ MMP-1/2/9, E-cadherin, and occluding Targeting ERK1/2 MAPK and NF-κB pathways	Beken et al. (2020)
		Diabetic wounds in rats	↓ VEGF, TGF-β, TNF-α, IL-1β/10 and MMP-9	Kant et al. (2021)
		Human HaCaT keratinocytes and HDMEC cells	↓ Inflammation, p65, ICAM−1 Targeting NF-κB signaling	Meng et al. (2024).
3	Taxifolin	Human dermal fibroblasts and epidermal keratinocytes	↓ Catalase, HO-1, quinone oxidoreductase, ROS and translocation of Nrf2	Rajnochová Svobodová et al. (2022)

(Continued)

Table 3.2 (Continued) Compounds Exhibiting Senotherapeutic Benefits on Skin

S.No.	*Compound*	*Model*	*Mechanism*	*Reference*
4	Dasatinib	Allergic dermatitis in mice	↓ IF-γ, TNF-α and cutaneous inflammatory response	Jung et al. (2013)
		Human melanocyte cells	↑ Melanin content Targeting ERK-CREB-MITF-tyrosinase signaling	Kang et al. (2020)
		C57Bl/6 mice wounds	↑ Fibrinogen, vascular permeability and re-epithelialization	Wichaiyo et al. (2023)
5	Quercetin + dasatinib	CAL27, human fibroblast and MCF cells, C3H mice and male Sprague Dawley rats	Cell cycle arrest at G1 phase, ↓ ulcers	H. Wang et al. (2020)
		Human dermal fibroblasts and mouse chimera model	↓ SASP	Takaya and Kishi (2024b)
6	Oleuropein and hydroxytyrosol	Human lung and neonatal human dermal fibroblasts	↓ p16, β-galactosidase activity, MMPs, IL-6, α-smooth-actin, COX-2 and NF-κB	Menicacci et al. (2017)
		Keratinocytes	↓ MMP and ROS	Maruki-Uchida et al. (2013)
7	Nectandrin B	Human dermal fibroblasts	↓ β-galactosidase activity, caveolin, $p16^{ink4a}$, p53, $p21^{waf1}$, cyclin D Targeting AMPK signaling	Jang et al. (2019)
8	Naringenin	UV-induced damage in hairless mice	↓ IL-6/1β/10 and TNF-α, glutathione reductase and Nrf2	Martinez et al. (2016)
9	Equol	UV-induced damage in hairless mice	↓ Epidermal hyperplasia, inflammation, and collagen	Reeve et al. (2005)
10	Gallic acid	Human dermal fibroblasts	↓ ROS, IL-6, MMP-1, TGF-1β and collagen	Hwang et al. (2014)
11	Ferulic acid	Human dermal fibroblasts	↓ Catalase, SOD, MMPs, p16, p21 and cell cycle arrest	Hahn et al. (2016)

12	Apigenin	HaCaT keratinocytes	↓ ROS targeting MAPK and NF-κB pathways	Das et al. (2013)
			↓ BAX, caspase-3	Britto et al. (2017)
13	Resibufogenin	Mice skin	↓ SASP, caspase-3	Takaya, Asou, and Kishi (2023)
14	Ligustilide	Mice Skin	↓ SASP, collagen	Takaya and Kishi (2024a)
15	Metformin	Human dermal fibroblasts and mesenchymal stem cells	↑ GPx7 and modulation of Nrf2	Fang et al. (2018)
16	Rapamycin	Human volunteers	↓ $p16^{INK4A}$ and collagen	Chung et al. (2019)
17	Tamatinib	Human dermal fibroblasts	↓ Caspase- and targeting MAPK and FAK signaling	Cho et al. (2020)
18	ABT-737	Epidermal cells	↓ SASP, $p16^{INK4A}$, p16, p21, HMGB1	Victorelli et al. (2019)
		Human psoriatic cells	↓ p21 and $p16^{INK4a}$ Targeting TET2-Th17 signaling	Zhu et al. (2024)
19	ABT-263/navitoclax	Mesenchymal stem cells	↓ Inflammatory cytokines, and DNA damage	Rothmiller et al. (2021)
		Fibroblast cells	↓ Inflammatory cytokines and MMPs	Takaya et al. (2023)
20	Niacinamide + hyaluronic acid	Women volunteers	↓ Fine lines, wrinkles; ↑ collagen, skin homogeneity	Bogdanowicz et al. (2024)

COX-2, cyclooxygenase-2; CREB, cAMP response element binding protein; DNA, deoxyribonucleic acid; ERK, extracellular signal-regulated kinase; HMGB1, high-mobility group box-1; HO-1, heme oxygenase-1; IL, interleukin; iNOS, inducible nitric oxide synthase; IκB, inhibitor of nuclear factor kappa B; JNK, Jun-N terminal kinase; MAPK, mitogen-activated protein kinase; MMP, matrix metalloproteinase; mRNA, messenger ribonucleic acid; NF-κB, nuclear factor kappa B; NO, nitric oxide; Nrf2, nuclear factor erythroid 2–related factor 2; PGE2, prostaglandin E2; ROS, reactive oxygen species; SASP, senescence-associated secretory phenotype; SOD, superoxide dismutase; TGF-β, tumor growth factor-β; TNF-α, tumor necrosis factor-α.

3.4 NATURAL COMPOUNDS

Several polyphenols and natural compounds have been documented to prevent inflammation and oxidative stress–induced cellular senescence. It is widely recognized that antioxidants naturally occurring in biological substrates help preserve cellular stemness by mitigating oxidative stress and preventing damage to cellular components. Most likely, the effect is observed through decrease in SASP and modulation of pro-survival signaling.

Pathogenesis of skin ailments is primarily associated with inflammation and oxidative stress. The flavonol fisetin was found to be effective against UV-induced collagen degradation in human fibroblast cells. Fisetin (5–25 μM) decreased the levels of ROS, prostaglandin E2 (PGE2), nitric oxide (NO) and suppressed the activity of cyclooxygenase-2 (COX-2) and MMPs induced by irradiation. The flavonol also attenuated the upregulated expressions of UV-induced MAPK, JNK, ERK, p38, p65, nuclear factor kappa B (NF-κB) and inhibitor of nuclear factor kappa B (IκB). In addition to this, fisetin also reduced the CREB (cAMP response element binding protein)-Ser-133 phosphorylation and modulated the P13/AKT/CREB pathway. The results suggested a photoprotective effect of fisetin in skin fibroblasts (Chiang et al. 2015). Similar photoprotective effects of fisetin were observed by Wu et al. in a preclinical study on BALB/c hairless mice. Cutaneous application of fisetin (50 μM) for 10 weeks suppressed hyperplasia and inhibited the expressions of COX-2, MMPs and nuclear factor erythroid 2-related factor (Nrf2). The expression of protein filaggrin was elevated that countered the UV irradiation–mediated skin disruption (Wu et al. 2017). Another study also displayed the protective effects of fisetin on human keratinocyte HaCaT cells. Fisetin (1–20 μM) elevated the protein expression and heme oxygenase (HO)-1 mRNA and decreased the expressions of COX-2 and iNOS while suppressing the levels of PGE2, IL-6/1β and NO. The outcome also showed suppression of NF-κB activity in TNF-α–treated HaCaT cells and translocation of Nrf2 to the nuclei by fisetin. And fisetin increased the phosphorylation of AKT, suggesting its role in the P13K/AKT pathway (Seo and Jeong 2015).

Quercetin, a flavonoid tyrosine-kinase inhibitor with antioxidant capacity, was given (1% by weight) in the diet to C3H/HeN female mice and decreased the accumulation of collagen and attenuated TGF-β signaling. It also decreased radiation-induced skin fibrosis in fibroblast cells (Horton et al. 2013). Quercetin was evaluated for its senolytic property in human dermal fibroblast cells. Quercetin treatment reduced the upregulated expressions of LPL and KCNE2 genes that also modulated proteins p53 and $p16^{INK4A}$ and the antioxidant enzymes catalase and superoxide dismutase (SOD). These results suggested restorative capacity of quercetin in cellular senescence in human dermal fibroblasts (HDFs) (Sohn et al. 2018). Quercetin was also acknowledged as an agent against skin aging. In human skin tissues, it reversed the UV irradiation–mediated elevated MMP-1 and COX-2 levels. In addition, it inhibited the AP-1 and NF-κB function in the tissues. Further, these anti-aging effects were identified due to quercetin's ability to target Janus kinase 2 (JAK2) and protein kinase C delta (PKCδ) signaling that mediate skin inflammation (E. J. Shin et al. 2019). Quercetin exhibited its anti-inflammatory potential in skin lesion similar to atopic dermatitis in human keratinocytes HaCaT cells. Administration for 8 days caused a decrease in expressions of interferon-γ, TNF-α, IL-6/4, CC17 and CC22 along with altered expression of the lnc RNA gene lnc-C7orf30–2 (Hou et al. 2019). In the following year, another study on the same model also showed a decrease in inflammation and downregulation of mRNA expressions of E-cadherin, occludin, MMP-1, MMP-2 and MMP-9. In addition to the above effects, the researchers found these effects to be mediated by NF-κB and ERK1/2 MAPK and pathways that led to healing of the wound (Beken et al. 2020). Quercetin 0.3% ointment was found effective against diabetic wounds in rats. The regeneration and repair of wounds was associated to a decrease in VEGF, TGF-β, TNF-α, IL-1β/10 and MMP-9 (Kant et al. 2021). In a recent study, quercetin effectively improved inflammatory rosacea in HaCaT and HDMEC cells. It significantly alleviated inflammation by targeting the p65, ICAM-1 and NF-κB pathway (Meng et al. 2024). Taxifolin, a structurally related flavonoid to quercetin, was evaluated for its effect on UV-induced skin damage on HDF and epidermal keratinocytes. The results showed that a concentration of 75 μM suppressed the antioxidant enzymes catalase, quinone oxidoreductase and HO-1. The antioxidant effect was confirmed with prevention of ROS generation, caspase activity, DNA break and stimulation of Nrf2 translocation in the HDF cells (Rajnochová Svobodová et al. 2022).

External application of dasatinib with LCB03–0110 attenuated the symptoms of allergic contact dermatitis in mice. A decrease in epidermal thickness, inflammatory cytokines like interferon-γ, IL-1β and TNF-α was observed that suppressed the cutaneous inflammatory response (Jung et al. 2013). Dasatinib increased the melanin content in human melanocyte cells through tyrosinase activity. The cellular differentiation of melanocytes was observed due to stimulation of cascade of ERK-CREB-MITF-tyrosinase signaling (Kang et al. 2020). Dasatinib 0.1% and 0.2% ointment application for 10 days to C57Bl/6 mice enhanced wound healing. The healing was an attribute of decreased inflammation, vascular hyperpermeability, re-epithelialization, increased fibrinogen and angiogenic effect of dasatinib (Wichaiyo et al. 2023). Quercetin in combination with dasatinib (50 mg/kg and 5 mg/kg, respectively) substantially reduced the cellular senescence in CAL27, human fibroblasts and MCF cells by inducing cell cycle arrest at G1 phase. The drugs decreased the ulcers mediated by radiations preclinically in C3H mice (female) and Sprague Dawley rats (male) (H. Wang et al. 2020). The combined treatment of dasatinib with quercetin was shown to be protective in another study on HDFs and mouse chimera models. Treatment with oral gavage for 30 days to animals suppressed the senescence induced by radiation and doxorubicin treatment. The drug treatment alleviated the cellular senescence through suppression of SASP and benefited skin aging (Takaya and Kishi 2024b).

Extra virgin oil poses several health benefits and protection against inflammation. The phenolic compounds present in the oil like oleuropein and hydroxytyrosol

(HT) have anti-oxidative capacity and are investigated for their senolytic potential. In human lung (MRC5) and neonatal HDF, aglycone 1 μM HT or 10 μM oleuropein were evaluated for their effect on cellular senescence after treatment for 4–6 weeks. Both compounds reduced the p16 expression and number of β-galactosidase–positive cells. Further, a decrease in senescence markers like MMPs, IL-6, α-smooth-actin, COX-2 and NF-κB was also observed with phenolic treatment in the cells, while the inflammation due to exposure to TNF-α was completely abolished indicating the efficacy of oils in suppressing senescence-associated inflammation (Menicacci et al. 2017). These compounds upregulated the levels of glutathione in UV-induced oxidative stress in the keratinocytes. The treatment also altered the MMP-1 levels and decreased ROS generation, suggesting the role of these compounds in modulating photoaging in cells (Maruki-Uchida et al. 2013).

Lignan, nectandrin B from *Myristica fragrans* increased the cell viability in HDFs. Nectandrin B reduced the activity of senescence markers like caveolin, $p16^{ink4a}$, p53, $p21^{waf1}$, cyclin D and activity of β-galactosidase. These effects were attributed to AMP-activated protein kinase (AMPK) signaling in addition to decrease in ROS. These results suggested protective effects of nectandrin B against cellular senescence to alleviate skin aging (Jang et al. 2019). Naringenin, when applied topically, protected the hairless mice from UV-induced inflammation, skin damage and oxidative stress. The results showed decrease in edema, cytokines like IL-6/1β/10 and TNF-α. Further, a decrease in mRNA expressions of glutathione peroxidase-1, glutathione reductase and Nrf2 along with increased expression of HO-1 was also observed. This showed preventive role of naringenin against UV irradiation induced skin senescence (Martinez et al. 2016). The effect of equol was tested on photoaging in UV irradiation exposure to hairless mice. Equol (10 μM), when applied externally to animals for 30 weeks, reversed epidermal hyperplasia, increased elastotic deposits, increased dermal mast cells, reduced collagen and dermal deposition of glycosaminoglycans. There alterations with equol exhibited its immunoprotective and anti-inflammatory properties to protect skin (Reeve et al. 2005).

Hwang et al. investigated the effect of phenolic compound gallic acid against photoaging in vitro in HDFs and in hairless mice. The results showed that gallic acid suppressed the elevated ROS, IL-6, MMP-1 and type-1 collagen in UV-irradiated HDFs. While the treatment regulated elastin levels, decreased MMP-1, TGF-1β that modulated the skin thickness, dryness and wrinkle formation in the animals. These results showed the potential capacity of gallic acid in reversing aging induced by UV irradiation (Hwang et al. 2014). In another research design, ferulic acid was investigated to identify its effect in UV-induced damage in HDFs. Pretreatment of cells with ferulic acid inhibited the cell cycle arrest, altered mRNA levels of catalase, SOD, MMPs, p16 and p21 levels, suggesting its significance in repairing DNA and decreasing cellular senescence of damaged skin (Hahn et al. 2016).

Photodamaged keratinocytes were preserved from damage to retain normal epithelia with the natural compound baicalin through its antioxidant effects (S.-C. Wang et al. 2013). Antioxidant polyphenol from *Lycopodium clavatum*, apigenin prevented DNA damage and protected UV-irradiated HaCaT keratinocytes and animals. The flavonoid reduced formation of free radicals and downregulated the MAPK and NF-κB communication (Das et al. 2013). Apigenin (15μM) also showed its protective effects in HDF cells to protect them from UV related damage. It prevented the generation of apoptotic genes BAX and caspase-3 and prevented skin damage (Britto et al. 2017). Toad venom, from traditional Chinese medicine, resibufogenin also exhibits senotherapeutic effects. It precisely causes senescent cell death and significantly suppresses SASP without affecting proliferative cells. Senescent cells were targeted via caspase-3–mediated apoptosis in mice. This compound improved the symptoms of skin aging and showed benefits against skin-associated senescent cells (Takaya, Asou, and Kishi 2023). Ligustilide, a major component of the herbal medicine *Angelica acutiloba*, was also found to enhance cell death of senescent cells, exhibiting therapeutic benefit. It significantly decreased SASP and increased the density of dermal collagen protein and adipose tissue content in mouse skin (Takaya and Kishi 2024a).

These studies highlight the potential of several natural compounds that have benefited skin by decreasing the burden of senescent cells.

3.5 SEMI-SYNTHETIC/SYNTHETIC COMPOUNDS

Besides the potential of natural substances, research has demonstrated the potency of compounds from semi-synthetic and synthetic origin in controlling senescence.

Fang et al. reported a decrease in senescent cells by the anti-diabetic drug metformin in human fibroblasts and mesenchymal stem cells. Levels of glutathione peroxidase 7 (GPx7) present in endoplasmic reticulum were found reduced in senescent cells. Metformin (100 μm) upregulated the expression of GPx7 present in the endoplasmic reticulum and enhanced the lifespan of cells. It also improved the concentration of Nrf2 in worms. Metformin was found effectual for pro-longevity signaling (Fang et al. 2018).

Targeted treatment of senescence was observed with overexpressed CD9 receptors-rapamycin nano formulation. The rapamycin loaded on lactose-wrapped calcium carbonate nanoparticles (CD9-Lac/$CaCO_3$/Rapa) targeted the β-galactosidase. This formulation decreased senescence as evidenced through a decrease in expression of p53/p21/CD9/cyclin D1 and activity of β-galactosidase. It also improved the proliferative capacity and migration of old cells by decreasing the inflammatory markers IL-1β/6 (Thapa et al. 2017). In a clinical trial with 36 participants over 40 years of age, rapamycin was tested for its potential to alleviate age-associated skin changes like decrease in dermal tissues and photoaging. A significantly higher level of collagen and lower levels of $p16^{INK4A}$ proteins was found. Rapamycin also improved the appearance of the skin by decreasing cellular senescence (Chung et al. 2019).

Tamatinib (R406), a novel senolytic agent significantly controlled the replicative senescence in diploid HDF. Tamatinib was found to induce the intrinsic apoptotic pathway mediated by capase-9. It also regulated the cell survival through inhibition of MAPK and focal adhesion kinase (FAK) (Cho et al. 2020).

The compound ABT-737, an inhibitor of BCL-2, BCL-XL and BCL-W, decreased the DNA damage–induced senescence in the lungs and in the epidermal cells. It improved the homeostasis of melanocytes through alteration of SASP, telomere functioning and decrease in senescent markers like $p16^{INK4A}$, p16, p21 and HMGB1. It also controlled the activation of ROS. This improved the basal keratinocyte proliferation that limited the skin aging process (Victorelli et al. 2019). Zhu et al. explored the role of senolytics in alleviating psoriasis in human psoriatic cells. ABT-737 was prepared as a gel for evaluation of its efficacy in imiquimod-induced psoriatic lesions. The lesions displayed an increase in expressions of p21 and $p16^{INK4a}$ in $CD4^+$ T cells. These classical markers were significantly decreased after topical application of senolytic gel. Additionally, attenuation of α and β chains of T cell receptor and methylcytosine dioxygenase 2 (TET2) was also observed. The results suggested the role of senolytic ABT-737 gel for treatment of psoriatic lesion through TET2-Th17 pathway (Zhu et al. 2024).

Another senolytic, navitoclax (ABT-263), was investigated for senotherapeutic behavior in skin-related cellular senescence. It improved the altered morphological changes, decreased DNA damage and pro-inflammatory cytokines in senescent cells induced by sulfur mustard in mesenchymal stem cells. The senescent removal capacity upholds it as a potential agent for chronic wound healing (Rothmiller et al. 2021). ABT-263 also showed therapeutic potential against skin aging. In senescent fibroblast cells, it exhibited a decrease in age-related hallmarks and secretory phenotypes like ILs and MMPs and eliminated the senescent cells (Takaya et al. 2023).

Senomorphic activity of a formulation with vitamin B3 or niacinamide (6%) and hyaluronic acid was tested for its benefits on skin aging. Forty-four healthy women volunteers (38–55 years) applied the formula once for 8 weeks on the face, neckline, and neck. After 8 weeks a significant radiance, improvement in complexion, smoothness and skin plumpness was observed along with a decrease in fine lines and wrinkles. The application of the formula also enhanced skin homogeneity, dermal density and collagen content in volunteers, suggesting its protective capacity against UV-associated damage (Bogdanowicz et al. 2024).

3.6 CONCLUSION AND FUTURE DIRECTIONS

Cellular senescence is primarily an anti-proliferative mechanism. However, buildup of senescent cells causes dysfunction of tissue metabolism. Studies have confirmed that cellular senescence occurs due to telomere attrition, increased oxidative stress, mitochondrial dysfunction, activation of oncogenes and metabolic imbalance. The senescent cells play a dual role of providing benefit in conditions like wound healing or cancer while being detrimental for repair and regeneration of tissues due to inflammation and matrix degradation.

In dermatological conditions also, cellular senescence plays a crucial role. The skin, being the largest organ, responds to internal and external stimuli it dispenses as an interesting target to understand cellular senescence and role of senotherapeutic compounds. It also provides an opportunity to investigate to discover newer drugs targeting senescence. Several senotherapeutic agents from natural and synthetic origin have displayed their efficacy in decreasing inflammation and improving skin regeneration. However, the precise target that affects skin integrity is still under investigation, though mostly the senescent burden is reduced by SASP- and SCAP-related pathways. Senolytics remove the senescent cells while senomorphics appear to help overcome the damaging effects of senescent cells. Several preclinical models establish the efficacy of senolytics, but senomorphics require long-term administration to establish their efficacy. Senescent pathways are being targeted via innovative tools. However, validation from clinical trials would allow better integration and management of therapy with skin-related disorders.

A considerable future challenge for skin-related therapy is to critically identify the origin and impact of senescent cells. Aging is a major factor that impact skin health, and removal of senescent cells is delayed with aging skin. Factors that are directly secreted and the communication of cells with the microenvironment is important for senotherapy. In addition, short-term and long-term effects of the therapy are yet to be established for its translation for clinical studies. The newer opportunities for the therapy shall be harnessed for their transformative role in skin benefits.

REFERENCES

Ahmed, Faraha, and Razia Khanam. 2023. "Senolytics in Brain Disorders: A Novel Pharmacological Approach to Control Cellular Senescence and Oxidative Stress." In *Adaptation under Stressful Environments through Biological Adjustments and Interventions*, 327–342. Singapore: Springer Nature Singapore. https://doi.org/10.1007/978-981-99-7652-2_20.

Azazmeh, Narmen, Benjamin Assouline, Eitan Winter, Shmuel Ruppo, Yuval Nevo, Alexander Maly, Karen Meir, et al. 2020. "Chronic Expression of P16INK4a in the Epidermis Induces Wnt-Mediated Hyperplasia and Promotes Tumor Initiation." *Nature Communications* 11 (1): 2711. https://doi.org/10.1038/s41467-020-16475-3.

Beken, Burcin, Riza Serttas, Mehtap Yazicioglu, Kader Turkekul, and Suat Erdogan. 2020. "Quercetin Improves Inflammation, Oxidative Stress, and Impaired Wound Healing in Atopic Dermatitis Model of Human Keratinocytes." *Pediatric Allergy, Immunology, and Pulmonology* 33 (2): 69–79. https://doi.org/10.1089/ped.2019.1137.

Bogdanowicz, Patrick, Paul Bensadoun, Maïté Noizet, Benoît Béganton, Armony Philippe, Sandrine Alvarez-Georges, Gautier Doat, et al. 2024. "Senomorphic Activity of a Combination of Niacinamide and Hyaluronic Acid: Correlation with Clinical Improvement of Skin Aging." *Scientific Reports* 14 (1): 16321. https://doi.org/10.1038/s41598-024-66624-7.

Borchers, Annette, and Tomas Pieler. 2010. "Programming Pluripotent Precursor Cells Derived from Xenopus Embryos to Generate Specific Tissues and Organs." *Genes* 1 (3): 413–426. https://doi.org/10.3390/genes1030413.

Branchet, M.C., S. Boisnic, C. Frances, and A.M. Robert. 1990. "Skin Thickness Changes in Normal Aging Skin." *Gerontology* 36 (1): 28–35. https://doi.org/10.1159/000213172.

Britto, S. Mary, D. Shanthakumari, B. Agilan, T. Radhiga, G. Kanimozhi, and N. Rajendra Prasad. 2017. "Apigenin Prevents Ultraviolet-B Radiation Induced Cyclobutane Pyrimidine Dimers Formation in Human Dermal Fibroblasts." *Mutation Research/Genetic Toxicology and Environmental Mutagenesis* 821 (September): 28–35. https://doi.org/10.1016/j.mrgentox.2017.06.002.

Bulbiankova, Darya, Rocío Díaz-Puertas, Francisco Javier Álvarez-Martínez, María Herranz-López, Enrique Barrajón-Catalán, and Vicente Micol. 2023a. "Hallmarks and Biomarkers of Skin Senescence: An Updated Review of Skin Senotherapeutics." *Antioxidants (Basel, Switzerland)* 12 (2). https://doi.org/10.3390/antiox12020444.

Bulbiankova, Darya, Rocío Díaz-Puertas, Francisco Javier Álvarez-Martínez, María Herranz-López, Enrique Barrajón-Catalán, and Vicente Micol. 2023b. "Hallmarks and Biomarkers of Skin Senescence: An Updated Review of Skin Senotherapeutics." *Antioxidants* 12 (2): 444. https://doi.org/10.3390/antiox12020444.

Chiang, Hsiu-Mei, Shih-Yun Chan, Yin Chu, and Kuo-Ching Wen. 2015. "Fisetin Ameliorated Photodamage by Suppressing the Mitogen-Activated Protein Kinase/Matrix Metalloproteinase Pathway and Nuclear Factor-KB Pathways." *Journal of Agricultural and Food Chemistry* 63 (18): 4551–4560. https://doi.org/10.1021/jf502500t.

Chin, Toby, Xin Er Lee, Pei Yi Ng, Yaelim Lee, and Oliver Dreesen. 2023. "The Role of Cellular Senescence in Skin Aging and Age-Related Skin Pathologies." *Frontiers in Physiology* 14 (November). https://doi.org/10.3389/fphys.2023.1297637.

Cho, Hyun-Ji, Eun Jae Yang, Joon Tae Park, Jae-Ryong Kim, Eok-Cheon Kim, Kyong-Jin Jung, Sang Chul Park, and Young-Sam Lee. 2020. "Identification of SYK Inhibitor, R406 as a Novel Senolytic Agent." *Aging* 12 (9): 8221–8240. https://doi.org/10.18632/aging.103135.

Chung, Christina Lee, Ibiyonu Lawrence, Melissa Hoffman, Dareen Elgindi, Kumar Nadhan, Manali Potnis, Annie Jin, et al. 2019. "Topical Rapamycin Reduces Markers of Senescence and Aging in Human Skin: An Exploratory, Prospective, Randomized Trial." *GeroScience* 41 (6): 861–869. https://doi.org/10.1007/s11357-019-00113-y.

Cristofalo, Vincent J., Antonello Lorenzini, R.G. Allen, Claudio Torres, and Maria Tresini. 2004. "Replicative Senescence: A Critical Review." *Mechanisms of Ageing and Development* 125 (10–11): 827–848. https://doi.org/10.1016/j.mad.2004.07.010.

Csekes, Erika, and Lucia Račková. 2021. "Skin Aging, Cellular Senescence and Natural Polyphenols." *International Journal of Molecular Sciences* 22 (23): 12641. https://doi.org/10.3390/ijms222312641.

Dańczak-Pazdrowska, Aleksandra, Justyna Gornowicz-Porowska, Adriana Polańska, Violetta Krajka-Kuźniak, Maciej Stawny, Aleksandra Gostyńska, Błażej Rubiś, et al. 2023. "Cellular Senescence in Skin-Related Research: Targeted Signaling Pathways and Naturally Occurring Therapeutic Agents." *Aging Cell* 22 (6). https://doi.org/10.1111/acel.13845.

Das, Sreemanti, Jayeeta Das, Avijit Paul, Asmita Samadder, and Anisur Rahman Khuda-Bukhsh. 2013. "Apigenin, a Bioactive Flavonoid from Lycopodium Clavatum, Stimulates Nucleotide Excision Repair Genes to Protect Skin Keratinocytes from Ultraviolet B-Induced Reactive Oxygen Species and DNA Damage." *Journal of Acupuncture and Meridian Studies* 6 (5): 252–262. https://doi.org/10.1016/j.jams.2013.07.002.

Domaszewska-Szostek, Anna, Monika Puzianowska-Kuźnicka, and Alina Kuryłowicz. 2021. "Flavonoids in Skin Senescence Prevention and Treatment." *International Journal of Molecular Sciences* 22 (13): 6814. https://doi.org/10.3390/ijms22136814.

Fang, Jingqi, Jiping Yang, Xun Wu, Gangming Zhang, Tao Li, Xi'e Wang, Hong Zhang, Chih-Chen Wang, Guang-Hui Liu, and Lei Wang. 2018. "Metformin Alleviates Human Cellular Aging by Upregulating the Endoplasmic Reticulum Glutathione Peroxidase 7." *Aging Cell* 17 (4). https://doi.org/10.1111/acel.12765.

Fitsiou, Eleni, Tanya Pulido, Judith Campisi, Fatouma Alimirah, and Marco Demaria. 2021. "Cellular Senescence and the Senescence-Associated Secretory Phenotype as Drivers of Skin Photoaging." *Journal of Investigative Dermatology* 141 (4): 1119–1126. https://doi.org/10.1016/j.jid.2020.09.031.

Hahn, Hyung Jin, Ki Bbeum Kim, Seunghee Bae, Byung Gon Choi, Sungkwan An, Kyu Joong Ahn, and Su Young Kim. 2016. "Pretreatment of Ferulic Acid Protects Human Dermal Fibroblasts against Ultraviolet A Irradiation." *Annals of Dermatology* 28 (6): 740. https://doi.org/10.5021/ad.2016.28.6.740.

Hayflick, L., and P.S. Moorhead. 1961. "The Serial Cultivation of Human Diploid Cell Strains." *Experimental Cell Research* 25 (3): 585–621. https://doi.org/10.1016/0014-4827(61)90192-6.

Horton, Jason A., Fei Li, Eun Joo Chung, Kathryn Hudak, Ayla White, Kristopher Krausz, Frank Gonzalez, and Deborah Citrin. 2013. "Quercetin Inhibits Radiation-Induced Skin Fibrosis." *Radiation Research* 180 (2): 205. https://doi.org/10.1667/RR3237.1.

Hou, Dian-Dong, Wei Zhang, Ya-Li Gao, Yu-Zhe Sun, He-Xiao Wang, Rui-Qun Qi, Hong-Duo Chen, and Xing-Hua Gao. 2019. "Anti-Inflammatory Effects of Quercetin in a Mouse Model of MC903-Induced Atopic Dermatitis." *International Immunopharmacology* 74 (September): 105676. https://doi.org/10.1016/j.intimp.2019.105676.

Huang, Weijun, LaTonya J. Hickson, Alfonso Eirin, James L. Kirkland, and Lilach O. Lerman. 2022. "Cellular Senescence: The Good, the Bad and the Unknown." *Nature Reviews Nephrology* 18 (10): 611–627. https://doi.org/10.1038/s41581-022-00601-z.

Hwang, Eunson, Sang-Yong Park, Hyun Ji Lee, Tae Youp Lee, Zheng-Wang Sun, and Tae Hoo Yi. 2014. "Gallic Acid Regulates Skin Photoaging in UVB-Exposed Fibroblast and Hairless Mice." *Phytotherapy Research* 28 (12): 1778–1788. https://doi.org/10.1002/ptr.5198.

Jang, Hyun-Jin, Kyeong Eun Yang, Won Keun Oh, Song-I Lee, In-Hu Hwang, Kyung-Tae Ban, Hwa-Seung Yoo, Jong-Soon Choi, Eui-Ju Yeo, and Ik-Soon Jang. 2019. "Nectandrin B-Mediated Activation of the AMPK Pathway Prevents Cellular Senescence in Human Diploid Fibroblasts by Reducing Intracellular ROS Levels." *Aging* 11 (11): 3731–3749. https://doi.org/10.18632/aging.102013.

Jung, S.H., X. Sun, W.-S. Ryu, and B.-S. Yang. 2013. "Topical Administration of the Pan-Src Kinase Inhibitors, Dasatinib and LCB 03-0110, Prevents Allergic Contact Dermatitis in Mice." *British Journal of Dermatology* 168 (1): 112–119. https://doi.org/10.1111/bjd.12069.

Kanaki, Theodora, Evgenia Makrantonaki, and Christos C. Zouboulis. 2016. "Biomarkers of Skin Aging." *Reviews in Endocrine and Metabolic Disorders* 17 (3): 433–442. https://doi.org/10.1007/s11154-016-9392-x.

Kang, Bogyeong, Yeongeun Kim, Tae Jun Park, and Hee Young Kang. 2020. "Dasatinib, a Second-Generation Tyrosine Kinase Inhibitor, Induces Melanogenesis via ERK-CREB-MITF-Tyrosinase Signaling in Normal Human Melanocytes." *Biochemical and Biophysical Research Communications* 523 (4): 1034–1039. https://doi.org/10.1016/j.bbrc.2020.01.051.

Kant, Vinay, Babu Lal Jangir, Maneesh Sharma, Vinod Kumar, and Vinay G. Joshi. 2021. "Topical Application of Quercetin Improves Wound Repair and Regeneration in Diabetic Rats." *Immunopharmacology and Immunotoxicology* 43 (5): 536–553. https://doi.org/10.1080/08923973.2021.1950758.

Kim, Eok Cheon, and Jae Ryong Kim. 2019. "Senotherapeutics: Emerging Strategy for Healthy Aging and Age-Related Disease." *BMB Reports* 52 (1): 47–55. https://doi.org/10.5483/BMBREP.2019.52.1.293.

Kim, William Y., and Norman E. Sharpless. 2006. "The Regulation of INK4/ARF in Cancer and Aging." *Cell* 127 (2): 265–275. https://doi.org/10.1016/j.cell.2006.10.003.

Lee, Young In, Sooyeon Choi, Won Seok Roh, Ju Hee Lee, and Tae-Gyun Kim. 2021. "Cellular Senescence and Inflammaging in the Skin Microenvironment." *International Journal of Molecular Sciences* 22 (8): 3849. https://doi.org/10.3390/ijms22083849.

Martinez, Renata M., Felipe A. Pinho-Ribeiro, Vinicius S. Steffen, Thais C. C. Silva, Carla V. Caviglione, Carolina Bottura, Maria J. V. Fonseca, et al. 2016. "Topical Formulation Containing Naringenin: Efficacy against Ultraviolet B Irradiation-Induced Skin Inflammation and Oxidative Stress in Mice." *PloS One* 11 (1): e0146296. https://doi.org/10.1371/journal.pone.0146296.

Maruki-Uchida, Hiroko, Ikuko Kurita, Kenkichi Sugiyama, Masahiko Sai, Kazuhisa Maeda, and Tatsuhiko Ito. 2013. "The Protective Effects of Piceatannol from Passion Fruit (*Passiflora Edulis*) Seeds in UVB-Irradiated Keratinocytes." *Biological and Pharmaceutical Bulletin* 36 (5): 845–849. https://doi.org/10.1248/bpb.b12-00708.

Meng, Xin, Yangfan Li, Fan Wang, Tao Li, Ben Wang, Qian Wang, Juan Long, Hongfu Xie, Yiya Zhang, and Ji Li. 2024. "Quercetin Attenuates Inflammation in Rosacea by Directly Targeting P65 and ICAM-1." *Life Sciences* 347 (June): 122675. https://doi.org/10.1016/j.lfs.2024.122675.

Menicacci, Beatrice, Caterina Cipriani, Francesca Margheri, Alessandra Mocali, and Lisa Giovannelli. 2017. "Modulation of the Senescence-Associated Inflammatory Phenotype in Human Fibroblasts by Olive Phenols." *International Journal of Molecular Sciences* 18 (11): 2275. https://doi.org/10.3390/ijms18112275.

Passos, João F., Gabriele Saretzki, Shaheda Ahmed, Glyn Nelson, Torsten Richter, Heiko Peters, Ilka Wappler, et al. 2007. "Mitochondrial Dysfunction Accounts for the Stochastic Heterogeneity in Telomere-Dependent Senescence." *PLoS Biology* 5 (5): e110. https://doi.org/10.1371/journal.pbio.0050110.

Payne, Drew. 2020. "Skin Integrity in Older Adults: Pressure-Prone, Inaccessible Areas of the Body." *British Journal of Community Nursing* 25 (1): 22–26. https://doi.org/10.12968/bjcn.2020.25.1.22.

Pils, Vera, Nadja Ring, Karla Valdivieso, Ingo Lämmermann, Florian Gruber, Markus Schosserer, Johannnes Grillari, and Mikolaj Ogrodnik. 2021. "Promises and Challenges of Senolytics in Skin Regeneration, Pathology and Ageing." *Mechanisms of Ageing and Development* 200 (December): 111588. https://doi.org/10.1016/j.mad.2021.111588.

Puizina-Ivić, Neira. 2008. "Skin Aging." *Acta Dermatovenerologica Alpina, Pannonica, et Adriatica* 17 (2): 47–54.

Rajnochová Svobodová, Alena, Alena Ryšavá, Kateřina Čížková, Lenka Roubalová, Jitka Ulrichová, Jiří Vrba, Bohumil Zálešák, and Jitka Vostálová. 2022. "Effect of the Flavonoids Quercetin and Taxifolin on UVA-Induced Damage to Human Primary Skin Keratinocytes and Fibroblasts." *Photochemical & Photobiological Sciences: Official Journal of the European Photochemistry Association and the European Society for Photobiology* 21 (1): 59–75. https://doi.org/10.1007/s43630-021-00140-9.

Reeve, Vivienne E., Sitarina Widyarini, Diane Domanski, Elaine Chew, and Karen Barnes. 2005. "Protection Against Photoaging in the Hairless Mouse by the Isoflavone Equol." *Photochemistry and Photobiology* 81 (6): 1548–1553. https://doi.org/10.1562/2005-07-26-RA-624.

Reilly, David M., and Jennifer Lozano. 2021. "Skin Collagen through the Lifestages: Importance for Skin Health and Beauty." *Plastic and Aesthetic Research* 8: 2. https://doi.org/10.20517/2347-9264.2020.153.

Rothmiller, Simone, Niklas Jäger, Nicole Meier, Thimo Meyer, Adrian Neu, Dirk Steinritz, Horst Thiermann, et al. 2021. "Chronic Senescent Human Mesenchymal Stem Cells as Possible Contributor to the Wound Healing Disorder after Exposure to the Alkylating Agent Sulfur Mustard." *Archives of Toxicology* 95 (2): 727–747. https://doi.org/10.1007/s00204-020-02946-5.

Russell-Goldman, Eleanor, and George F. Murphy. 2020. "The Pathobiology of Skin Aging." *The American Journal of Pathology* 190 (7): 1356–1369. https://doi.org/10.1016/j.ajpath.2020.03.007.

Seo, Seung-Hee, and Gil-Saeng Jeong. 2015. "Fisetin Inhibits TNF-α-Induced Inflammatory Action and Hydrogen Peroxide-Induced Oxidative Damage in Human Keratinocyte HaCaT Cells through PI3K/AKT/Nrf-2-Mediated Heme Oxygenase-1 Expression." *International Immunopharmacology* 29 (2): 246–253. https://doi.org/10.1016/j.intimp.2015.11.014.

Shah, Parisha P., Greg Donahue, Gabriel L. Otte, Brian C. Capell, David M. Nelson, Kajia Cao, Varun Aggarwala, et al. 2013. "Lamin B1 Depletion in Senescent Cells Triggers Large-Scale Changes in Gene Expression and the Chromatin Landscape." *Genes & Development* 27 (16): 1787–1799. https://doi.org/10.1101/gad.223834.113.

Shin, Eun Ju, Ji Su Lee, Seungpyo Hong, Tae-Gyu Lim, and Sanguine Byun. 2019. "Quercetin Directly Targets JAK2 and PKCδ and Prevents UV-Induced Photoaging in Human Skin." *International Journal of Molecular Sciences* 20 (21). https://doi.org/10.3390/ijms20215262.

Shin, J., J.-H. Kim, and E.K. Kim. 2012. "Repeated Exposure of Human Fibroblasts to UVR Induces Secretion of Stem Cell Factor and Senescence." *Journal of the European Academy of Dermatology and Venereology* 26 (12): 1577–1580. https://doi.org/10.1111/j.1468-3083.2011.04223.x.

Sohn, Eun-Ju, Jung Min Kim, Se-Hui Kang, Joseph Kwon, Hyun Joo An, Jung-Suk Sung, Kyung A Cho, Ik-Soon Jang, and Jong-Soon Choi. 2018. "Restoring Effects of Natural Anti-Oxidant Quercetin on Cellular Senescent Human Dermal Fibroblasts." *The American Journal of Chinese Medicine* 46 (4): 853–873. https://doi.org/10.1142/S0192415X18500453.

Takaya, Kento, Toru Asou, and Kazuo Kishi. 2023. "Identification of Resibufogenin, a Component of Toad Venom, as a Novel Senolytic Compound in Vitro and for Potential Skin Rejuvenation in Male Mice." *Biogerontology* 24 (6): 889–900. https://doi.org/10.1007/s10522-023-10043-0.

Takaya, Kento, Tatsuyuki Ishii, Toru Asou, and Kazuo Kishi. 2023. "Navitoclax (ABT-263) Rejuvenates Human Skin by Eliminating Senescent Dermal Fibroblasts in a Mouse/Human Chimeric Model." *Rejuvenation Research* 26 (1): 9–20. https://doi.org/10.1089/rej.2022.0048.

Takaya, Kento, and Kazuo Kishi. 2024a. "Ligustilide, A Novel Senolytic Compound Isolated from the Roots of *Angelica Acutiloba*." *Advanced Biology* (January). https://doi.org/10.1002/adbi.202300434.

Takaya, Kento, and Kazuo Kishi. 2024b. "Combined Dasatinib and Quercetin Treatment Contributes to Skin Rejuvenation through Selective Elimination of Senescent Cells in Vitro and in Vivo." *Biogerontology* 25 (4): 691–704. https://doi.org/10.1007/s10522-024-10103-z.

Thapa, Raj Kumar, Hanh Thuy Nguyen, Jee-Heon Jeong, Jae Ryong Kim, Han-Gon Choi, Chul Soon Yong, and Jong Oh Kim. 2017. "Progressive Slowdown/Prevention of Cellular Senescence by CD9-Targeted Delivery of Rapamycin Using Lactose-Wrapped Calcium Carbonate Nanoparticles." *Scientific Reports* 7 (1): 43299. https://doi.org/10.1038/srep43299.

Thompson, Elizabeth L., Louise E. Pitcher, Laura J. Niedernhofer, and Paul D. Robbins. 2022. "Targeting Cellular Senescence with Senotherapeutics: Development of New Approaches for Skin Care." *Plastic and Reconstructive Surgery* 150 (October): 12S–19S. https://doi.org/10.1097/PRS.0000000000009668.

Victorelli, Stella, Anthony Lagnado, Jessica Halim, Will Moore, Duncan Talbot, Karen Barrett, James Chapman, et al. 2019. "Senescent Human Melanocytes Drive Skin Ageing via Paracrine Telomere Dysfunction." *The EMBO Journal* 38 (23). https://doi.org/10.15252/embj.2019101982.

Wang, Audrey S., and Oliver Dreesen. 2018. "Biomarkers of Cellular Senescence and Skin Aging." *Frontiers in Genetics* 9 (August). https://doi.org/10.3389/fgene.2018.00247.

Wang, Huilan, Ziwen Wang, Yu Huang, Yue Zhou, Xiaowu Sheng, Qingzhi Jiang, Yawei Wang, Peng Luo, Min Luo, and Chunmeng Shi. 2020. "Senolytics (DQ) Mitigates Radiation Ulcers by Removing Senescent Cells." *Frontiers in Oncology* 9 (February). https://doi.org/10.3389/fonc.2019.01576.

Wang, Shou-Cheng, Sue-Fung Chen, Yi-Min Lee, Chin-Liang Chuang, Da-Tian Bau, and Song-Shei Lin. 2013. "Baicalin Scavenges Reactive Oxygen Species and Protects Human Keratinocytes against UVC-Induced Cytotoxicity." *In Vivo (Athens, Greece)* 27 (6): 707–714.

Wichaiyo, Surasak, Saovaros Svasti, Arnatchai Maiuthed, Pattarawit Rukthong, Arman Syah Goli, and Noppawan Phumala Morales. 2023. "Dasatinib Ointment Promotes Healing of Murine Excisional Skin Wound." *ACS Pharmacology & Translational Science* 6 (7): 1015–1027. https://doi.org/10.1021/acsptsci.2c00245.

Wlaschek, Meinhard, Pallab Maity, Evgenia Makrantonaki, and Karin Scharffetter-Kochanek. 2021. "Connective Tissue and Fibroblast Senescence in Skin Aging." *Journal of Investigative Dermatology* 141 (4): 985–992. https://doi.org/10.1016/j.jid.2020.11.010.

Wu, Po-Yuan, Jia-Ling Lyu, Yi-Jung Liu, Ting-Yi Chien, Hao-Cheng Hsu, Kuo-Ching Wen, and Hsiu-Mei Chiang. 2017. "Fisetin Regulates Nrf2 Expression and the Inflammation-Related Signaling Pathway to Prevent UVB-Induced Skin Damage in Hairless Mice." *International Journal of Molecular Sciences* 18 (10): 2118. https://doi.org/10.3390/ijms18102118.

Wyles, Saranya P., Parisa Dashti, Tamar Pirtskhalava, Burak Tekin, Christina Inman, Lilian Sales Gomez, Anthony B. Lagnado, et al. 2023. "A Chronic Wound Model to Investigate Skin Cellular Senescence." *Aging* (April). https://doi.org/10.18632/aging.204667.

Zhu, Huan, Jiao Jiang, Ming Yang, Mingming Zhao, Zhenghao He, Congli Tang, Cailing Song, et al. 2024. "Topical Application of a BCL-2 Inhibitor Ameliorates Imiquimod-Induced Psoriasiform Dermatitis by Eliminating Senescent Cells." *Journal of Dermatological Science* (June). https://doi.org/10.1016/j.jdermsci.2024.06.002.

Chapter 4

Senotherapeutics in Cancer

Gurpreet Kaur, Ishita Kakkar, Yashasvi Sharma, Saurabh Mittal, Sonal Setya, and Sushama Talegaonkar

4.1 INTRODUCTION

Senotherapeutics is an emerging strategy focused on eliminating senescent cells to enhance health span in addition to combating conditions associated with aging (Kim & Kim, 2019). Senescent cells accumulate with age, contributing to tissue aging and various chronic diseases (Park & Shin, 2022). Senotherapeutics are systematically categorized into senolytics, designed to precisely target and remove accumulated senescent cells; and senomorphics, intended to modulate their functions while simultaneously delaying the progression of senescence (Kim & Kim, 2019; Robbins et al., 2021). These interventions have shown promise in animal models, alleviating disease across various organ systems and improving physical function (Robbins et al., 2021). Both synthetic agents and natural compounds have been proposed as senotherapeutics, with initial clinical trials suggesting potential translatability to humans. However, caution is warranted due to potential side effects, particularly with senolytic agents. Natural senolytic compounds may offer advantages in terms of lower toxicity, although their precise modes of action demand deeper investigation (Boccardi & Mecocci, 2021). Recent research has focused on targeting surface proteins of senescence-associated cells, which has emerged as a key strategy for advancing senolytic therapies. They function by inhibiting the senescence-associated secretory phenotype (SASP) and facilitating immune-mediated clearance of senescent cells, potentially offering novel strategies for extending health span and treating age-related tissue degradation (Rossi & Abdelmohsen, 2021).

The development of senotherapeutics—therapies targeting senescent cells—has provided new hope for counteracting senescence-driven complications in cancer. Senotherapeutics are typically categorized into two mechanistic classes: senolytics and senomorphics (Bousset & Gil, 2022). Senolytic agents, such as navitoclax, target anti-apoptotic pathways that are upregulated in senescent cellular environments, inducing apoptosis selectively within these cells. For instance, navitoclax inhibits BCL-2, a key protein that prevents apoptosis in senescent cells, thereby allowing the immune system to clear them (Domen et al., 2022). Senomorphics,

DOI: 10.1201/9781003493969-4

on the other hand, do not eliminate senescent cells but instead modulate the harmful aspects of their SASP. Drugs like rapamycin and metformin have been shown to suppress the release of pro-inflammatory activity linked to the SASP, thereby reducing tumor-promoting effects linked with senescence-associated cells without killing the senescent cells themselves (Prasanna et al., 2021). This strategy is particularly advantageous when senescent cells serve a beneficial function in preventing abnormal cellular growth in early-stage cancers.

A primary obstacle to effective cancer therapy is the persistence of senescent cells within the tumor microenvironment (TME). Senescent stromal cells, immune cells, and even endothelial cells within the TME secrete factors that remodel the extracellular matrix, promote angiogenesis, and suppress immune surveillance (Prasanna et al., 2021). This contributes to a more aggressive tumor phenotype, fostering both primary tumor growth and metastasis.

Eliminating senescent cells from the TME through senotherapeutics can potentially reverse this pro-tumorigenic environment. For example, studies have shown that the use of senolytic drugs in mouse models of cancer not only reduces tumor size but also enhances the efficacy of immune checkpoint inhibitors by restoring immune function within the tumor (Zhang et al., 2023).This suggests that targeting senescence within the TME could be a powerful adjunct to current immunotherapy strategies.

4.2 CELLULAR SENESCENCE AND ITS ROLE IN CANCER

4.2.1 Cancer and Cellular Senescence

Cancer is one of the most complex diseases, characterized by its unchecked cellular proliferation, invasion into surrounding tissues, and resistance to treatment. Over the past few decades, the traditional methods of treating cancer have encompassed surgical intervention, cytotoxic therapy, and radiotherapy, yet these methods often fail to eliminate all malignant cells, leading to recurrence and metastasis. Ongoing progress in deciphering the mechanisms of cellular senescence have illuminated an innovative therapeutic avenue known as senotherapeutics, which seeks to target senescent cells that accumulate during cancer progression or in response to therapy.

The concept of cellular senescence was first identified by Hayflick and Moorhead, who demonstrated that normal human cells divide a limited number of times prior to permanently adopting a durable growth-arrested state without triggering apoptosis (Li et al., 2023; Myrianthopoulos et al., 2019). In aging and cancer, senescence, once considered solely a protective barrier against tumor development, is now recognized to play a more complex role. In cancer therapy, cellular senescence functions as a double-edged sword. On the one side, it halts the precancerous or damaged cells from proliferating, thereby preventing malignant

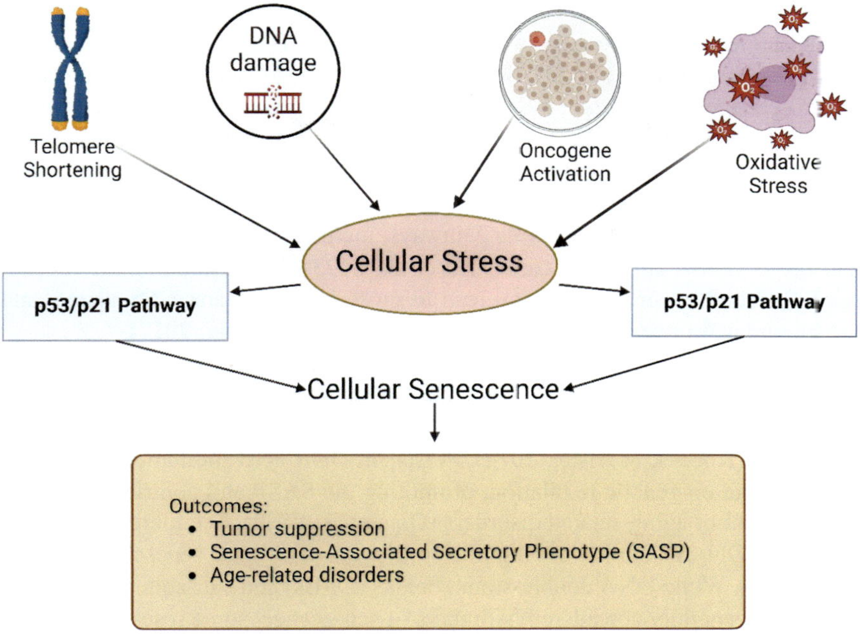

Figure 4.1 Pathways and triggers of cellular senescence.

Source: Lucas et al. (2023).

transformation. Conversely, the SASP, which is a collection of pro-inflammatory cytokines, growth factors, and proteases secreted by senescent cells, can promote tumorigenesis (Malayaperumal et al., 2023; Sánchez-Díaz et al., 2022) (Figure 4.1).

The accumulation of senescent cells in tissues with advancing age may contribute to the progression of age-related disorders (Provinciali et al., 2013) The balance between apoptosis and senescence is crucial in both cancer and the aging process, with carcinogenesis associated with a reduced ability to trigger these responses, while aging tissues show increased senescent cell accumulation. Recent discoveries suggest that pro-senescence strategies may have applications in cancer prevention therapy (Cerella et al., 2016). Understanding the mechanisms governing apoptosis and cellular senescence is essential for developing effective anticancer and anti-aging strategies (Cerella et al., 2016; Provinciali et al., 2013).

4.2.2 Mechanisms of Cellular Senescence

Cellular senescence is characterized by a permanent cessation of cell division induced by a range of stressors such as telomere attrition and physiological stress signals (Gire, 2005; Kumari & Jat, 2021). The regulation of senescence is predominantly governed by the p53/p21 and p16INK4a/pRB signaling pathways, and sustained overexpression of these elements can trigger the onset of senescence (Zarneshan et al., 2023). Senescent cells undergo functional and morphological changes, developing a SASP that can impact tissue function (Kumari & Jat, 2021; Regulski, 2017). Aging and age-related disorders may be exacerbated by the accumulation of senescent cells, even though senescence acts as a tumor-suppressive mechanism (Gire, 2005; Regulski, 2017). The process involves complex interactions between multiple pathways, including cyclin-dependent kinases and the DREAM complex (Zarneshan et al., 2023). Understanding the mechanisms of cellular senescence may lead to more effective cancer treatments and interventions for age-related conditions (Gire, 2005; Regulski, 2017).

Cellular senescence is also closely linked to DNA damage response (DDR) and genomic instability (Lee & Ong, 2021; Qian et al., 2023). The DDR pathway, with p53 as a key protein, may contribute to senescence, repair of DNA, or death of the cell (Korwek & Alster, 2014). Persistent DDR activation alters chromatin structure and epigenetic regulation, promoting the SASP and contributing to the development of aging-related disorders (Qian et al., 2023). Telomere erosion and ribosomal DNA instability are significant triggers of cellular senescence (Lee & Ong, 2021). While DNA double-strand breaks (DSBs) and subsequent DDR activation are generally considered hallmarks of senescence, some research suggests that senescence can occur without DDR or damage to DNA (Bielak-Zmijewska et al., 2018).

Another mechanism associated with cellular senescence is significant metabolic and epigenetic changes. Senescent cells exhibit altered mitochondrial function, perturbed growth signaling pathways, and high metabolic rates despite their non-dividing state (Nacarelli & Sell, 2017). These metabolic alterations may be crucial for inducing and maintaining senescence (Nakao et al., 2020). Senescent cells also undergo chromatin rearrangement and autophagy modulation while producing a SASP that influences various normal and disease-associated processes (Herranz & Gil, 2018). The relationship between senescence and metabolism is bidirectional, with metabolic states influencing senescence and SASP, which in turn can drive metabolic dysfunction (Wiley & Campisi, 2021). Interventions targeting metabolism or senescent cells, such as rapamycin treatment and methionine restriction, may break this degenerative feedback cycle and potentially mitigate the age-promoting effects of cellular senescence (Nacarelli & Sell, 2017; Wiley & Campisi, 2021).

4.2.3 The Dual Role of Cellular Senescence in Cancer: A Tumor-Suppressive Barrier and Tumor-Promoting Factor

Cellular senescence exhibits paradoxical functions in the development and management of cancer. Initially recognized as a tumor suppressor mechanism by suppressing the activity of the cell cycle (Schosserer et al., 2017; Yang et al., 2021),

Table 4.1 Roles of Cellular Senescence in Physiological and Pathological Processes

Process	*Description*	*Key Molecules/Pathways Involved*
1. Wound healing	Cellular senescence promotes wound closure by differentiation of fibroblasts into myofibroblasts.	PDGF-AA, myofibroblasts
2. Fetus development	Cellular senescence plays a role in fetal development.	Wnt, TGF-β
3. Tumor cell proliferation and migration	Senescent cells can secrete factors like MMP, IL-1β, and VEGF, influencing tumor growth and migration.	MMP, IL-1β, VEGF, oncogene-induced senescence (OIS)
4. Immunosuppressive signaling	Senescent cancer cells suppress the activity of key immune cells like T-cells, NK cells, macrophages, and plasma cells.	PGE2, immunosuppressive signaling

Source: Lucas et al. (2023).

senescence can also promote cancer progression through SASP (Prieto & Baker, 2019; Yasuda et al., 2023). SASP contributes to growth of tumors, resistance to therapy, and metastasis by creating an immunosuppressive microenvironment (Yang et al., 2021; Yasuda et al., 2023). Inducing senescence in tumor cells for cancer treatment can improve outcomes, but unintended senescence in healthy cells may trigger inflammation and cancer relapse. The progressive accrual of senescent cells in aged tissues further complicates the dual role, as it can fuel the progression of aging-linked cancers (Schosserer et al., 2017). Comprehending the complex dynamics is essential for formulating effective cancer treatments that target harmful senescent cells while preserving beneficial aspects of senescence (Yasuda et al., 2023) (Table 4.1).

Senescence acts as a tumor-suppressive barrier through pathways such as oncogene-induced senescence (OIS), where oncogenic signaling from mutations in RAS or MYC drives cells into senescence to prevent tumorigenesis (Zhang et al., 2023). This is particularly relevant in early-stage cancers, where senescence functions as a crucial fail-safe mechanism. Senescent cell accumulation in tissues, however, may eventually promote the progression of tumors. The SASP factors secreted by senescent cells, including IL-6, IL-1β, and TNF-α, contribute to an inflammatory environment that facilitates tumor growth and immune evasion (Schmitt et al., 2022).

The TME is closely linked to the pro-tumorigenic effects of senescent cells. In the TME, senescent cells, particularly those induced by chemotherapy or radiotherapy, can alter the extracellular matrix, promote angiogenesis, and create an immunosuppressive niche (Balducci et al., 2024). These modifications encourage treatment resistance in addition to promoting the survival of malignant cells, leading to cancer recurrence (Zhang et al., 2023).

4.2.4 Impact of the SASP on the TME

As discussed, the SASP exhibits dual roles, exerting both tumor-promoting and tumor-suppressive effects, which underscores its intricate influence within the TME. One important characteristic of senescent cells is the SASP, which is defined by the production of several substances, such as growth factors, chemokines, and cytokines (Cuollo et al., 2020; Takasugi et al., 2022). SASP can remodel surrounding tissues, modulate adjacent cells like stromal and immune cells, and influence immune responses. Persistent senescent cells in the TME can contribute to cancer progression, metastasis, and resistance to treatment, even if senescence serves as a barrier to tumor progression (D'Ambrosio & Gil, 2023; Takasugi et al., 2022).

The SASP's composition is regulated by various molecular mechanisms and can be modulated through genetic or pharmacological interventions. Their regulation occurs at multiple levels, involving chromatin remodeling, transcription factors like NF-κB, and mRNA translation (Lopes-Paciencia et al., 2019; Takasugi et al., 2022). Recent therapeutic strategies aim to eliminate senescent cells using senolytics or suppress the SASP composition using senomorphics to combat cancer and age-related diseases. Understanding the context-dependent nature of SASP and its effects on tumorigenesis opens new avenues for cancer therapy, including the potential use of senotherapy to target the SASP and senescent cells (Cuollo et al., 2020; Takasugi et al., 2022).

4.2.5 Therapy-Induced Senescence and Cancer Recurrence

Therapy-induced senescence (TIS) is a major problem in cancer treatment, as conventional treatments such as radiation and chemotherapy cause senescence in both malignant and healthy cells. While this may initially halt tumor growth, the persistent presence of therapy-induced senescent cells can contribute to cancer relapse and metastasis over time (Zhang et al., 2023). Through their SASP, these senescent cells provide a pro-tumorigenic microenvironment that promotes the survival of cancer cells that remain and eventually aids in their revival (Bousset & Gil, 2022).

Recent studies suggest that combining senolytic drugs with traditional chemotherapy may enhance cancer treatment efficacy by clearing both proliferative and senescent tumor cells. For example, senolytics and chemotherapy have been demonstrated to significantly enhance patient outcomes in preclinical models by preventing relapse (Balducci et al., 2024). This combinatorial approach holds promise as a future treatment paradigm, particularly for cancers that are prone to recurrence after initial treatment.

4.3 TYPES OF SENOTHERAPEUTICS

Senotherapeutics, developed to target and manage senescent cells, are typically distinguished into two primary types: senolytics, designed to specifically eliminate senescent cells; and senomorphics, which regulate the effects of senescent cells without inducing cell death. Each type holds promise in the therapeutic context of cancer, aging, and other degenerative diseases, with distinct mechanisms and roles that contribute to improved treatment outcomes.

4.3.1 Senolytics

Senolytics constitute a class of agents developed to selectively target and remove senescent cells from tissues. Senescent cells resist apoptosis—a natural, energy-dependent process of programmed cell death—by upregulating apoptosis-suppressing pathways. The SASP is a collection of inflammatory and matrix-degrading factors secreted by senescent cells which paradoxically facilitate their survival and persistence, which negatively impact neighboring cells and tissue health. Senolytics temporarily inhibit these anti-apoptotic pathways, triggering apoptosis in senescent cells with tissue-destructive SASP characteristics (Kirkland & Tchkonia, 2017). Based on the mechanism of action, senolytics can be generally divided into three primary types: (1) BCL family inhibitors, (2) PI3K/AKT/mTOR pathway inhibitors, and (3) FOXO regulators.

4.3.1.1 BCL Family Inhibitors

BCL-2 (B-cell lymphoma 2) is a family of proteins that includes essential regulators of apoptosis with both pro-apoptotic and anti-apoptotic members. In healthy cells, these proteins maintain a careful equilibrium to regulate cell survival and death. However, in senescent cells, the overexpression of anti-apoptotic proteins from the BCL-2 family allows cells to evade apoptosis, potentially leading to tumorigenesis and malignant transformation (Qian et al., 2023).

1. *Navitoclax (ABT-263 or ABT-737)*: Navitoclax is a bioavailable, orally administered agent known for its inhibitory action on the BCL-2 family protein. Originally derived from ABT-737 (also known as ABT-263), navitoclax binds and inhibits key anti-apoptotic proteins, including anti-apoptotic members of the BCL-2 family including BCL-W, BCL-2, BCL-XL (B-cell lymphoma–extra-large), thereby facilitating the selective clearance of senescent cells via programmed cell death. Preclinical studies show that navitoclax effectively reduces tumor progression and fibrosis, either as a monotherapy or combined with other therapeutic agents (Mohamad Anuar et al., 2020; Yamamoto et al., 2021). However, navitoclax's side effects, such as thrombocytopenia due to platelet BCL-XL dependence, remain a challenge and are being addressed through structural optimization and analog development.

2. *Other BCL inhibitors*: ABT-737, a precursor to navitoclax, was also developed as a potent BCL-2 inhibitor and showed significant senolytic activity, but it had limitations in oral bioavailability and solubility. The subsequent development of navitoclax addressed these limitations, improving clinical applicability (Zhang et al., 2021). Newer analogs like A-1331852 and A-1155463 further refine these therapeutic effects. A-1331852, a selective BCL-XL inhibitor, has been effective in inducing apoptosis in senescent cells with reduced toxicity to healthy cells, suggesting promising potential for clinical applications (Wang et al., 2020b). Additionally, panobinostat, a histone deacetylase inhibitor, shows senolytic effects by disrupting multiple cancer pathways and reversing epigenetic changes, offering a unique approach to target senescent cells in conditions like head and neck squamous cell carcinoma (HNSCC) and non-small cell lung cancer (NSCLC) (Wang et al., 2020a; Huang et al., 2019).

4.3.1.2 mTOR Pathway Inhibitors

mTOR pathway inhibitors are also referred to as a AKT/PI3K signaling pathway. The AKT/PI3K/mTOR signaling pathway serves a pivotal role by regulating various cellular activities including autophagy, senescence, and apoptosis (Fan et al., 2024). This pathway is often hyperactivated in cancer, contributing to tumor progression and resistance to conventional cancer therapies. Through suppression of mTOR signaling, senolytics can overcome the resistance, suppress cellular proliferation, and trigger programmed cell death in senescent cells, presenting it as an effective target for cancer treatment (Yang et al., 2019).

Dasatinib and quercetin (D + Q): This combination of drugs is widely used as a senolytic treatment. Dasatinib is a tyrosine kinase inhibitor used in leukemia treatment, which targets SRC/ABL1 kinases and the BCR-ABL1 fusion protein, the primary oncogene in chronic myeloid leukemia. Quercetin is a naturally occurring polyphenolic flavonoid commonly occurring in a wide range of vegetables and fruits with known bioactive properties. Together, dasatinib and quercetin act synergistically as senolytics, each contributing a distinct mechanism: dasatinib disrupts ephrin-mediated apoptosis suppression and inhibits tyrosine kinases, while quercetin inhibits several key survival pathways, including PI3K/AKT, BCL2/BCL2L1, and TP53/P21 pathways. The D + Q combination reduces the SASP, alleviates inflammation, and promotes apoptosis in senescent cells, particularly in various preclinical cancer models (Meiners et al., 2024).

4.3.1.3 FOXO4-DRI Peptides (FOXO4-D-Retro-Inverso)

The relationship between the transcription factor FOXO4 and TP53 (p53) serves as a vital role in maintaining senescence. The interaction between the transcription

Table 4.2 Mechanisms of Action for Key Senotherapeutics in Cancer Therapy

Category	*Senotherapeutic Agent*	*Mechanism of Action*	*Target Pathways*
Senolytics	Navitoclax (ABT-263)	Inhibits BCL-2 family proteins, inducing senescent cells to undergo programmed cell death	BCL-W, BCL-2, BCL-XL
	Dasatinib + quercetin	Dasatinib inhibits SRC/ABL1 kinases; quercetin blocks PI3K/AKT pathways, inducing apoptosis in senescent cells	SRC, ABL1, PI3K/AKT
	FOXO4-DRI	Disrupts FOXO4-p53 interaction, causing apoptosis in senescent cells	FOXO4, p53
Senomorphics	Rapamycin	Suppresses mTOR pathway, reducing SASP expression and SASP-driven inflammation	mTOR, SASP
	Metformin	Inhibits NF-κB signaling, modulating inflammatory cytokines to reduce SASP effects	NF-κB, SASP
	Ruxolitinib	Blocks JAK/STAT signaling, lowering pro-inflammatory SASP factors	JAK/STAT

Sources: Baker et al. (2021); Xu et al. (2018); Zarneshan et al. (2023).

factor FOXO4 and TP53 (p53) is crucial for maintaining senescence. Disrupting this interaction can trigger programmed cell death specifically in senescent cells. FOXO4-DRI is a synthetic peptide developed to interfere with the interaction between FOXO4 and p53, causing senescent cells to undergo apoptosis without affecting non-senescent cells.

Mechanism of action: FOXO4-DRI was engineered to imitate the TP53-binding region of FOXO4, which allows it to bind with TP53, displacing FOXO4 and triggering TP53-mediated apoptosis in senescent cells. FOXO4 is typically expressed in limited amounts in adult non-senescent cells, making it an ideal target for systemic senolytic therapy. Preclinical studies indicate that FOXO4-DRI reduces the number of senescent cells and improves health markers without significant toxicity, positioning it as a promising therapeutic for cancer as well as aging-related illness (Le et al., 2021) (Table 4.2).

4.3.1.3.1 Targeting TIS with Senolytics

Senescent cells that result from the accumulation of cancer therapies, known as TIS cells, pose a unique risk. The presence of TIS cells after treatments like chemotherapy or radiotherapy contributes to tumor relapse and disease progression. Senolytics can be utilized post-therapy to eliminate TIS cells, potentially reducing these adverse effects.

1. *Chromatin and gene expression vulnerabilities in senescent cells*: In senescent cells, alterations in chromatin structure lead to distinct gene expression patterns, including upregulated anti-apoptotic proteins. This vulnerability allows for the selective targeting of senescent cells using senolytics like navitoclax and ABT-737. Studies have shown that targeting BCL-2 family proteins with these agents effectively eliminates senescent cells, reducing the potential for tumor progression and resistance (Wang et al., 2022).
2. *Immune system-mediated senolysis*: The immunological response is influenced by the SASP through two distinct mechanisms. While some SASP factors promote inflammation, others can hinder the immune-mediated clearance of senescent cells. Research highlights that SASP components can stimulate immune responses that promote senescent cell clearance, thereby contributing to tissue homeostasis (Wang et al., 2022). For example, glutaminase 1 (GLS1) overexpression in senescent cells is critical for their survival. By increasing glutaminolysis, GLS1 neutralizes intracellular acidosis and protects against protein misfolding. Inhibition of GLS1, particularly using the GLS1 inhibitor BPTES, induces apoptosis and significantly reduces cancer cell viability, offering a senolytic approach via metabolic disruption (Imawari & Nakanishi, 2024).
3. *uPAR-specific CAR T cells in targeted senolysis*: Chimeric antigen receptor (CAR) T-cell therapies specifically target the urokinase-type plasminogen activator receptor (uPAR), which is upregulated on the surfaces of senescent cells. In both mouse models and in vitro studies, uPAR-targeted CAR T cells have demonstrated efficacy in eliminating senescent cells, particularly in lung cancer driven by MEK and CDK4/6 inhibitors. This approach demonstrates a dual benefit by enabling cancer treatment while clearing senescent cells, potentially preventing tumor relapse and improving immune responses (Imawari & Nakanishi, 2024).

4.3.2 Senomorphics

Senomorphics are small molecules designed to modulating the SASP, thereby inhibiting the detrimental effects of senescent cells. Unlike senolytics, which induce apoptosis in senescent cells, senomorphics work by selectively suppressing SASP factors, thereby slowing the progression of cellular senescence without triggering cell death (Lagoumtzi & Chondrogianni, 2021). This class of pharmacological agents, also referred to as gerosuppressors or senostatics, helps restore senescent cells to a less inflammatory state by targeting key signaling pathways and SASP components. Through these mechanisms, senomorphics reduce inflammation and tumor-promoting effects associated with senescence while preserving the beneficial roles senescent cells play in tumor suppression (Nehlin, 2023; Park & Shin, 2022).

Senomorphics encompass a range of therapeutic agents, including inhibitors of JAK/STAT pathway inhibitors, NF-κB and p38 MAPK, and ATM inhibitors. Some compounds, like rapamycin, function as senomorphics by suppressing the SASP, while others, such as fisetin, exhibit senomorphic effects in certain cell types but act as senolytics in others (Niedernhofer & Robbins, 2018). Key senomorphic agents and their respective pathways are detailed in the following sections.

4.3.2.1 NF-κB Pathway Inhibitors

The initiation and progression of cancer are primarily regulated by the nuclear factor kappa-light-chain-enhancer of activated B cells pathway (NF-κB pathway) (Hoesel & Schmid, 2013). NF-κB is a crucial component of signal transduction pathways that regulate inflammatory responses, immune activation, and cellular survival. NF-κB activation has been closely linked to malignant cell properties, influencing SASP factors that promote proliferation, apoptosis resistance, invasion, and metastasis in tumor cells.

Mechanism of NF-κB pathway activation: Activation of the NF-κB pathway is mediated through two main pathways: the canonical pathway, which involves the IκB kinase (IKK) complex; and the non-canonical pathway. The overactivation of these pathways leads to therapy resistance in various cancers, including resistance to chemotherapy, endocrine therapy, and immunotherapy.

Targeting NF-κB in cancer: A primary therapeutic approach for NF-κB inhibition involves blocking IKK activation, which prevents NF-κB from translocating to the cell's nucleus and initiating the transcription of SASP-associated genes. Metformin, for instance, inhibits IκB and IKKα/β phosphorylation, effectively preventing NF-κB nuclear translocation and SASP expression. Proteasome inhibitors have also been explored to prevent IκB degradation, stabilizing this inhibitory protein and blocking NF-κB activation (Li et al., 2024; Zhang et al., 2023). By targeting NF-κB signaling, these inhibitors enhance cancer cell sensitivity to treatments and potentially reduce therapy resistance, making them promising senomorphics in cancer therapy (Park & Shin, 2022).

4.3.2.2 p38 MAPK Pathway Inhibitors

Cellular stress, such as oncogenic, radiotherapy, and chemotherapy-induced stress activates the p38 mitogen-activated protein kinase (p38 MAPK) pathway. In the

TME, p38 MAPK promotes SASP-driven cytokine production, which fosters tumor development, invasiveness, and metastasis. One strategy to modify the pro-tumorigenic microenvironment and enhance cancer therapy efficacy is the targeted inhibition of p38 MAPK signaling.

p38 MAPK inhibition and cancer: By inhibiting p38 MAPK, senomorphics decrease the production of pro-survival, pro-angiogenic, and pro-inflammatory factors, creating a less favorable environment for tumor cell persistence. Ralimetinib (LY2228820 dimesylate) selectively targets and inhibits the isoforms α and β, and has shown promise in reducing SASP factors in the TME, thereby reducing cancer progression. Through modulation of this pathway, p38 MAPK inhibitors enhance the response to conventional therapies and improve prognosis for cancer patients (Patnaik et al., 2016).

4.3.2.3 STAT Pathway Inhibitors

The signal transducer and activator of transcription (STAT) pathway, also known as the Janus kinase (JAK) pathway, is implicated in numerous cancers. Hyperactivation of STAT or JAK signaling results in persistent inflammation, heightened SASP expression, and tumor-promoting effects, which are linked to unfavorable outcomes and increased tumor recurrence rates. This pathway is overactivated in several malignancies, including hematologic cancers in addition to non-hematologic cancers affecting organs including the lung, liver, and breast (Qureshy et al., 2020).

Targeting JAK/STAT in senescence: Due to the challenge of directly targeting STATs, JAK inhibitors are often employed to suppress JAK/STAT signaling. Ruxolitinib, a JAK1 and JAK2 inhibitor, blocks the ATP-binding sites of these kinases, thereby inhibiting cytokine and growth factor signaling associated with SASP production. Pro-inflammatory cytokines and chemokines are significantly reduced as a result of this inhibition, enhancing the sensitivity of cancer cells to therapy as well as reducing inflammatory responses in conditions such as myelofibrosis (Haq & Adnan, 2025).

4.3.2.4 ATM Pathway Inhibitors

The protein known as ataxia-telangiectasia mutated (ATM) is essential for repairing DSBs and regulation of cellular checkpoints, which are triggered in reaction to damage to DNA. ATM inhibitors target this repair pathway, rendering cancer cells more sensitive to DNA-damaging treatments and senescence-inducing therapies.

Role of ATM in senescence and cancer: ATM inhibition not only disrupts DNA repair but also improves mitochondrial function, promotes autophagy, and enhances metabolic reprogramming in senescent cells (Zhang et al., 2023). ATM inhibitors like KU-55933 and KU-60019 have demonstrated potential as senomorphics, particularly in combination with radiotherapy. KU-60019, for instance, selectively inhibits ATM kinase, enhancing the sensitivity of glioma cells to radiation by suppressing the DDR. These agents can also stabilize lysosomal and mitochondrial functions in senescent cells, preventing further tumor progression while mitigating SASP-driven inflammation (Biddlestone-Thorpe et al., 2013; Li & Yang, 2010; Sánchez-Díaz et al., 2022).

4.3.2.5 Additional Insights on Senomorphics in Cancer Therapy

Senomorphics offer a unique therapeutic strategy by suppressing SASP factors rather than eliminating senescent cells, thus preserving the potential antitumor functions of senescent cells in early-stage cancers. SASP inhibition has been shown to modulate immune responses and improve the oncogenic niche, potentially increasing the efficacy of complementary cancer therapies. For example, by reducing SASP-driven immune suppression, senomorphics may create a favorable environment for immunotherapies, including checkpoint inhibitors, to perform more effectively. Compounds like rapamycin, metformin, and ralimetinib highlight the versatility of senomorphics in targeting diverse pathways, making them a critical component of emerging cancer therapies.

4.4 TARGETING SENESCENT CELLS IN CANCER THERAPY USING SENOTHERAPEUTICS

Senotherapeutics represent an emerging category of therapeutic agents designed to manage senescence in cancer. This class includes two main types: senolytics, which selectively target and eradicate senescent cells; and senostatics (or senomorphics), which suppress the SASP, thereby preventing the harmful pro-inflammatory environment that these cells promote (Sánchez-Díaz et al., 2022). In the context of cancer, cellular senescence involves an irreversible cell cycle arrest accompanied by a multifaceted phenotype that includes metabolic shifts, chromatin reorganization, altered gene expression, and autophagy activation. This dual-nature response can initially suppress tumor formation but, over time, may promote tumor progression due to the persistent accumulation of SASP-expressing senescent cells (Zhang et al., 2023).

Integrating senotherapeutics into cancer treatment holds great promise for improving therapeutic efficacy and patient outcomes. Through targeted elimination, SASP inhibition, and immune enhancement, senotherapy offers innovative approaches to address the pro-tumorigenic effects of senescence in cancer (Mishra et al., 2023).

4.4.1 Approaches to Targeting Senescent Cells

Senotherapy in cancer treatment employs three primary strategies:

1. Targeted ablation of senescent cells using senolytics
2. SASP neutralization strategy (anti-SASP approach)
3. Enhancement of immune-mediated senescent cell clearance.

These strategies seek to mitigate the detrimental consequences of accumulated senescent cells, which can compromise cancer treatment efficacy and contribute to tumor recurrence.

4.4.1.1 Senolytic Agents for Selective Senescent Cell Elimination

Senolytics are agents that selectively disrupt anti-apoptotic pathways upregulated in senescent cells, inducing apoptosis specifically within this population. However, many senolytics exhibit limited selectivity, which can cause unintended damage to non-senescent cells. To improve targeting, recent advancements have introduced nanocapsule-based senolytics. These nanocapsules contain toxins or senolytic compounds within an enzyme-sensitive outer layer, which is activated by enzymes overexpressed in senescent cells. This strategy enables the release of senolytics exclusively within senescent cells, offering a higher degree of specificity and reducing off-target effects.

Natural compounds like quercetin and fisetin show senolytic activity but lack clear biological specificity, making them ideal candidates for nanocapsule delivery. Through this approach, senolytics target vital proteins associated with apoptosis, comprising BCL-2, BCL-XL, PI3K, AKT, and FOXO4, ensuring the selective elimination of SASP-expressing cells without extensive collateral damage (von Kobbe, 2019).

4.4.1.2 Anti-SASP Therapies to Neutralize SASP Effects

The SASP, also referred to as the senescence-messaging secretome (SMS), is a persistent pro-inflammatory program distinguished by the release of growth factors, chemokines, proteases, and cytokines. SASP significantly contributes to the adverse impact of senescence by creating an environment that encourages both inflammation and pro-tumorigenic progression (Cuollo et al., 2020). Multiple strategies have been explored to mitigate the effects of the SASP, including maintaining mitochondrial integrity, targeting autophagy, and modulating glucose metabolism.

Rapamycin, an mTOR inhibitor, suppresses IL-1α synthesis, thereby reducing IL-6 secretion from senescent cells and preventing tumor-promoting inflammation associated with SASP. Similarly, simvastatin inhibits CDC42, resulting in a reduction of IL-6 secretion and potentially enhancing the therapeutic response in breast cancer by counteracting SASP-driven resistance to chemoradiation. Targeting mitochondrial function and autophagy pathways offers an additional anti-SASP approach, with promising effects in preventing cancer progression associated with senescent cells (Wang et al., 2017).

4.4.1.3 Enhancing Immune Clearance of Senescent Cells

Elimination of senescent cells is a key immunological process essential for the effective regulation of cellular senescence. Immune cells, such as CD8+ T lymphocytes, natural killer (NK) cells, and macrophages, effectively eliminate senescent cells in young people, maintaining tissue homeostasis. The immune system's capacity to clear senescent cells declines with age due to reduced immune cell efficiency, leading to their accumulation and contributing to cancer development and other age-related illness (Reynolds et al., 2024).

Role of SASP in immune-mediated clearance: Senescent cells produce SASP factors that recruit immune cells to clear senescent cells from tissues For example, reactivation of p53 in hepatic tumors induces senescence, which is followed by the release of chemokines like CCL2, which selectively recruit immune cells like NK cells and macrophages. Since p53-induced SASP factors are essential for immune surveillance, their recruitment helps eliminate senescent cancer cells.

Additionally, the epigenetic regulator BRD4 modulates SASP gene enhancers and super-enhancers, which are essential for the immune-mediated clearance of senescent cells. BRD4 inhibition reduces SASP activity and impairs immune clearance, indicating that BRD4's regulation of SASP can be a valuable target for enhancing senotherapy in cancer (Kale et al., 2020).

4.4.2 Combination Therapies: Senotherapy with Chemotherapy and Radiotherapy

Combination therapies incorporating senotherapeutics with conventional cancer treatments can significantly enhance therapeutic outcomes. These regimens are designed to employ agents that not only combat cancer cells directly but also target the surrounding senescent environment to reduce recurrence and improve patient tolerance (Makin, 2018).

Synergistic chemotherapy-senotherapy combinations: TIS occurs when cancer treatments like chemotherapy or radiotherapy induce senescence in cancer cells, which can lead to tumor relapse. Senolytics, such as ABT263 or cardiac glycosides, have been employed both genetically and pharmacologically to eliminate TIS cells and have been effective in preventing tumor regrowth across several cancer models. Additionally, co-treatment with X AZD8055, an mTOR pathway blocker and XL413, a CDC7 inhibitor L413, has shown potent growth suppression in liver cancer, highlighting the potential of senolytic-based combination therapies to reduce tumor progression (Prasanna et al., 2021).

Metformin in radiotherapy enhancement: Metformin has demonstrated potential in enhancing radiotherapy efficacy. Studies indicate that metformin administration alongside radiation reduces relapse rates in prostate, esophageal, and rectal cancers. In mouse models, metformin enhances the sensitivity of NSCLC cells to radiation by increasing DNA damage signaling, arresting growth, and inhibiting mTOR signaling, which cumulatively promote apoptosis in cancer cells. In prostate cancer xenografts, metformin improves tumor oxygenation and enhances the efficacy of radiation, showcasing the promise of this synergistic approach in clinical oncology (Short et al., 2019).

4.4.3 Cellular Plasticity and Senescence Reversal

Emerging evidence suggests that senescent cells may regain proliferative capacity under specific conditions, a phenomenon known as cellular plasticity. Senescent cell's potential to re-enter the cell cycle and proliferate with potentially more aggressive characteristics poses a risk in cancer treatment. Recent findings underscore the importance of continuous senotherapeutic interventions to manage cellular plasticity and prevent senescent cells from contributing to tumor recurrence and metastasis.

Addressing cellular plasticity: Developing effective treatments requires an understanding of the mechanisms behind this plasticity. To illustrate, SASP-modulating agents can potentially reduce the likelihood of cellular reprogramming by lowering inflammatory and pro-survival signaling within the TME. Continued research on senescence reversal mechanisms offers the potential to develop strategies to prevent senescent cell reactivation and improve cancer therapy outcomes (Sánchez-Díaz et al., 2022).

4.5 APPLICATIONS OF TARGETING CELLULAR SENESCENCE

In cancer and other diseases, cellular senescence has a dual function: it stops damaged cells from proliferating, but senescent cells also release substances that might support tumor growth and contribute to age-related disorders. Senolytics, which destroy senescent cells, and senomorphics, which modulate the harmful SASP without killing the cells, are two examples of senotherapy techniques. This

Table 4.3 Preclinical Applications of Senotherapeutics in Cancer Therapy

Application Area	*Senotherapeutic Approach*	*Examples*	*Preclinical Outcome*
Enhancing chemotherapy	Senolytics combined with chemotherapy	ABT-263 (navitoclax)	Reduced tumor size, increased survival rates when combined with chemotherapy (e.g. in mouse models)
Modulating immune responses	Senolytics to improve immunotherapy efficacy	Dasatinib + quercetin	Enhanced T-cell activation, reducing tumor-supportive SASP in the tumor microenvironment (Xu et al., 2018)
Normalizing tumor microenvironment	Senomorphics to reduce SASP-related inflammation	Rapamycin, metformin	Suppression of SASP-induced inflammation, potentially improving tumor responses to standard treatments
Preventing cancer recurrence	Maintenance therapy with senolytics	ABT-263 (post-surgical treatment)	Lower tumor regrowth rates in preclinical models, highlighting preventive potential (Xu et al., 2018)

Sources: Xu et al. (2018); Prasanna et al. (2021); Zhang et al. (2023).

section delves into the applications of senotherapy across oncology and age-related disease contexts, highlighting the current progress and therapeutic potential of senolytics and senomorphics.

4.5.1 Applications of Senotherapeutics in Cancer

Cellular senescence significantly impacts cancer treatment. On one hand, the induction of senescence can hinder tumor proliferation, acting as a barrier against cancer progression; on the other hand, TIS can contribute to tumor recurrence due to the SASP. Senotherapy holds promise in addressing these complex roles of senescence within cancer therapy (Table 4.3).

4.5.1.1 Senolytics in Enhancing Conventional Cancer Therapies

By precisely identifying and eliminating senescent cells that arise from conventional cancer therapies such as radiation and chemotherapy, senolytic agents aim to enhance the overall efficacy of these treatments. Tumor growth may be aided by senescent cells that remain in the TME and contribute to immunological suppression and inflammation. Combining senolytics with standard treatments may counteract these effects, reducing tumor recurrence and improving outcomes.

For example, ABT-263 (navitoclax), a BCL-2 family inhibitor, has demonstrated effectiveness in animal studies by reducing tumor size when used alongside chemotherapy. Navitoclax disrupts the anti-apoptotic mechanisms that enable senescent cells to persist and, when paired with chemotherapy, has shown a substantial decrease in tumor burden and an improvement in survival rates (Zhai et al., 2020). This combined strategy highlights senolytics' potential in reducing the tumor-supportive inflammation caused by TIS.

4.5.1.2 Modulating Immune Responses in Cancer with Senotherapy

Senescent cells impair the effectiveness of immunotherapies, such as immune checkpoint inhibitors, by evading immune detection and potentially creating an immunosuppressive environment. By eliminating these immunosuppressive senescent cells, senolytics may enhance anti-tumor immunity. Studies suggest that depleting senescent cells may improve T-cell infiltration and activation, creating a more favorable environment for immune responses against tumors (Xu et al., 2018).

For instance, the combinatorial approach of dasatinib and quercetin—a common senolytic pairing—has shown potential in reducing the SASP and enhancing immune function within the TME, allowing immune cells to target and eradicate residual cells of cancer more effectively. This strategy holds significant potential for patients receiving immune checkpoint inhibitors, as it could enhance the activation of immune cells against cancerous cells.

4.5.1.3 Senomorphics for SASP Modulation and TME Control

Senomorphics offer a complementary approach to senolytics by modulating the SASP rather than eliminating senescent cells. By targeting pro-inflammatory and tumor-supportive factors within the SASP, senomorphics reduce the risk of adverse immune responses and may enhance treatment outcomes by normalizing the TME. Rapamycin, for example, is an mTOR inhibitor that decreases SASP expression, helping to prevent tumor-promoting inflammation without cell death, which is particularly useful when senescent cells retain some tumor-suppressive functions.

Other agents, such as metformin, also serve a function in SASP modulation by suppressing NF-κB signaling. This approach helps counteract SASP-driven immune suppression and inflammation, especially following radiotherapy, where SASP can otherwise support tumor recurrence and resistance. Reducing inflammation via SASP modulation could lead to better treatment efficacy and mitigate some of the therapy-associated complications linked to conventional cancer approaches.

4.5.1.4 *Preventing Cancer Recurrence through Senotherapeutics*

The key challenges in the therapy of cancer is the risk of recurrence, often due to residual senescent cells that secrete factors promoting tumor regrowth. Studies have shown that using senolytics after primary cancer treatments, such as surgery or chemotherapy, could lower recurrence rates. For example, ABT-263 administered post-surgically has been demonstrated to reduce tumor regrowth in animal models (Xu et al., 2018). This suggests a role for senotherapeutics as a preventive maintenance therapy that may improve long-term outcomes for cancer patients.

4.5.2 Other Applications of Senotherapeutics beyond Cancer

Beyond oncology, senotherapeutics holds promise in addressing aging and age-related conditions where senescent cell accumulation is a prevalent clinical characteristic. These applications span age-related degenerative diseases, immune function, and metabolic health (Figure 4.2).

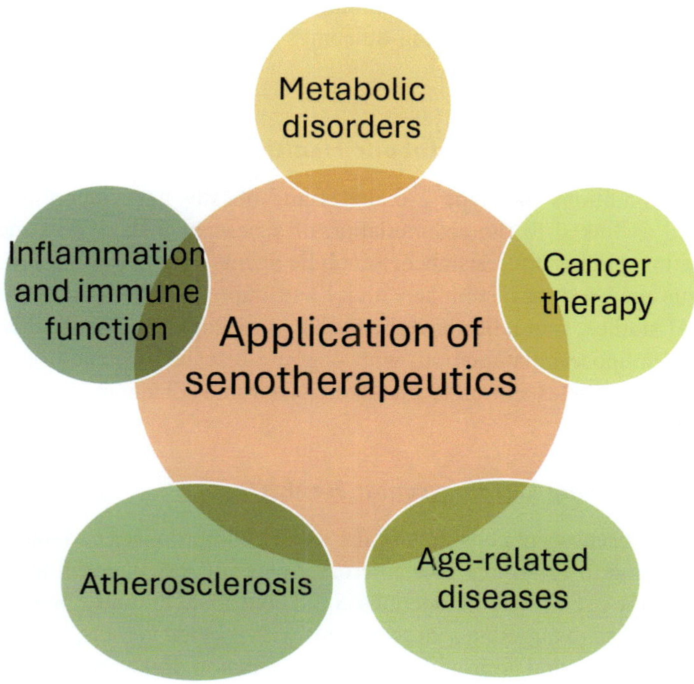

Figure 4.2 Applications of senotherapeutics.

4.5.2.1 Anti-Aging and Management of Age-Linked Diseases

Aging and age-associated diseases are intrinsically connected to cellular senescence. In preclinical studies, the elimination of senescent cells has been shown to hinder the progression of aging phenotypes along with extending health span. Baker et al. (2016) elucidated that removing senescent cells in murine models led to enhanced muscle function and reduced frailty. Clinical trials are now exploring senolytics like dasatinib and quercetin in age-related conditions, including osteoarthritis and chronic kidney disease, aiming to enhancing the well-being and life quality of aging populations.

4.5.2.2 Mitigating Chronic Inflammation and Enhancing Immune Function

The SASP contributes to chronic inflammation, exacerbating conditions like atherosclerosis, rheumatoid arthritis, and age-related tissue degeneration. By targeting senescent cells, senotherapy can reduce chronic inflammation, potentially leading to improved tissue function and immune health. Senolytic therapies in animal models have been shown to decrease inflammatory markers and enhance tissue repair, underscoring their therapeutic potential (Wang et al., 2021). Moreover, by clearing senescent cells, senotherapy may enhance immune responsiveness in older adults, improving outcomes like vaccine efficacy and general immunity.

4.5.2.3 Applications in Metabolic Health

Metabolic conditions like type 2 diabetes and obesity have increasingly been recognized as linked to the accumulation of senescent cells, where they drive inflammation and insulin resistance. Senolytic agents targeting these cells in adipose tissue may restore insulin sensitivity and improve metabolic outcomes. In preclinical studies, senolytics have been shown to improve glucose metabolism and reduce adipose inflammation, with ongoing research focusing on potential treatments for diabetes as well as metabolic syndrome (Zhang et al., 2021).

4.5.2.4 Improving Cardiovascular Health

The accrual of senescent cells in vascular tissues compromises endothelial activity, contributing to conditions like atherosclerosis and vascular stiffness. Studies recommend the use of senotherapeutics could contribute to improving cardiovascular health through targeting senescent cells within blood vessels, thereby reducing arterial stiffness and improving endothelial function. Baker et al. (2016) found that senolytics reduced markers of vascular aging in animal models, pointing to promising applications for senotherapy in managing cardiovascular diseases in humans.

4.6 CURRENT CHALLENGES IN TARGETING CELLULAR SENESCENCE

4.6.1 Complexity of Senescence Mechanisms

Understanding the complex mechanisms that drive cellular senescence presents a significant challenge. Key signaling pathways, including p16INK4a and p53, are crucial for the onset and with maintenance of senescence, yet their interactions with surrounding cellular and tissue environments remain incompletely understood. Detailed insights into these mechanisms are essential for developing senotherapeutics that selectively target or modulate senescent cells without affecting healthy tissues (Childs et al., 2017a).

4.6.2 Specificity of Senolytic Agents

The specificity of senolytics remains a challenge, as existing agents often lack the precision needed to selectively target senescent cells without impacting normal, healthy cells. Given the diversity in senescent cell populations across various tissues, developing universal biomarkers is difficult. Current research is working toward refining senolytic selectivity to mitigate off-target effects and improve therapeutic outcomes (Xu et al., 2018).

4.6.3 Prolonged Therapeutic Safety and Efficacy

The prolonged safety and efficacy of senolytic and senomorphic treatments are critical concerns. While preclinical studies show promise, potential risks like impaired tissue regeneration and unintended consequences on normal cell function need thorough exploration. More extensive research is essential to ensure these treatments are viable for prolonged use in humans (Baker et al., 2016).

4.6.4 Regulatory and Ethical Considerations

Senotherapeutics in clinical practice brings regulatory and ethical challenges. Designing clinical trials that can accurately assess senotherapeutic efficacy and safety in age-related and cancer treatment settings is complex. Moreover, ethical considerations around equitable access and the implications of such therapies on healthcare disparities must be addressed to ensure fair access to senotherapeutic treatments (Kirkland & Tchkonia, 2017).

4.6.5 Public Perception and Acceptance

The use of senescence-targeting therapies to potentially extend health spans could face public skepticism. Communicating the scientific basis and potential benefits and risks associated with senotherapeutics is crucial for public acceptance.

Transparent engagement with both the medical community and the general public can foster confidence in senotherapy (Kirkland et al., 2020).

4.7 CLINICAL TRIALS

Clinical trials assess the safety and efficacy of new treatments, with senotherapeutics, like senolytics, gaining interest in cancer therapy. Recent clinical trials are summarized in Table 4.4.

4.8 FUTURE DIRECTIONS IN SENOTHERAPEUTICS

4.8.1 Biomarker Development for Precision Targeting

Developing biomarkers that can accurately distinguish between senescent and non-senescent cells is pivotal, especially given the heterogeneous nature of cellular senescence. Future research should refine biomarkers for different senescence types across tissues to improve therapeutic precision and outcomes (Li et al., 2023).

4.8.2 Optimizing Timing and Dosing

Optimal timing and dosing strategies are essential to balance therapeutic benefits with potential risks, as senescent cells may have protective roles in certain contexts, such as preventing the proliferation of pre-malignant cells. Careful consideration of timing, especially in early-stage cancers, is necessary to avoid unintended consequences (Prasanna et al., 2021; Zhang et al., 2023).

4.8.3 Advancements of Drug Delivery

Innovative drug delivery systems, including nanotechnology, offer promising pathways for enhancing the specificity and safety of senotherapeutics. These systems could enable targeted drug release directly to senescent cells, minimizing systemic effects and increasing therapeutic efficacy (Baker et al., 2021).

4.8.4 Integrating Senotherapy with Conventional Treatments

Integrating senotherapeutics with existing treatments of the cancer, including cytotoxic therapy and immune-based cancer therapy, has the potential to maximize the treatment efficacy. Senotherapeutics may reduce the buildup of TIS within the TME, allowing for improved immune function and responsiveness to treatments like immune checkpoint inhibitors (Xu et al., 2018).

Table 4.4 Recent Clinical Trials of Senotherapeutic Agents and Their Results

S.No.	*Clinical Trials Registration No.*	*Study Type*	*Senotherapeutic Agent*	*Evident Findings*	*Results*
1	NCT00445198	Interventional	Navitoclax (ABT-263)	A study involving 47 patients, including 29 diagnosed with either pulmonary carcinoid or small cell lung cancer, reported primary toxicities such as diarrhea, nausea, vomiting, and fatigue, predominantly classified as grade 1 or 2. For Bcl-2 amplification, pro-gastrin-releasing peptide was recognized as a marker.	Navitoclax is considered safe and easily tolerated, with dosage-dependent thrombocytopenia being the most frequently reported side effect.
2	NCT00481091	Interventional	Navitoclax (ABT-263)	The lymphoma study includes 17 participants, 3 of whom completed various dosage levels. A grade 3 dose-limiting toxicity (DLT) was observed in the 160 mg group, leading to an expansion of that cohort to 6 participants. Two patients with bulky SLL/CLL experienced tumor reductions after the fourth and second treatment cycles, respectively, and are continuing their treatment. ABT-263 led to a dose-dependent decrease in platelet counts, with 1 participant developing thrombocytopenia.	ABT-263 is an orally available small molecule that inhibits Bcl-2 family proteins and shows potential effectiveness against lymphoid malignancies.

(*Continued*)

Table 4.4 (Continued) Compounds Exhibiting Senotherapeutic Benefits on Skin

S.No.	*Clinical Trials Registration No.*	*Study Type*	*Senotherapeutic Agent*	*Evident Findings*	*Results*
3	NCT01440504	Observational	ABT-737	In 14/25 tumors, treatment to ABT-737 resulted in 20% to 80% of cancer cells undergoing apoptosis (median caspase-3/5 30%). ABT-737 alone exhibited much more effective treatment.	ABT-737, ATMi, chloroquine, navitoclax, ATRi, BV-6, PX-866, fisetin, and artesunate demonstrate senolytic properties, effectively promoting cell death in senescent cells while working synergistically with Bcl-2 inhibitors.
4	NCT02891278	Interventional	Sertraline	Sertraline, a selective serotonin reuptake inhibitor, was identified to inhibit CDC7.365, a kinase involved in cell cycle regulation.	Sertraline demonstrated selective cytotoxicity against senescent hepatocellular carcinoma cells, indicating potential senolytic activity.
5	NCT00650910	Interventional	Cardiac glycoside (digoxin)	Status: Recruiting	N/A
6	NCT03928210	Interventional	Cardiac glycoside (digoxin)	Nine patients exhibiting CTC clusters participated in the study. Digoxin treatment decreased cluster size in 8 patients (88.9%) and the fraction of circulating tumor cell (CTC) clusters versus single CTCs in 6 of them (66.7%). The effect was evident for both homotypic as well as heterotypic clusters. The course of therapy was well tolerated, and all patients followed the protocol with no complications.	DICCT presents the initial human evidence suggesting that digoxin can partially break down clusters of CTCs in patients with metastatic breast cancer at safe and well-tolerated dosages. Future studies are being organized to explore Na/K-ATPase inhibitors and assess patient outcomes.

7	NCT02717455	Intervention	Panobinostat	This study involved 19 subjects with evaluable dose-finding results, with thrombocytopenia and neutropenia as dose-limiting toxicities, and 34 eligible subjects with 29/34 evaluable, with DLTs reported.	For children with progressive DIPG/ DMG, the MTD for panobinostat was 10 mg/m^2 per dose, administered 3 times a week for 3 consecutive weeks. In a similar group prior to progression, the MTD was 22 mg/m^2 per dose, given 3 times a week with 1 week off. In both dosing regimens, myelosuppression was the most frequently observed toxic event.
8	NCT05893472	Interventional	Venetoclax	Ongoing study	N/A
9	NCT05893472	Interventional	ABT-263	ABT-263 showed early activity in resistant or relapsed lymphoid malignancies in a phase I clinical trial; nevertheless, toxicities linked with ABT-263, such as a decrease in circulating platelet count due to Bcl-XL inhibition, are assumed to be mechanism based.	After ADT, senescent PCa cells are destroyed with senolytic navitoclax (ABT-263) and prevent androgen-independent proliferation. PARPi causes senescence towards breast cancer cells and ovarian cancer cells, making them susceptible to senolytic drugs.
10	NCT02591095	Interventional	ABT-263	The study found no correlation between the expression of Mcl-1, Bim, or P-ERK with clinical response which also reported a 22.7% 3-month PFS and 16 total responders. The most common adverse effect that caused 8 people to stop their medication was thrombocytopenia.	While not linked to the levels of Mcl-1, Bim, or P-ERK, navitoclax monotherapy showed modest efficacy but did not result in intolerable toxicity.
11	NCT00788684	Interventional	ABT-263	Ongoing study	N/A

4.8.5 Expanding Clinical Trials and Research

Extensive clinical trials across various cancer types and age demographics are crucial to realizing the full potential of senotherapeutics. Rigorous testing will help validate the safety and efficacy of these therapies, particularly for diverse populations (Bousset & Gil, 2022).

4.9 CONCLUSION

Senotherapeutics represents a groundbreaking approach in cancer therapy by targeting the complex contributions of cellular senescence to tumor advancement and suppression. Through selective depletion in conjunction with modulation of senescent cells, senolytics and senomorphics show significant potential in clinical response in the treatment of cancer. However, such a dual function of cellular senescence in both preventing and promoting tumor growth adds complexity to developing safe and effective therapies. Future directions in senotherapeutics should emphasize biomarker development, drug specificity, and a deeper understanding of long-term effects. The promise of senotherapeutics lies in advancing these therapies through ongoing research, improving their safety profiles, and integrating them with existing cancer treatments. With these advancements, senotherapeutics could become a valuable tool in managing age-related diseases and enhancing cancer therapies, potentially extending health span and improving quality of life.

REFERENCES

Baker, D. J., et al. (2021). Targeting senescent cells in cancer: A therapeutic strategy. *Nature Reviews Cancer*, 21(5), 307–322. https://doi.org/10.1038/s41571-020-00449-x

Baker, D. J., Petersen, R. C., & J. T. (2016). Cellular senescence: A key contributor to aging and age-related diseases. *Nature Reviews Molecular Cell Biology*, 17(7), 445–458. https://doi.org/10.1038/nrm.2016.22

Balducci, L., Falandry, C., & Monfardini, S. (2024). Senotherapy, cancer, and aging. *Journal of Geriatric Oncology*, 15(4). https://doi.org/10.1016/j.jgo.2023.101671

Biddlestone-Thorpe, L., Sajjad, M., Rosenberg, E., Beckta, J. M., Valerie, N. C. K., Tokarz, M., Adams, B. R., Wagner, A. F., Khalil, A., Gilfor, D., Golding, S. E., Deb, S., Temesi, D. G., Lau, A., O'Connor, M. J., Choe, K. S., Parada, L. F., Lim, S. K., Mukhopadhyay, N. D., & Valerie, K. (2013). ATM kinase inhibition preferentially sensitizes p53-mutant glioma to ionizing radiation. *Clinical Cancer Research*, 19(12), 3189–3200. https://doi.org/10.1158/1078-0432.CCR-12-3408

Bielak-Zmijewska, A., Mosieniak, G., & Sikora, E. (2018). Is DNA damage indispensable for stress-induced senescence? *Mechanisms of Ageing and Development*, 170. https://doi.org/10.1016/j.mad.2017.08.004

Boccardi, V., & Mecocci, P. (2021). Senotherapeutics: Targeting senescent cells for the main age-related diseases. *Mechanisms of Ageing and Development*, 197. https://doi.org/10.1016/j.mad.2021.111526

Bousset, L., & Gil, J. (2022). Targeting senescence as an anticancer therapy. *Molecular Oncology*, 16(21). https://doi.org/10.1002/1878-0261.13312

Cerella, C., Grandjenette, C., Dicato, M., & Diederich, M. (2016). Roles of apoptosis and cellular senescence in cancer and aging. *Current Drug Targets*, 17(4). https://doi.org/10.2174/1389450116666150202155915

Childs, B. G., Durik, M., & Baker, D. J. (2017a). Cellular senescence in aging and age-related disease: from mechanisms to therapy. *Nature Reviews Molecular Cell Biology*, 18(12), 779–793. https://doi.org/10.1038/nrm.2017.115

Cuollo, L., Antonangeli, F., Santoni, A., & Soriani, A. (2020). The senescence-associated secretory phenotype (Sasp) in the challenging future of cancer therapy and age-related diseases. *Biology*, 9(12). https://doi.org/10.3390/biology9120485

D'Ambrosio, M., & Gil, J. (2023). Reshaping of the tumor microenvironment by cellular senescence: An opportunity for senotherapies. *Developmental Cell*, 58(12). https://doi.org/10.1016/j.devcel.2023.05.010

Domen, A., Deben, C., Verswyvel, J., Flieswasser, T., Prenen, H., Peeters, M., Lardon, F., & Wouters, A. (2022). Cellular senescence in cancer: Clinical detection and prognostic implications. *Journal of Experimental and Clinical Cancer Research*, 41(1). https://doi.org/10.1186/s13046-022-02555-3

Fan, Z., Tong, Y., Yang, Z., Wang, S., Huang, T., Yang, D., Ni, Q., Zhang, M., Li, D., Yang, M., & Fan, X. (2024). Inhibitor PF-04691502 works as a senolytic to regulate cellular senescence. *Experimental Gerontology*, 186, 112359. https://doi.org/10.1016/j.exger.2024.112359

Gire, V. (2005). Senescence: A telomeric limit to immortality or a cellular response to physiologic stresses? *Medecine/Sciences*, 21(5). https://doi.org/10.1051/medsci/2005215491

Haq, M., & Adnan, G. (2025). Ruxolitinib. In *StatPearls*. StatPearls Publishing. http://www.ncbi.nlm.nih.gov/books/NBK570600/

Herranz, N., & Gil, J. (2018). Mechanisms and functions of cellular senescence. *Journal of Clinical Investigation*, 128(4). https://doi.org/10.1172/JCI95148

Hoesel, B., & Schmid, J. A. (2013). The complexity of NF-κB signaling in inflammation and cancer. *Molecular Cancer*, 12(1), 86. https://doi.org/10.1186/1476-4598-12-86

Huang, M., Zhang, J., Yan, C., Li, X., Zhang, J., & Ling, R. (2019). Small molecule HDAC inhibitors: Promising agents for breast cancer treatment. *Bioorganic Chemistry*, 91, 103184. https://doi.org/10.1016/j.bioorg.2019.103184

Imawari, Y., & Nakanishi, M. (2024). Senescence and senolysis in cancer: The latest findings. *Cancer Science*, 115(7), 2107–2116. https://doi.org/10.1111/cas.16184

Kale, A., Sharma, A., Stolzing, A., Desprez, P.-Y., & Campisi, J. (2020). Role of immune cells in the removal of deleterious senescent cells. *Immunity & Ageing*, 17(1), 16. https://doi.org/10.1186/s12979-020-00187-9

Kim, E. C., & Kim, J. R. (2019). Senotherapeutics: Emerging strategy for healthy aging and age-related disease. *BMB Reports*, 52(1). https://doi.org/10.5483/BMBRep.2019.52.1.293

Kirkland, J. L., & Tchkonia, T. (2017). Senolytic drugs: Towards the clinic. *Nature Reviews Drug Discovery*, 16(5), 321–322. https://doi.org/10.1038/nrd.2017.44

Kirkland, J. L., et al. (2020). Senolytics and senomorphics: Towards a comprehensive approach to target senescence. *Nature Reviews Drug Discovery*, 19(11), 777–778. https://doi.org/10.1038/d41573-020-00182-4

Korwek, Z., & Alster, O. (2014). The role of the DNA damage response in apoptosis and cell senescence. *Postepy Biochemii*, 60(2).

Kumari, R., & Jat, P. (2021). Mechanisms of cellular senescence: Cell cycle arrest and senescence associated secretory phenotype. *Frontiers in Cell and Developmental Biology*, 9. https://doi.org/10.3389/fcell.2021.645593

Lagoumtzi, S. M., & Chondrogianni, N. (2021). Senolytics and senomorphics: Natural and synthetic therapeutics in the treatment of aging and chronic diseases. *Free Radical Biology and Medicine*, 171, 169–190. https://doi.org/10.1016/j.freeradbiomed.2021.05.003

Lee, J. W., & Ong, E. B. B. (2021). Genomic instability and cellular senescence: Lessons from the budding yeast. *Frontiers in Cell and Developmental Biology*, 8. https://doi.org/10.3389/fcell.2020.619126

Li, Y., & Yang, D.-Q. (2010). The ATM inhibitor KU-55933 suppresses cell proliferation and induces apoptosis by blocking Akt in cancer cells with overactivated Akt. *Molecular Cancer Therapeutics*, 9(1), 113–125. https://doi.org/10.1158/1535-7163.MCT-08-1189

Li, Y., Zhao, B., Peng, J., Tang, H., Wang, S., Peng, S., Ye, F., Wang, J., Ouyang, K., Li, J., Cai, M., & Chen, Y. (2024). Inhibition of NF-κB signaling unveils novel strategies to overcome drug resistance in cancers. *Drug Resistance Updates*, 73, 101042. https://doi.org/10.1016/j.drup.2023.101042

Li, Z., Tian, M., Wang, G., Cui, X., Ma, J., Liu, S., Shen, B., Liu, F., Wu, K., Xiao, X., & Zhu, C. (2023). Senotherapeutics: An emerging approach to the treatment of viral infectious diseases in the elderly. *Frontiers in Cellular and Infection Microbiology*, 13. https://doi.org/10.3389/fcimb.2023.1098712

Lopes-Paciencia, S., Saint-Germain, E., Rowell, M. C., Ruiz, A. F., Kalegari, P., & Ferbeyre, G. (2019). The senescence-associated secretory phenotype and its regulation. *Cytokine*, 117. https://doi.org/10.1016/j.cyto.2019.01.013

Lucas, V., Cavadas, C., & Aveleira, C. A. (2023). Cellular senescence: From mechanisms to current biomarkers and senotherapies. *Pharmacological Reviews*, 75(4). https://doi.org/10.1124/pharmrev.122.000622

Makin, G. (2018). Principles of chemotherapy. *Paediatrics and Child Health*, 28(4), 183–188. https://doi.org/10.1016/j.paed.2018.02.002

Malayaperumal, S., Marotta, F., Kumar, M. M., Somasundaram, I., Ayala, A., Pinto, M. M., Banerjee, A., & Pathak, S. (2023). The emerging role of senotherapy in cancer: A comprehensive review. *Clinics and Practice*, 13(4). https://doi.org/10.3390/clinpract13040076

Meiners, F., Hinz, B., Boeckmann, L., Secci, R., Sueto, S., Kuepfer, L., Fuellen, G., & Barrantes, I. (2024). Computational identification of natural senotherapeutic compounds that mimic dasatinib based on gene expression data. *Scientific Reports*, 14(1), 6286. https://doi.org/10.1038/s41598-024-55870-4

Mishra, S., Raval, M., Kachhawaha, A. S., Tiwari, B. S., & Tiwari, A. K. (2023). Chapter Eight—Aging: Epigenetic modifications. In V. Singh & I. Mani (Eds.), *Progress in Molecular Biology and Translational Science* (Vol. 197, pp. 171–209). Academic Press. https://doi.org/10.1016/bs.pmbts.2023.02.002

Mohamad Anuar, N. N., Nor Hisam, N. S., Liew, S. L., & Ugusman, A. (2020). Clinical review: Navitoclax as a pro-apoptotic and anti-fibrotic agent. *Frontiers in Pharmacology*, 11. https://doi.org/10.3389/fphar.2020.564108

Myrianthopoulos, V., Evangelou, K., Vasileiou, P. V. S., Cooks, T., Vassilakopoulos, T. P., Pangalis, G. A., Kouloukoussa, M., Kittas, C., Georgakilas, A. G., & Gorgoulis, V. G. (2019). Senescence and senotherapeutics: A new field in cancer therapy. *Pharmacology and Therapeutics*, 193. https://doi.org/10.1016/j.pharmthera.2018.08.006

Nacarelli, T., & Sell, C. (2017). Targeting metabolism in cellular senescence, a role for intervention. *Molecular and Cellular Endocrinology*, 455. https://doi.org/10.1016/j.mce.2016.08.049

Nakao, M., Tanaka, H., & Koga, T. (2020). Cellular senescence variation by metabolic and epigenomic remodeling. *Trends in Cell Biology*, 30(12). https://doi.org/10.1016/j.tcb.2020.08.009

Nehlin, J. O. (2023). Senolytic and senomorphic interventions to defy senescence-associated mitochondrial dysfunction. *Advances in Protein Chemistry and Structural Biology*, 136, 217–247. https://doi.org/10.1016/bs.apcsb.2023.02.020

Niedernhofer, L. J., & Robbins, P. D. (2018). Senotherapeutics for healthy ageing. *Nature Reviews Drug Discovery*, 17(5), 377–377. https://doi.org/10.1038/nrd.2018.44

Park, J., & Shin, D. W. (2022). Senotherapeutics and their molecular mechanism for improving aging. *Biomolecules and Therapeutics*, 30(6). https://doi.org/10.4062/biomolther.2022.114

Patnaik, A., Haluska, P., Tolcher, A. W., Erlichman, C., Papadopoulos, K. P., Lensing, J. L., Beeram, M., Molina, J. R., Rasco, D. W., Arcos, R. R., Kelly, C. S., Wijayawardana, S. R., Zhang, X., Stancato, L. F., Bell, R., Shi, P., Kulanthaivel, P., Pitou, C., Mulle, L. B., . . . Goetz, M. P. (2016). A first-in-human phase I study of the oral p38 MAPK inhibitor, ralimetinib (LY2228820 Dimesylate), in patients with advanced cancer. *Clinical Cancer Research: An Official Journal of the American Association for Cancer Research*, 22(5), 1095–1102. https://doi.org/10.1158/1078-0432.CCR-15-1718

Prasanna, P. G., Citrin, D. E., Hildesheim, J., Ahmed, M. M., Venkatachalam, S., Riscuta, G., Xi, D., Zheng, G., Deursen, J. van, Goronzy, J., Kron, S. J., Anscher, M. S., Sharpless, N. E., Campisi, J., Brown, S. L., Niedernhofer, L. J., O'Loghlen, A., Georgakilas, A. G., Paris, F., . . . Coleman, C. N. (2021). Therapy-induced senescence: Opportunities to improve anticancer therapy. *Journal of the National Cancer Institute*, 113(10). https://doi.org/10.1093/jnci/djab064

Prieto, L. I., & Baker, D. J. (2019). Cellular senescence and the immune system in cancer. *Gerontology*, 65(5). https://doi.org/10.1159/000500683

Provinciali, M., Cardelli, M., Marchegiani, F., & Pierpaoli, E. (2013). Impact of cellular senescence in aging and cancer. *Current Pharmaceutical Design*, 19(9). https://doi.org/10.2174/1381612811319090017

Qian, J., Zhou, X., Tanaka, K., & Takahashi, A. (2023). Alteration in the chromatin landscape during the DNA damage response: Continuous rotation of the gear driving cellular senescence and aging. *DNA Repair*, 131. https://doi.org/10.1016/j.dnarep.2023.103572

Qureshy, Z., Johnson, D. E., & Grandis, J. R. (2020). Targeting the JAK/STAT pathway in solid tumors. *Journal of Cancer Metastasis and Treatment*, 6, 27.

Regulski, M. J. (2017). Cellular senescence: What, why, and how. *Wounds*, 29(6).

Reynolds, L. E., Maallin, S., Haston, S., Martinez-Barbera, J. P., Hodivala-Dilke, K. M., & Pedrosa, A.-R. (2024). Effects of senescence on the tumour microenvironment and response to therapy. *The FEBS Journal*, 291(11), 2306–2319. https://doi.org/10.1111/febs.16984

Robbins, P. D., Jurk, D., Khosla, S., Kirkland, J. L., Lebrasseur, N. K., Miller, J. D., Passos, J. F., Pignolo, R. J., Tchkonia, T., & Niedernhofer, L. J. (2021). Senolytic drugs: Reducing senescent cell viability to extend health span. *Annual Review of Pharmacology and Toxicology*, 61. https://doi.org/10.1146/annurev-pharmtox-050120-105018

Rossi, M., & Abdelmohsen, K. (2021). The emergence of senescent surface biomarkers as senotherapeutic targets. *Cells*, 10(7). https://doi.org/10.3390/cells10071740

Sánchez-Díaz, L., Espinosa-Sánchez, A., Blanco, J. R., & Carnero, A. (2022). Senotherapeutics in cancer and HIV. *Cells*, 11(7). https://doi.org/10.3390/cells11071222

Schmitt, C. A., Wang, B., & Demaria, M. (2022). Senescence and cancer—role and therapeutic opportunities. *Nature Reviews Clinical Oncology*, 19(10). https://doi.org/10.1038/s41571-022-00668-4

Schosserer, M., Grillari, J., & Breitenbach, M. (2017). The dual role of cellular senescence in developing tumors and their response to cancer therapy. *Frontiers in Oncology*, 7(November). https://doi.org/10.3389/fonc.2017.00278

Short, S., Fielder, E., Miwa, S., & von Zglinicki, T. (2019). Senolytics and senostatics as adjuvant tumour therapy. *EBioMedicine*, 41, 683–692. https://doi.org/10.1016/j.ebiom.2019.01.056

Takasugi, M., Yoshida, Y., & Ohtani, N. (2022). Cellular senescence and the tumour microenvironment. *Molecular Oncology*, 16(18). https://doi.org/10.1002/1878-0261.13268

von Kobbe, C. (2019). Targeting senescent cells: Approaches, opportunities, challenges. *Aging*, 11(24), 12844–12861. https://doi.org/10.18632/aging.102557

Wang, B., Kohli, J., & Demaria, M. (2020a). Senescent cells in cancer therapy: Friends or foes? *Trends in Cancer*, 6(10), 838–857. https://doi.org/10.1016/j.trecan.2020.05.004

Wang, C., et al. (2021). The effects of senescent cell clearance on immune responses in aging. *Nature Aging*, 1, 310–320. https://doi.org/10.1038/s43587-021-00019-4

Wang, L., Doherty, G. A., Judd, A. S., Tao, Z.-F., Hansen, T. M., Frey, R. R., Song, X., Bruncko, M., Kunzer, A. R., Wang, X., Wendt, M. D., Flygare, J. A., Catron, N. D., Judge, R. A., Park, C. H., Shekhar, S., Phillips, D. C., Nimmer, P., Smith, M. L., . . . Souers, A. J. (2020b). Discovery of A-1331852, a first-in-class, potent, and orally-bioavailable BCL-XL inhibitor. *ACS Medicinal Chemistry Letters*, 11(10), 1829–1836. https://doi.org/10.1021/acsmedchemlett.9b00568

Wang, L., Lankhorst, L., & Bernards, R. (2022). Exploiting senescence for the treatment of cancer. *Nature Reviews Cancer*, 22(6), 340–355. https://doi.org/10.1038/s41568-022-00450-9

Wang, R., Yu, Z., Sunchu, B., Shoaf, J., Dang, I., Zhao, S., Caples, K., Bradley, L., Beaver, L. M., Ho, E., Löhr, C. V., & Perez, V. I. (2017). Rapamycin inhibits the secretory phenotype of senescent cells by a Nrf2-independent mechanism. *Aging Cell*, 16(3), 564–574. https://doi.org/10.1111/acel.12587

Wiley, C. D., & Campisi, J. (2021). The metabolic roots of senescence: Mechanisms and opportunities for intervention. *Nature Metabolism*, 3(10). https://doi.org/10.1038/s42255-021-00483-8

Xu, M., et al. (2018). Senolytic therapy alleviates atherosclerosis in mice. *Nature*, 575(7781), 652–658. https://doi.org/10.1038/s41586-019-1774-4

Yamamoto, M., Sanomachi, T., Suzuki, S., Togashi, K., Sugai, A., Seino, S., Sato, A., Okada, M., & Kitanaka, C. (2021). Gemcitabine radiosensitization primes irradiated malignant meningioma cells for senolytic elimination by navitoclax. *Neuro-Oncology Advances*, 3(1), vdab148. https://doi.org/10.1093/noajnl/vdab148

Yang, J., Liu, M., Hong, D., Zeng, M., & Zhang, X. (2021). The paradoxical role of cellular senescence in cancer. *Frontiers in Cell and Developmental Biology*, 9. https://doi.org/10.3389/fcell.2021.722205

Yang, J., Nie, J., Ma, X., Wei, Y., Peng, Y., & Wei, X. (2019). Targeting PI3K in cancer: Mechanisms and advances in clinical trials. *Molecular Cancer*, 18(1), 26. https://doi.org/10.1186/s12943-019-0954-x

Yasuda, T., Baba, H., & Ishimoto, T. (2023). Cellular senescence in the tumor microenvironment and context-specific cancer treatment strategies. *FEBS Journal*, 290(5). https://doi.org/10.1111/febs.16231

Zarneshan, S. N., Fakhri, S., Bachtel, G., & Bishayee, A. (2023). Exploiting pivotal mechanisms behind the senescence-like cell cycle arrest in cancer. *Advances in Protein Chemistry and Structural Biology*, 135. https://doi.org/10.1016/bs.apcsb.2022.11.007

Zhai, C., et al. (2020). Senolytic ABT-263 enhances the efficacy of chemotherapy in preclinical cancer models. *Cancer Research*, 80(12), 2598–2608. https://doi.org/10.1158/0008-5472.CAN-19-3355

Zhang, L., Pitcher, L. E., Prahalad, V., Niedernhofer, L. J., & Robbins, P. D. (2023). Targeting cellular senescence with senotherapeutics: Senolytics and senomorphics. *FEBS Journal*, 290(5), 1362–1383. https://doi.org/10.1111/febs.16350

Zhang, Y., et al. (2021). Senolytics improve metabolic health in obese mice. *Nature Metabolism*, 3(5), 698–711. https://doi.org/10.1038/s42255-021-00405-3

Chapter 5

Senotherapeutics in Aging and Age-Associated Disorders

Saima Zameer and Divya Vohora

5.1 INTRODUCTION

According to the World Health Organization (WHO), the number of people aged 60 and above worldwide is projected to double by 2050 (Zheng et al. 2024). The advancement in healthcare facilities such as availability of vaccines and awareness about sanitation have improved the quality of life and extended life expectancy, which co-occurs with age-related disorders. Aging is a complex and widespread biological process marked by the gradual and irreversible decline in physical functions across various organ systems, resulting from exposure to a wide range of stressors. Aging leads to a decreased ability of the organism to adapt to its environment, diminishing the regenerative capacity of tissues and organs throughout the body. As a result, this vulnerability increases the risk of developing various age-related diseases, including diabetes, cancer, cardiovascular conditions, musculoskeletal issues, neurodegenerative disorders (López-Otín et al. 2013; Kennedy et al. 2014; Hernández Cordero et al. 2022), idiopathic pulmonary fibrosis, and glaucoma (McHugh and Gil 2018). Moreover, with the advancement of age especially after 60 years, many people have comorbidities and require combined potential therapies to alleviate the disease symptoms (Ding et al. 2023) Consequently, it is crucial to understand the therapies for age-related clinical manifestations preceding the understanding of the aging process. In 1956, the free radical theory of aging proposed that aging results due to free radicals released from cellular metabolism (Harman 1956). Subsequently, research has been conducted to leverage mechanisms underlying the aging process.

The aging process is driven by a gradual and continuous decline in the body's ability to manage and respond to various biological stresses, leading to reduced function and diminished capacity for tissue repair and regeneration (L. Zhang, Pitcher, et al. 2023). Moreover, there are three categories of aging hallmarks: (1) primary, causative factors for age-linked damage; (2) antagonistic, hallmarks which generate in responses to age-linked decline; and (3) integrative, the results of these responses and key factors influencing the aging phenotypes. Senescence refers to the cellular process that halts the proliferation of aged or damaged cells. While senescence has critical physiological roles in maintaining tissue homeostasis

 DOI: 10.1201/9781003493969-5

and normal development (D. Muñoz-Espín et al. 2013; Daniel Muñoz-Espín and Serrano 2014), it is considered one of the antagonistic hallmarks of the aging process and contributes to the onset of a diverse range of age-associated disorders.

5.2 ACTIVATORS AND HALLMARKS OF SENESCENCE

Senescence is a heterogenous process that arises due to insults triggered by increasing age, such as environmental, epigenetic, and genetic manipulations, leading to gradual suppression of physiological cell functions (van Deursen 2014; Lagoumtzi and Chondrogianni 2021; Guo et al. 2022). Disruption in nutrient signaling and proteostasis are the other hallmarks of aging which crosstalk with senescence responses. Furthermore, there is a wide range of activators for senescence including oncogene activation, reactive oxygen species (ROS), mitochondrial dysfunction, and telomere length shortening. These activators transform healthy cells into senescent cells (SnC), which can provoke the consequential age-associated causal factors including chronic inflammation and stem cell exhaustion (McHugh and Gil 2018) that could be considered senescence hallmarks. While there are no standard hallmarks to identify senescence, a combination of multiple hallmarks can be used to demonstrate this phenotype (Mylonas and O'Loghlen 2022). Some of the characteristic features of senescence are senescence-specific secretomes, stable cell cycle arrest, altered metabolism and cellular morphology, cytoplasmic chromatin fragments (CCF), and senescence-associated heterochromatin foci (SAHF). The increase in senescence-associated-β-galactosidase (SA-β-gal) activity is also one of the key senescence markers. SA-β-gal, which is a lysosomal hydrolase, can be identified by staining cells with X-gal, which turns blue in presence of β-galactosidase (Valieva et al. 2022). Additionally, SnC exhibit the increased expression of $p16^{Ink4a}$ and $p21^{Cip1/Waf}$, which are cyclin-dependent kinase inhibitors that play a key role in cell cycle arrest (Wagner and Wagner 2022). Despite these markers, senescence-associated secretory phenotype (SASP) generated through vesicles, and proteins are also one of the key hallmarks of senescence. SASP contains bioactive lipids, pro-inflammatory agents such as cytokines, chemokines, and factors which mediate paracrine or autocrine signaling within SnC (Childs et al. 2017; Birch and Gil 2020). The detection of senescence can be achieved by identifying a combination of these markers using various techniques like immunohistochemistry, Western blot, and ELISA (Figure 5.1).

5.3 ROLE OF SENESCENCE IN AGING AND ASSOCIATED DISORDERS

With aging, SnC accumulate in different tissues and contribute to age-related degeneration through various mechanisms. One of the significant ways is inflammation, as SASP factors trigger chronic inflammation which can exacerbate tissue

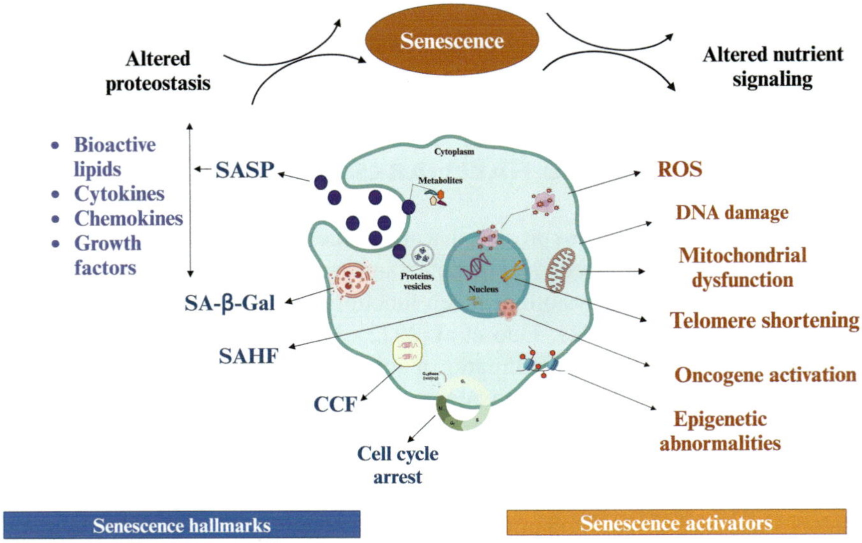

Figure 5.1 The figure depicts the activators and hallmarks of cellular senescence. Multiple factors, including generation of reactive oxygen species, mitochondrial dysfunction, and activation of oncogenes, contribute to the transformation of healthy cells into senescent cells. Additionally, factors such as DNA damage, epigenetic alterations, and telomere shortening are the primary determinants of aging. Some of these factors can trigger senescence, which subsequently leads to aging and age-related diseases in response to damage, including inflammation, proteostasis dysfunction, and disrupted nutrient signaling. CCF, cytoplasmic chromatin fragment; ROS, reactive oxygen species; SASP, senescence-associated secretory phenotypes; SA-β-gal, senescence-associated-β-galactosidase; SAHF, senescence-associated heterochromatin foci. The figure is generated in Biorender.

damage. Additionally, SnC impair tissue regeneration and function leading to tissue dysfunction over time. Furthermore, these cells are implicated in various age-linked diseases including cancer (Y. Kim et al. 2024) and cardiovascular (Kalies et al. 2024), musculoskeletal (Fielding et al. 2023) and neurodegenerative diseases (McHugh and Gil 2018; Zheng et al. 2024). How senescence and its mechanisms contribute to these age-linked diseases is summarized in Table 5.1.

5.4 SENOTHERAPEUTICS IN AGE-RELATED DISORDERS

Addressing the challenges posed by the increasing number of elderly individuals across the globe is of prime importance. The substantial rise in the proportion of people aged 65 years or above, including centenarians, poses significant social and economic burdens. Aging is not classified as a disease; rather, it is widespread and progressive decline in physiological functions over time, which exaggerates

Table 5.1 Age-Related Diseases and Associated Senescence Mechanisms

Age-Related Disease	*Disease Mechanism*	*Senescence Mechanism*	*Reference*
		Cardiovascular Disease	
Myocardial infarction	Ischemia and reperfusion injury	Senescence-like phenotype in cardiomyocytes	Tang, Li, and Chen (2020)
Atherosclerosis	Endothelial dysfunction, plaque formation, inflammation	Senescence-associated β-galactosidase (SA-β-gal) activity, telomere shortening	Ali et al. (2024); Yin and Pickering (2023)
Cardiac fibrosis	Excessive extracellular matrix deposition	Metabolic changes, epigenetic alteration	Xie et al. (2023); Shao, Liu, and Zuo (2022)
		Musculoskeletal Disease	
Sarcopenia	Loss of muscle mass and strength	SASP, $p53/p21^{CIP1}$, and $p16^{INK4a}/pRB$ pathways	He et al. (2021)
Osteoarthritis	Joint inflammation, cartilage degradation	Altered mitotic activity and telomere length	Surmachevska and Rubio (2023)
		Cancer	
Prostate cancer	Uncontrolled cell growth, hormone regulation disruption	Expression of the SASP, epigenetic alterations like nuclear envelop alteration, senescence-associated heterochromatin foci (SAHF), $p16^{INK4a}/pRb$ and $p53/p21^{WAF1/CIP1}$ pathway, androgen-deprivation–induced senescence	Kallenbach et al. (2022); Yong Zhang, Dong, et al. (2018)
General (ex-breast, lung, etc.)	Metastasis, uncontrolled cell growth	DNA damage response (DDR), senescence-associated proliferation arrest (SAPA), upregulated SA-β-gal activity, deposition of lipofuscin, angiogenesis, migration invasiveness, activation of immune surveillance, oncogene-induced senescence	Schmitt, Wang, and Demaria (2022); Milanovic et al. (2018); Xiao et al. (2023)

(*Continued*)

Table 5.1 (Continued) Age-Related Diseases and Associated Senescence Mechanisms

Age-Related Disease	*Disease Mechanism*	*Senescence Mechanism*	*Reference*
		Neurodegenerative Disease	
Alzheimer's disease (AD)	Amyloid beta (Aβ) plaque formation, tau protein containing neurofibrillary tangles	p16 and p21 upregulation, SA-β-gal activity, cell cycle repressors activation (p16, p21, p53), DNA damage response, reactive oxygen species (ROS), SASP, telomere deficiency	P. Zhang et al. (2019)
Parkinson's disease (PD)	Alpha-synuclein aggregation, Lewy body formation	SASP factors, senescence in pericyte due to p16 activation, mitochondrial dysfunction, p21 activation	Russo and Riessland (2022); Garretti et al. (2019); Yamazaki et al. (2016)
Huntington's disease (HD)	Huntingtin protein aggregation, neuronal loss	Telomere shortening, epigenetic alterations, mitochondrial dysfunction, genomic instability, p53/p21 signaling	Aziz and Weydt (2018); Horvath et al. (2016); Machiela and Southwell (2020)
Multiple sclerosis (MS)	Demyelination, immune mediated CNS attack	$p16^{INK4a}$ expressed senescent cells, telomere attrition, immune-mediated senescence, DNA methylation	Yang et al. (2024); Yinan Zhang, Atkinson, et al. (2023)
Amyotrophic lateral sclerosis (ALS)	TDP-43 proteinopathy, motor neuron degeneration	Oxidative stress, DNA damage, telomere shortening, p21 upregulation, higher SA-β-gal expression	Melo Pereira, Ribeiro, and Logarinho (2019); Birger et al. (2019)

our vulnerability to a broad range of age-associated health issues (Austad 2016). Experimentally, it has been demonstrated that dietary restrictions profoundly retard aging process. Nonetheless, there are ample other causative factors, as evidenced by epidemiological data sets, which trigger the process of aging and subsequently lead to the onset of numerous chronic diseases. In a similar vein, it is essential to understand the biological mechanisms driving the aging process and identify the therapeutic targets in order to alleviate the age-related diseases. The geroscience hypothesis states "any intervention which decelerate the aging process will concurrently either retard the onset or alleviate diverse age-related diseases," which has been supported by substantial amount of evidence in different organism model systems (Sierra 2016; Chaib, Tchkonia, and Kirkland 2022). Moreover, targeting any one of the biological mechanisms underlying the aging process and its associated diseases can impact many others, supporting a unified theory of a fundamental aging mechanism (Tchkonia, Palmer, and Kirkland 2021).

In 2011, Baker and colleagues demonstrated the direct association of senescence with age-associated diseases in a mice model. They proposed that eliminating SnC could enhance health span and delay or attenuate physiological dysfunctions and their consequences (E.C. Kim and Kim 2019). Therefore, clearing SnC or ameliorating its effects could be a promising approach to treat age-associated diseases (Baker et al. 2016). In this context, three main approaches have been developed to target these cells: (1) senolytics, which specifically eliminate SnC or induce their destruction; (2) senomorphics, which mitigate the adverse effects of SASPs to achieve senostasis; and (3) senescence targeting immunotherapeutics.

5.4.1 Senolytics

Senolytics are designed to trigger apoptosis in SnC while sparing healthy cells. This selectivity is achieved through various mechanisms which affect the unique survival pathways present in SnC. These cells often upregulate anti-apoptotic pathways to evade cell death, and one of the key strategies of senolytics is to disrupt these pathways, thereby promoting apoptosis. Additionally, these cells have altered metabolic states as compared to the non-SnC. Senolytics exploit these metabolic differences to selectively induce cell death (Baar et al. 2017; Kirkland and Tchkonia 2017). Senolytics have been increasingly studied as a potential approach to alleviate senescence and age-related diseases. Diverse range of senolytics have been investigated such as inhibitors for protein tyrosine kinase, Bcl-2 inhibitors, p53 binding, foxhead box protein 04 (FOXO4), histone deacetylase (HDAC), UBX0101 (Niedernhofer and Robbins 2018), and heat shock protein 90 (HSP90) (Zhu et al. 2015, 2016; Baar et al. 2017; Jeon et al. 2017; Samaraweera et al. 2017; Xu et al. 2018). Senolytics came into play when Zhu and colleagues demonstrated the gene expression changes between SnC and healthy cells, highlighting an enhanced expression of anti-apoptotic biomarkers such as components of PI3K/Akt, the Bcl-2 family, and others. Subsequently, they screened 46 drug molecules having the potential to selectively eliminate SnC in vitro. They observed that combining a protein kinase inhibitor dasatinib with the plant flavonoid quercetin hastened apoptosis of SnC in Ercc1-/Δ-progeroid, irradiated and aged mice, as well as ameliorated age-linked symptoms. These findings emphasized the dasatinib and quercetin combination as one of the pioneering senolytic treatments. Dasatinib effectively eliminated senescent preadipocytes and is clinically used in cancer treatment, while quercetin, which targets the PI3K/AKT pathways and BCL-2, removed mesenchymal stem cells derived from mouse bone marrow and senescent endothelial SnC (Zhu et al. 2015). As a result, several in vivo studies have been conducted to validate the effectiveness of this treatment against senescence and senescence-induced age-related diseases including insulin resistance, skeletal muscle dysfunction, hepatic steatosis, physical dysfunction, and neurodegeneration (Xu et al. 2018; Wissler Gerdes et al. 2020). The combination of dasatinib and quercetin is presently being investigated in clinical trials for different age-related diseases such as kidney disease, pulmonary fibrosis, adult cancer, skeletal health issues, and Alzheimer's disease (Park and Shin 2022).

The overexpression of Bcl-2 family proteins in SnC blocks apoptosis, suggesting that targeting and inhibiting these anti-apoptotic proteins could serve as a promising strategy for senolytic therapy (Chang et al. 2016; Zhu et al. 2016). Compounds such as ABT-263 (known as navitoclax), A1155463, A1331852, and ABT-737 have shown senolytic activity in cell culture and in animal models (Yosef et al. 2016; Zhu et al. 2017). Navitoclax was observed to eliminate senescent human lung fibroblasts (Zhu et al. 2016) and rejuvenate muscle and blood-forming stem cells in mice (Chang et al. 2016; Miura et al. 2022). It cleared foam cell macrophages in atherosclerotic lesions but caused bone loss in aged mice (Garrido et al. 2022). Moreover, ABT-737, which is another senolytic, targeted SnC in various tissues and stimulated hair follicle stem cell proliferation (Yosef et al. 2016). A1331852 and A115546 selectively cleared irradiation-induced SnC (Zhu et al. 2017). Besides the protein kinases, FOXO4 plays a key role in enhancing the viability of SnC by facilitating p53's nuclear localization and its involvement in apoptotic pathways (C. Zhang, Xie, et al. 2020; Baar et al. 2017). To this context, Baar and colleagues developed the FOXO4-DRI peptide to disrupt the interaction between FOXO4 and p53, promoting the relocation of p53 to the cytoplasm and triggering caspase-3/7-dependent apoptosis in SnC, such as human lung fibroblasts. This peptide inhibitor in different mouse models of aging was cited to alleviate renal dysfunction and restore hair density (Baar et al. 2017). Simultaneously, FOXO4-DRI has been shown to induce cell death in aging Leydig cells within the testes and help delay the development of hypogonadism (C. Zhang, Xie, et al. 2020). These notions unveiled the FOXO4-p53 as a promising target for mitigating senescence and associated disorders. In addition to FOXO4, p53 has an affinity towards its negative regulator known as MDM2, an E3 ligase. In vivo models of osteoarthritis suggested the inhibitor of MDM2/p53 protein complex as a potential senolytic agent. UBX0101 targeted this protein complex and effectively removed SnC from the joint tissues and surrounding membranes, enhancing chondrocyte cartilage formation and reducing post-traumatic osteoarthritis in mice (Jeon et al. 2017). UBX0101 was the first senolytic to advance into phase I clinical trials, but it failed to meet the endpoints in phase II. Nonetheless, there are HDAC inhibitors which could be a potential therapy to improve cancer metastasis. Panobinostat is one of the FDA-approved HDAC inhibitors which promotes acetylation of histone H3, reduces expression of Bcl-xl, and in turn induces senescence in different cancer cell lines (Samaraweera et al. 2017).

HSP90 is an ATP-driven chaperone essential for protein stabilization and folding. It is essential for maintaining proteostasis within the cells and facilitating the activity of a variety of proteins, such as those involved in signal transduction, stress responses, and the regulation of the cell cycle (C. Hu et al. 2022). HSP90 interacts with co-chaperones and client proteins to form complexes that ensure the proper functioning, folding, and processing of critical cellular machinery, thereby supporting overall cellular homeostasis (K. Lee et al. 2021). These proteins are essential for the activation of some steroid receptors and kinases (Lu et al. 2014) and contribute to the development of several diseases by modulating programmed cell death (B. Hu et al. 2020). The complex of HSP90 with client proteins is considered a critical target to treat diseases. However, HSP90 inhibitors have emerged as one of the promising therapies to block this complex formation (Mielczarek-Lewandowska, Hartman, and Czyz 2020; Sang et al. 2018). These inhibitors have been evidenced to exert an anti-tumor effect, and some of the members of this family, such as geldanamycin (GDA), which was developed in the early 1990s, and its derivatives 17-allylamino-17-demethoxy-geldanamycin (17-AAG) and alvespimycin, have been investigated in clinical trials (Z. Zhang, Jing, et al. 2020; Bao et al. 2009). GDA and its derivatives interfere with ATPase activity and hinder the interaction between HSP90 and its client proteins, resulting in the degradation of these proteins and disruption of cellular functions (Gorska et al. 2012). 17-DMAG interrupts the binding of Akt to HSP90 and induces apoptosis in SnC. These HSP90 inhibitors had emerged as senolytic agents following screening of 97 drug candidates in $Ercc1^{-/-}$ mouse embryonic fibroblasts (MEFs). In vivo and in vitro datasets evidenced that these inhibitors induce apoptosis of irradiation or oxidative stress–induced senescence in different cells such as mesenchymal stem cells, human fibroblasts (W-38, IMR-90), and others, prolongs lifespan, and delays age-associated disease onset (Fuhrmann-Stroissnigg et al. 2017).

In addition to synthetic senolytics, there are different plant-based compounds which degrade SnC. Fisetin is one of the flavonoids which is structurally similar to quercetin and has neuroprotective, anticancer, anti-inflammatory, and antioxidant properties (Fuhrmann-Stroissnigg et al. 2017). Fisetin regulates diverse a range of signaling pathways such as nuclear factor kappa B (NF-κB) and NRF2 (Chiang et al. 2015; Pal et al. 2015). This plant-based senolytic triggers irradiation and oxidation-induced senescence in epithelial cells derived from human umbilical veins (HUVECs) and reduces markers of cellular aging in aged mice (Zhu et al. 2017; Yousefzadeh et al. 2018). Fisetin is under clinical trials for conditions such as osteoarthritis and chronic kidney diseases (Park and Shin 2022).

Correspondingly, it is evident that a natural alkaloid called piperlongumine induces apoptosis in human fibroblasts by blocking the PI3K/Akt/mTOR pathway and increases the generation of reactive oxygen species (ROS) (Wang et al. 2016). It is also demonstrated to have a binding affinity to the oxidation resistance 1 (OXR1) protein which degrades anti-oxidant enzymes (X. Zhang, Zhang, et al. 2018). Different senolytics are listed in Table 5.2.

5.4.2 Senomorphics

Senomorphics is another key senotherapeutic which modifies the phenotype of SnC, restoring them to healthy state by interfering with senoinflammation or inflammaging induced by SASP without triggering apoptosis (Kirkland and Tchkonia 2017; Lagoumtzi and Chondrogianni 2021). These agents modulate pathways linked to senescence such as NF-κB, IL-1α, MAPKs, and the mTOR pathway (Yun et al. 2018; Birch and Gil 2020; Lagoumtzi and Chondrogianni 2021). Senomorphics are similar to anti-senescence or anti-aging molecules including activators for telomerase (Liu, Zhao, and Luo 2017), sirtuin (Hubbard and Sinclair 2014), autophagy (Nakamura and Yoshimori 2018), and proteasomes (Chondrogianni et al. 2015), as well as antioxidants (Si and Liu 2014), mTOR inhibitors (Lamming et al. 2013), and anti-inflammatory agents to target inflammaging or senoinflammation (Soto-Gamez and Demaria 2017). In this chapter we will focus on agents with senomorphic potential, utilizing specific markers of senescence, including SA-β-gal and SASP in different experimental settings. The transcription factor NF-κB plays a vital role in mediating aging-related processes, including the response to DNA damage and regulation of insulin, SIRT, mTOR, and FOXO (Tilstra et al. 2011). NF-κB is a key target of senomorphics, as supported by various datasets. Inhibition of the NF-κB activating kinase called IKK by 8K-NBD peptide reduces senescence and age-linked pathologies in a progeroid mouse with a defective Ercc1 gene (Tilstra et al. 2012). Additionally, SASP in SnC, which is modulated by Janus kinase signal transducers and activators of transcription (JAK/STAT), is another potential target for senomorphics (Novakova et al. 2010). Mechanistically, the phosphorylated JAK tyrosine kinase triggers STAT3 phosphorylation and activates the Bcl-2 family and interleukin receptors (Banerjee and Resat 2016). Moreover, STAT3 consistently promotes NF-κB during chronic inflammation (Liang et al. 2013). Consequently, the inhibition of JAK was evidenced to potentially suppress SASP in SnC and tumor cells (Toso et al. 2014). In conjunction to such reports, ruxolitinib, an inhibitor of JAK1/2, was approved for myelofibrosis treatment (Harrison, Talpaz, and Mead 2016) and was demonstrated to improve insulin sensitivity and ameliorates lipotoxicity and fat loss in aged mice. This JAK1/2 inhibitor reduces senoinflammation in senescent models, age-related pathologies, and enhances physical activity (Xu et al. 2015; Xu et al. 2015).

Furthermore, ataxia-telangiectasia mutated (ATM) kinase triggered by DNA double-strand breaks modulates senescence (Fausti et al. 2013). This kinase inhibitor

Table 5.2 Types of Senolytics

Senolytics	*Mechanism*	*Drugs*	*Experimental Model*	*References*
Bcl-2 family inhibitors	SCAPs	Dasatinib (D) + quercetin (Q)	Ercc$^{-1/\Delta}$ and aged C57B/L6 mice Preadipocytes/HUVECs	Zhu et al. (2015); Xu et al. (2018)
	Inhibit BCL-2, BCL-XL, BCL-W	ABT-263 (navitoclax) ABT-737	C57B/6J, p16–3MR transgenic mouse model Ercc$^{-/-}$ mouse embryonic fibroblasts (MEFs) Preadipocytes/HUVECs IMR-90 fibroblasts Osteoarthritic chondrocytes	Chang et al. (2016); Miura et al. (2022); Sharma et al. (2020)
	Inhibit BCL-XL	A-1155463 A-1331852	HUVECs IMR-90 fibroblasts	Zhu et al. (2017)
p53 targets	Disrupt MDM2/p53 interaction	UBX0101 RG7112 (RO5045337)	p16::3MR mice Osteoarthritis mouse model	Jeon et al. (2017); Tovar et al. (2013)
	Disrupt FOXO4-p53 interaction	FOXO4-DRI	Xpd$^{TFD/TTD}$, p16::3MR mice Leydig cells IMR-90 fibroblasts	Baar et al. (2017); Z. Zhang, Jing, et al. (2020)
HSP90 inhibitors	Inhibit HSP90 Disrupt HSP90-AKT interaction	Geldanamycin Ganetespib 17-AAG (tanespimycin) 17-DMAG (alvespimycin)	Ercc1$^{-/-}$ mice MEFs	Fuhrmann-Stroissnigg et al. (2017)
Natural products and their analogs	Downregulate Nrf2 and NF-κB pathways	o-Vanillin (curcumin metabolite) Curcumin	Human intervertebral disc (IVD) cells	Cherif et al. (2019)
	The mechanism is not certain, but it modulates unclear, OXR1, NF-κB	Piperlongumine and its analogs	WI-38	Wang et al. (2016); Yong Zhang, Dong, et al. (2018)

(Continued)

Table 5.2 (Continued) Types of Senolytics

Senolytics	*Mechanism*	*Drugs*	*Experimental Model*	*References*
	The mechanism is not clear, it alkalizes lysosome and elevate sROS levels and exacerbates mitophagy deficiency to induce apoptosis	GL-V9	Breast cancer cells Replication-induced senescent MEF cells Malignant T-cell lines MMTV-PyMT mice	Zheng et al. (2024)
Galactose modified pro-drugs	SA-β-gal	Pro-drug A (JHB75B) SSK1 5FURGa Nav-Gal		
Cardiac glycosides	Inhibit Na^+/K^+-ATPase, upregulate BCL2-family protein NOXA	Ouabain Digoxin	Cell lines like primary bronchial/tracheal epithelial cell, MEF, IMR90 ER-RAS cells, etc.	Guerrero et al. (2019)
	Inhibit Na^+/K^+-ATPase	Bufalin K-Strophanthus Procellariids A Strophanthidin	Immunodeficient nude NMRInu/nu mice	Guerrero et al. (2019); Triana-Martínez et al. (2019)
PROTACs	Degrade BRD4	ARV825	Hepatocellular carcinoma (HCC) mouse mode Different cell lines like MEFs	Wakita et al. (2020)
	Degrade BCL-XL	PZ15227	Aged mice	Baar et al. (2017)
Miscellaneous senolytics	Reduce mitochondrial membrane potential, inhibit OXPHOS	MitoTam (mitochondria-targeted tamoxifen)	Cell lines such as human breast carcinoma cell line MCF7 Lung-derived fibroblast cell line (HFP-1) Balb/c and transgenic FVB/N c-neu mice	Samaraweera et al. (2017); L. Zhang, Pitcher et al. (2023)

Inhibitor of c-IAP1, c-IAP2, and XIAP	AT-406	Sprague Dawley (SD) rats
Syk inhibitor, FAK and p38MAPK	Tamatinib (R406)	Model of diploid human dermal fibroblasts (HDFs)
Induce autophagy and glycolysis	Azithromycin Roxithromycin	MRC-5 human fibroblasts cell line
PPARa agonist	Fenofibrate	Human chondrocytes
Histone deacetylase inhibitor	Panobinostat	Non-small cell lung cancer (NSCLC) and head and neck squamous cell carcinoma (HNSCC) cell lines

named KU-60019 has demonstrated senomorphic potential by restoring lysosome/autophagy functions and facilitating changes in cellular metabolism (Kang et al. 2017). Ongoing research aims to explore the novel therapies and repurpose existing drugs to impede SnC generation and age-related pathologies. In context of repurposing, metformin, an established anti-diabetic therapy, has been shown to efficiently inhibit SASP followed by diminishing the expression of interleukins and chemokines (Moiseeva et al. 2013). It also demonstrated senomorphic activity by abolishing the IκB and its kinase phosphorylation, thereby inhibiting activity of NF-κB. Metformin is currently undergoing clinical studies as a potential advanced therapeutic option for slowing down age-related changes (Kulkarni, Gubbi, and Barzilai 2020). Furthermore, an in vivo data set has shown metformin's potential to recover the SnC in lens epithelium through activation of adenosine 5′-monophosphate protein kinase (AMPK) (Chen et al. 2022). MDM2 inhibitors such as nutlin-3a and MI-63 were also highlighted as another important approach to target SnC. These inhibitors have been shown to reduce cytokine levels and SASP factors, while also inhibiting the growth of tumor cells in genotoxin-induced senescence (Wiley et al. 2018). Nonetheless, there are several additional senomorphic targets to mitigate senescence and associated symptoms. A lamin A protein called progerin acquires a telomere shortening, leading to the senescence of healthy and normal human fibroblast in Hutchinson-Gilford progeria syndrome (HGPS) (Cao et al. 2011). Senomorphics exhibit a protective role in such senescence-induced pathologies. Akin to this, JH4 was shown to serve as a senomorphic agent in an HGPS mouse model by interfering in lamin A/C and progerin binding, ameliorating age-related pathological consequences and senescence markers including SA-β-gal activity and growth arrest in HGPS (S.J. Lee et al. 2016).

Another approach to reprogramming SnC into young, functional cells may involve the use of neutralizing antibodies targeting SASP factors, including cytokines. It has been suggested that targeting the cytokines and their receptors may diminish the SASP expression during senescence. Numerous studies have demonstrated that the neutralizing anti-human IL-1α monoclonal antibody provides protective benefits in conditions like inflammation and diabetes (Park and Shin 2022). Simultaneously, neutralizing monoclonal antibodies (MABs) against IL-6 and IL-8 (CXC motif chemokine), another important SASP for immunosuppression and tumor proliferation, were also acknowledged as a potential target for SnC and associated symptoms. Olokizumab (an IL-6 targeting MAB) was shown to effectively hinder STAT signaling and diminish the senescence-associated symptoms of arthritis in primates (Kuilman et al. 2008) (Table 5.3), while ABX-IL-8 (MAB for IL-8) was evidenced to reduce the growth rate in various cancer xenograft models (Waugh and Wilson 2008). Nonetheless, several plant-based compounds like quercetin-3-O-β-D-glucuronide, (−)-loliolide, and quercetagetin 3,4′-dimethyl ether were also examined for their potential to modify the phenotype of SnC (Park and Shin 2022). Simultaneously, miRNAs and growth factors have also been demonstrated to exert an anti-aging or senomorphic effect in HDF and HUVEC cells and in various in vivo models (Bae et al. 2019).

Table 5.3 Types of Senomorphics

Mechanism	*Drugs*	*Experimental Models*	*References*
Decreases NF-κB activity	8K-NBD peptide KU-60019	$Ercc^{-/-}$ MEFs $Ercc^{-/\Delta}$ mice	Tilstra et al. (2012); Kang et al. (2017)
Alters JAK1/2 family	Ruxolitinib	Preadipocytes Aged C57BL/6 mice	Xu et al. (2015)
Decreases NF-κB and enhances AMPK activity	Metformin	IMR-90 fibroblasts Raw 264.7 cells Lens epithelial cells from aged C57BL/6 mice	Moiseeva et al. (2013); Chen et al. (2022)
Inhibits MDM2	Nutlin-3a (MI-63)	HCA2 foreskin IMR-90/WI-38 fibroblasts	Wiley et al. (2018)
Reduces IL-6 and STAT3 levels	Mab-IL-6.8 Ab (Olokizumab)	Different cell lines such as human hepatocytes HUVECs, HepG2 cells IMR-90 fibroblasts Cynomolgus monkey arthritis model	Kuilman et al. (2008)
Attenuates IL-1α activity	MABp1 Ab	HCA2 foreskin	Park and Shin (2022)

5.4.3 Senescence-Targeting Immunotherapeutics

Senescence activates immune responses, which subsequently facilitate the clearance of SnC to help maintain homeostasis. Along with the removal or destruction of SnC and changes to their phenotypes, strengthening the immunological functions is another key approach to reducing senescence and associated diseases. The elimination of SnC is essential in regulating tissue homeostasis, including processes like hepatic fibrosis, wound healing, and the development of the embryo and placenta. However, inadequate SnC clearance, often caused by altered immune responses, can lead to their accumulation in various tissues and contribute to aging and related complications (Park and Shin 2022; E.C. Kim and Kim 2019).

Immune cell populations like macrophages, NK cells, and $CD8^+$ T cells, have the ability to identify and remove SnC (Salminen 2021). The accumulation of senescent immune cells might be reduced with targeted antibodies capable of recognizing senescence-specific surface markers. Moreover, identification of these surface markers is vital. For instance, CD44 expression, a gene associated with cell binding and senescence, is increased in the aorta endothelium of aging rat. Antibodies against CD44 have been shown to induce significant decrease in the monocyte's recruitment to lesions in endothelial SnC (L. Zhang, Yang, et al. 2023).

Additionally, NK cells recognize the receptor of CD58/ICAM1 on SnC (Vicente et al. 2016) while CD26/(DPP4) was found on the surface of fibroblasts in replicative senescence (K.M. Kim et al. 2017). Kim and colleagues (2017) also demonstrated that DPP4 facilitates antibody-dependent cell-mediated cytotoxicity, aiding NK cells in recognizing and eliminating SnC. Their work suggests that DPP4 could serve as a potential target for immunotherapeutic strategies (K.M. Kim et al. 2017). Furthermore, macrophages can identify modified membrane receptors, such as lipids and glycans, present on SnC through receptors like IgM and CD36. Enhancing the binding capacity of these receptors, combined with targeted T cell therapies aimed at senescence-associated molecules, offers a promising approach for cancer treatment (Park and Shin 2022).

Nonetheless, a promising strategy to rejuvenate SnC of the immune system involves reversing their dysfunctional behavior. As individuals age, there is a decline in the activity of critical immune cells such as NK and T cells. Immunotherapies targeting these cells have the potential to alleviate the effects of senescence. One key factor contributing to the aging process is the activation of AMPK, a protein involved in nutrient sensing. Interestingly, inhibiting the activity of AMPK has been shown to enhance the performance of immune cells that have undergone age-related changes (Di Mitri et al. 2011). Additionally, targeting p38 signaling in aging CD8+ T cells can promote both their expansion and the function of mitochondria (Henson et al. 2014). The reduction of CD28 expression is a well-known feature of aging in CD8+ T cells, but increasing CD28 levels or stimulating T cell activation via alternative receptors may reverse this aging effect (Vicente et al. 2016). These findings highlight the importance of various immune cells in delaying diseases linked to the accumulation of SnC.

5.5 CONCLUSION

The role of cellular senescence in aging and related diseases is becoming increasingly apparent. Current research efforts focus on addressing cell aging and reducing its harmful effects. This chapter examines the key activators and distinguishing features of senescence while emphasizing therapeutic strategies known as senotherapeutics. These interventions are designed to either eliminate SnC (senolytics) or modify their phenotypic expression to achieve a stable, non-detrimental state (senomorphics). Furthermore, immunotherapy approaches have proven to be a promising method for promoting the removal of SnC, thereby alleviating disease-related symptoms. These treatment strategies have considerable potential to promote healthy aging and prevent the onset of age-related diseases. Although several senotherapeutics have shown positive results in preclinical trials with few or no adverse effects, comprehensive long-term studies are essential to fully understand their implications and ensure their safe and effective use in both the treatment and prevention of aging and age-related disorders.

REFERENCES

Ali, Ilyas, Hongliang Zhang, Syed Aqib Ali Zaidi, and Guangqian Zhou. 2024. "Understanding the intricacies of cellular senescence in atherosclerosis: Mechanisms and therapeutic implications." *Ageing Res Rev* 96: 102273. https://www.sciencedirect.com/science/article/pii/S1568163724000916.

Austad, Steven N. 2016. "The geroscience hypothesis: Is it possible to change the rate of aging?" *Adv Geroscience*: 1–36.

Aziz, N. A., and P. Weydt. 2018. "Telomere length as a modifier of age-at-onset in Huntington disease: A two-sample Mendelian randomization study." *J Neurol* 265 (9): 2149–2151. https://doi.org/10.1007/s00415-018-8972-y.

Baar, M. P., R. M. C. Brandt, D. A. Putavet, J. D. D. Klein, K. W. J. Derks, B. R. M. Bourgeois, S. Stryeck, Y. Rijksen, H. van Willigenburg, D. A. Feijtel, I. van der Pluijm, J. Essers, W. A. van Cappellen, IJcken W. F. van, A. B. Houtsmuller, J. Pothof, R. W. F. de Bruin, T. Madl, J. H. J. Hoeijmakers, J. Campisi, and P. L. J. de Keizer. 2017. "Targeted apoptosis of senescent cells restores tissue homeostasis in response to chemotoxicity and aging." *Cell* 169 (1): 132–147.e16. https://doi.org/10.1016/j.cell.2017.02.031.

Bae, Y. U., Y. Son, C. H. Kim, K. S. Kim, S. H. Hyun, H. G. Woo, B. A. Jee, J. H. Choi, H. K. Sung, H. C. Choi, S. Y. Park, J. H. Bae, K. O. Doh, and J. R. Kim. 2019. "Embryonic stem cell-derived mmu-miR-291a-3p inhibits cellular senescence in human dermal fibroblasts through the TGF-β receptor 2 pathway." *J Gerontol A Biol Sci Med Sci* 74 (9): 1359–1367. https://doi.org/10.1093/gerona/gly208.

Baker, Darren J., Bennett G. Childs, Matej Durik, Melinde E. Wijers, Cynthia J. Sieben, Jian Zhong, Rachel A. Saltness, Karthik B. Jeganathan, Grace Casaclang Verzosa, Abdulmohammad Pezeshki, Khashayarsha Khazaie, Jordan D. Miller, and Jan M. van Deursen. 2016. "Naturally occurring p16Ink4a-positive cells shorten healthy lifespan." *Nature* 530 (7589): 184–189. https://doi.org/10.1038/nature16932.

Banerjee, K., and H. Resat. 2016. "Constitutive activation of STAT3 in breast cancer cells: A review." *Int J Cancer* 138 (11): 2570–2578. https://doi.org/10.1002/ijc.29923.

Bao, R., C. J. Lai, D. G. Wang, H. Qu, L. Yin, B. Zifcak, X. Tao, J. Wang, R. Atoyan, M. Samson, J. Forrester, G. X. Xu, S. DellaRocca, M. Borek, H. X. Zhai, X. Cai, and C. Qian. 2009. "Targeting heat shock protein 90 with CUDC-305 overcomes erlotinib resistance in non-small cell lung cancer." *Mol Cancer Ther* 8 (12): 3296–3306. https://doi.org/10.1158/1535-7163.Mct-09-0538.

Birch, J., and J. Gil. 2020. "Senescence and the SASP: Many therapeutic avenues." *Genes Dev* 34 (23–24): 1565–1576. https://doi.org/10.1101/gad.343129.120.

Birger, A., I. Ben-Dor, M. Ottolenghi, T. Turetsky, Y. Gil, S. Sweetat, L. Perez, V. Belzer, N. Casden, D. Steiner, M. Izrael, E. Galun, E. Feldman, O. Behar, and B. Reubinoff. 2019. "Human iPSC-derived astrocytes from ALS patients with mutated C9ORF72 show increased oxidative stress and neurotoxicity." *EBioMedicine* 50: 274–289. https://doi.org/10.1016/j.ebiom.2019.11.026.

Cao, K., C. D. Blair, D. A. Faddah, J. E. Kieckhaefer, M. Olive, M. R. Erdos, E. G. Nabel, and F. S. Collins. 2011. "Progerin and telomere dysfunction collaborate to trigger cellular senescence in normal human fibroblasts." *J Clin Invest* 121 (7): 2833–2844. https://doi.org/10.1172/jci43578.

Chaib, Selim, Tamar Tchkonia, and James L. Kirkland. 2022. "Cellular senescence and senolytics: the path to the clinic." *Nat Med* 28 (8): 1556–1568. https://doi.org/10.1038/s41591-022-01923-y.

Chang, J., Y. Wang, L. Shao, R. M. Laberge, M. Demaria, J. Campisi, K. Janakiraman, N. E. Sharpless, S. Ding, W. Feng, Y. Luo, X. Wang, N. Aykin-Burns, K. Krager, U. Ponnappan, M. Hauer-Jensen, A. Meng, and D. Zhou. 2016. "Clearance of senescent cells by ABT263 rejuvenates aged hematopoietic stem cells in mice." *Nat Med* 22 (1): 78–83. https://doi.org/10.1038/nm.4010.

Chen, Mengmeng, Yushan Fu, Xu Wang, Ruitong Wu, Dongmei Su, Nan Zhou, and Yanhua Qi. 2022. "Metformin protects lens epithelial cells against senescence in a naturally aged mouse model." *Cell Death Discov* 8 (1): 8. https://doi.org/10.1038/s41420-021-00800-w.

Cherif, H., D. G. Bisson, P. Jarzem, M. Weber, J. A. Ouellet, and L. Haglund. 2019. "Curcumin and o-Vanillin exhibit evidence of senolytic activity in human IVD cells in vitro." *J Clin Med* 8 (4). https://doi.org/10.3390/jcm8040433.

Chiang, H. M., S. Y. Chan, Y. Chu, and K. C. Wen. 2015. "Fisetin ameliorated photodamage by suppressing the mitogen-activated protein kinase/matrix metalloproteinase pathway and nuclear factor-κB pathways." *J Agric Food Chem* 63 (18): 4551–4560. https://doi.org/10.1021/jf502500t.

Childs, B. G., M. Gluscevic, D. J. Baker, R. M. Laberge, D. Marquess, J. Dananberg, and J. M. van Deursen. 2017. "Senescent cells: An emerging target for diseases of ageing." *Nat Rev Drug Discov* 16 (10): 718–735. https://doi.org/10.1038/nrd.2017.116.

Chondrogianni, N., K. Voutetakis, M. Kapetanou, V. Delitsikou, N. Papaevgeniou, M. Sakellari, M. Lefaki, K. Filippopoulou, and E. S. Gonos. 2015. "Proteasome activation: An innovative promising approach for delaying aging and retarding age-related diseases." *Ageing Res Rev* 23 (Pt A): 37–55. https://doi.org/10.1016/j.arr.2014.12.003.

Di Mitri, D., R. I. Azevedo, S. M. Henson, V. Libri, N. E. Riddell, R. Macaulay, D. Kipling, M. V. Soares, L. Battistini, and A. N. Akbar. 2011. "Reversible senescence in human CD4+CD45RA+CD27- memory T cells." *J Immunol* 187 (5): 2093–2100. https://doi.org/10.4049/jimmunol.1100978.

Ding, J., K. Lohman, A. Molina, O. Delbono, A. Bertoni, S. Shea, W. Post, X. Guo, R. G. Barr, A. W. Manichaikul, J. S. Pankow, J. I. Rotter, I. Hoeschele, S. B. Kritchevsky, and Y. Liu. 2023. "The association between aging-related monocyte transcriptional networks and comorbidity burden: The Multi-Ethnic Study of Atherosclerosis (MESA)." *Geroscience* 45 (1): 197–207. https://doi.org/10.1007/s11357-022-00608-1.

Fausti, F., S. Di Agostino, M. Cioce, P. Bielli, C. Sette, P. P. Pandolfi, M. Oren, M. Sudol, S. Strano, and G. Blandino. 2013. "ATM kinase enables the functional axis of YAP, PML and p53 to ameliorate loss of Werner protein-mediated oncogenic senescence." *Cell Death Differ* 20 (11): 1498–509. https://doi.org/10.1038/cdd.2013.101.

Fielding, Roger A., Elizabeth J. Atkinson, Zaira Aversa, Thomas A. White, Amanda A. Heeren, Michelle M. Mielke, Steven R. Cummings, Marco Pahor, Christiaan Leeuwenburgh, and Nathan K. LeBrasseur. 2023. "Biomarkers of cellular senescence predict the onset of mobility disability and are reduced by physical activity in older adults." *J Gerontol: Series A* 79 (3). https://doi.org/10.1093/gerona/glad257.

Fuhrmann-Stroissnigg, Heike, Yuan Yuan Ling, Jing Zhao, Sara J. McGowan, Yi Zhu, Robert W. Brooks, Diego Grassi, Siobhan Q. Gregg, Jennifer L. Stripay, Akaitz Dorronsoro, Lana Corbo, Priscilla Tang, Christina Bukata, Nadja Ring, Mauro Giacca, Xuesen Li, Tamara Tchkonia, James L. Kirkland, Laura J. Niedernhofer, and Paul D. Robbins. 2017. "Identification of HSP90 inhibitors as a novel class of senolytics." *Nat Commun* 8 (1): 422. https://doi.org/10.1038/s41467-017-00314-z.

Garretti, F., D. Agalliu, C. S. Lindestam Arlehamn, A. Sette, and D. Sulzer. 2019. "Autoimmunity in parkinson's disease: The role of α-synuclein-specific T cells." *Front Immunol* 10: 303. https://doi.org/10.3389/fimmu.2019.00303.

Garrido, A. M., A. Kaistha, A. K. Uryga, S. Oc, K. Foote, A. Shah, A. Finigan, N. Figg, L. Dobnikar, H. Jørgensen, and M. Bennett. 2022. "Efficacy and limitations of senolysis in atherosclerosis." *Cardiovasc Res* 118 (7): 1713–1727. https://doi.org/10.1093/cvr/cvab208.

Gorska, M., U. Popowska, A. Sielicka-Dudzin, A. Kuban-Jankowska, W. Sawczuk, N. Knap, G. Cicero, and F. Wozniak. 2012. "Geldanamycin and its derivatives as Hsp90 inhibitors." *Front Biosci (Landmark Ed)* 17 (6): 2269–2277. https://doi.org/10.2741/4050.

Guerrero, A., N. Herranz, B. Sun, V. Wagner, S. Gallage, R. Guiho, K. Wolter, J. Pombo, E. E. Irvine, A. J. Innes, J. Birch, J. Glegola, S. Manshaei, D. Heide, G. Dharmalingam, J. Harbig, A. Olona, J. Behmoaras, D. Dauch, A. G. Uren, L. Zender, S. Vernia, J. P. Martínez-Barbera, M. Heikenwalder, D. J. Withers, and J. Gil. 2019. "Cardiac glycosides are broad-spectrum senolytics." *Nat Metab* 1 (11): 1074–1088. https://doi.org/10.1038/s42255-019-0122-z.

Guo, Jun, Xiuqing Huang, Lin Dou, Mingjing Yan, Tao Shen, Weiqing Tang, and Jian Li. 2022. "Aging and aging-related diseases: From molecular mechanisms to interventions and treatments." *Signal Transduct Target Ther* 7 (1): 391. https://doi.org/10.1038/s41392-022-01251-0.

Harman, D. 1956. "Aging: A theory based on free radical and radiation chemistry." *J Gerontol* 11 (3): 298–300. https://doi.org/10.1093/geronj/11.3.298.

Harrison, C. N., M. Talpaz, and A. J. Mead. 2016. "Ruxolitinib is effective in patients with intermediate-1 risk myelofibrosis: A summary of recent evidence." *Leuk Lymphoma* 57 (10): 2259–2267. https://doi.org/10.1080/10428194.2016.1195501.

He, Y., W. Xie, H. Li, H. Jin, Y. Zhang, and Y. Li. 2021. "Cellular senescence in sarcopenia: Possible mechanisms and therapeutic potential." *Front Cell Dev Biol* 9: 793088. https://doi.org/10.3389/fcell.2021.793088.

Henson, S. M., A. Lanna, N. E. Riddell, O. Franzese, R. Macaulay, S. J. Griffiths, D. J. Puleston, A. S. Watson, A. K. Simon, S. A. Tooze, and A. N. Akbar. 2014. "p38 signaling inhibits mTORC1-independent autophagy in senescent human CD8$^+$ T cells." *J Clin Invest* 124 (9): 4004–4016. https://doi.org/10.1172/jci75051.

Hernández Cordero, A. I., C. X. Yang, J. Yang, S. Horvath, T. Shaipanich, J. MacIsaac, D. T. S. Lin, M. S. Kobor, S. Guillemi, M. Harris, W. Lam, S. Lam, J. Montaner, S. F. P. Man, D. D. Sin, and J. M. Leung. 2022. "Airway aging and methylation disruptions in HIV-associated chronic obstructive pulmonary disease." *Am J Respir Crit Care Med* 206 (2): 150–160. https://doi.org/10.1164/rccm.202106-1440OC.

Horvath, S., P. Langfelder, S. Kwak, J. Aaronson, J. Rosinski, T. F. Vogt, M. Eszes, R. L. Faull, M. A. Curtis, H. J. Waldvogel, O. W. Choi, S. Tung, H. V. Vinters, G. Coppola, and X. W. Yang. 2016. "Huntington's disease accelerates epigenetic aging of human brain and disrupts DNA methylation levels." *Aging (Albany NY)* 8 (7): 1485–512. https://doi.org/10.18632/aging.101005.

Hu, B., S. Zhang, W. Liu, P. Wang, S. Chen, X. Lv, D. Shi, K. Ma, B. Wang, Y. Wu, and Z. Shao. 2020. "Inhibiting heat shock protein 90 protects nucleus pulposus-derived stem/progenitor cells from compression-induced necroptosis and apoptosis." *Front Cell Dev Biol* 8: 685. https://doi.org/10.3389/fcell.2020.00685.

Hu, C., J. Yang, Z. Qi, H. Wu, B. Wang, F. Zou, H. Mei, J. Liu, W. Wang, and Q. Liu. 2022. "Heat shock proteins: Biological functions, pathological roles, and therapeutic opportunities." *MedComm* (2020) 3 (3): e161. https://doi.org/10.1002/mco2.161.

Hubbard, B. P., and D. A. Sinclair. 2014. "Small molecule SIRT1 activators for the treatment of aging and age-related diseases." *Trends Pharmacol Sci* 35 (3): 146–154. https://doi.org/10.1016/j.tips.2013.12.004.

Jeon, Ok Hee, Chaekyu Kim, Remi-Martin Laberge, Marco Demaria, Sona Rathod, Alain P. Vasserot, Jae Wook Chung, Do Hun Kim, Yan Poon, and Nathaniel David. 2017. "Local clearance of senescent cells attenuates the development of post-traumatic osteoarthritis and creates a pro-regenerative environment." *Nat Med* 23 (6): 775–781.

Kalies, Katrin, Kai Knöpp, Leonie Wurmbrand, Laura Korte, Jochen Dutzmann, Claudia Pilowski, Susanne Koch, and Daniel Sedding. 2024. "Isolation of circulating endothelial cells provides tool to determine endothelial cell senescence in blood samples." *Sci Rep* 14 (1): 4271. https://doi.org/10.1038/s41598-024-54455-5.

Kallenbach, Julia, Golnaz Atri Roozbahani, Mehdi Heidari Horestani, and Aria Baniahmad. 2022. "Distinct mechanisms mediating therapy-induced cellular senescence in prostate cancer." *Cell Biosci* 12 (1): 200. https://doi.org/10.1186/s13578-022-00941-0.

Kang, H. T., J. T. Park, K. Choi, Y. Kim, H. J. C. Choi, C. W. Jung, Y. S. Lee, and S. C. Park. 2017. "Chemical screening identifies ATM as a target for alleviating senescence." *Nat Chem Biol* 13 (6): 616–623. https://doi.org/10.1038/nchembio.2342.

Kennedy, B. K., S. L. Berger, A. Brunet, J. Campisi, A. M. Cuervo, E. S. Epel, C. Franceschi, G. J. Lithgow, R. I. Morimoto, J. E. Pessin, T. A. Rando, A. Richardson, E. E. Schadt, T. Wyss-Coray, and F. Sierra. 2014. "Geroscience: Linking aging to chronic disease." *Cell* 159 (4): 709–713. https://doi.org/10.1016/j.cell.2014.10.039.

Kim, E. C., and J. R. Kim. 2019. "Senotherapeutics: Emerging strategy for healthy aging and age-related disease." *BMB Rep* 52 (1): 47–55. https://doi.org/10.5483/BMBRep.2019.52.1.293.

Kim, K. M., J. H. Noh, M. Bodogai, J. L. Martindale, X. Yang, F. E. Indig, S. K. Basu, K. Ohnuma, C. Morimoto, P. F. Johnson, A. Biragyn, K. Abdelmohsen, and M. Gorospe. 2017. "Identification of senescent cell surface targetable protein DPP4." *Genes Dev* 31 (15): 1529–1534. https://doi.org/10.1101/gad.302570.117.

Kim, Yeonju, Yeji Jang, Mi-Sung Kim, and Chanhee Kang. 2024. "Metabolic remodeling in cancer and senescence and its therapeutic implications." *Trends Endocrinol Metab* 35 (8): 732–744. https://doi.org/10.1016/j.tem.2024.02.008.

Kirkland, J. L., and T. Tchkonia. 2017. "Cellular senescence: A translational perspective." *EBioMedicine* 21: 21–28. https://doi.org/10.1016/j.ebiom.2017.04.013.

Kuilman, T., C. Michaloglou, L. C. Vredeveld, S. Douma, R. van Doorn, C. J. Desmet, L. A. Aarden, W. J. Mooi, and D. S. Peeper. 2008. "Oncogene-induced senescence relayed by an interleukin-dependent inflammatory network." *Cell* 133 (6): 1019–1031. https://doi.org/10.1016/j.cell.2008.03.039.

Kulkarni, A. S., S. Gubbi, and N. Barzilai. 2020. "Benefits of metformin in attenuating the hallmarks of aging." *Cell Metab* 32 (1): 15–30. https://doi.org/10.1016/j.cmet.2020.04.001.

Lagoumtzi, S. M., and N. Chondrogianni. 2021. "Senolytics and senomorphics: Natural and synthetic therapeutics in the treatment of aging and chronic diseases." *Free Radic Biol Med* 171: 169–190. https://doi.org/10.1016/j.freeradbiomed.2021.05.003.

Lamming, D. W., L. Ye, D. M. Sabatini, and J. A. Baur. 2013. "Rapalogs and mTOR inhibitors as anti-aging therapeutics." *J Clin Invest* 123 (3): 980–989. https://doi.org/10.1172/jci64099.

Lee, K., A. C. Thwin, C. M. Nadel, E. Tse, S. N. Gates, J. E. Gestwicki, and D. R. Southworth. 2021. "The structure of an Hsp90-immunophilin complex reveals cochaperone recognition of the client maturation state." *Mol Cell* 81 (17): 3496–3508.e5. https://doi.org/10.1016/j.molcel.2021.07.023.

Lee, S. J., Y. S. Jung, M. H. Yoon, S. M. Kang, A. Y. Oh, J. H. Lee, S. Y. Jun, T. G. Woo, H. Y. Chun, S. K. Kim, K. J. Chung, H. Y. Lee, K. Lee, G. Jin, M. K. Na, N. C. Ha, C. Bárcena, J. M. Freije, C. López-Otín, G. Y. Song, and B. J. Park. 2016. "Interruption of progerin-lamin A/C binding ameliorates Hutchinson-Gilford progeria syndrome phenotype." *J Clin Invest* 126 (10): 3879–3893. https://doi.org/10.1172/jci84164.

Liang, Jie, Masayuki Nagahashi, Eugene Y. Kim, Kuzhuvelil B. Harikumar, Akimitsu Yamada, Wei-Ching Huang, Nitai C. Hait, Jeremy C. Allegood, Megan M. Price, Dorit Avni, Kazuaki Takabe, Tomasz Kordula, Sheldon Milstien, and Sarah Spiegel. 2013. "Sphingosine-1-phosphate links persistent STAT3 activation, chronic intestinal inflammation, and development of colitis-associated cancer." *Cancer Cell* 23 (1): 107–120. https://www.sciencedirect.com/science/article/pii/S1535610812004928.

Liu, P., H. Zhao, and Y. Luo. 2017. "Anti-aging implications of astragalus membranaceus (Huangqi): A well-known Chinese tonic." *Aging Dis* 8 (6): 868–886. https://doi.org/10.14336/ad.2017.0816.

López-Otín, C., M. A. Blasco, L. Partridge, M. Serrano, and G. Kroemer. 2013. "The hallmarks of aging." *Cell* 153 (6): 1194–1217. https://doi.org/10.1016/j.cell.2013.05.039.

Lu, X. A., X. Wang, W. Zhuo, L. Jia, Y. Jiang, Y. Fu, and Y. Luo. 2014. "The regulatory mechanism of a client kinase controlling its own release from Hsp90 chaperone machinery through phosphorylation." *Biochem J* 457 (1): 171–183. https://doi.org/10.1042/bj20130963.

Machiela, E., and A. L. Southwell. 2020. "Biological aging and the cellular pathogenesis of huntington's disease." *J Huntingtons Dis* 9 (2): 115–128. https://doi.org/10.3233/jhd-200395.

McHugh, D., and J. Gil. 2018. "Senescence and aging: Causes, consequences, and therapeutic avenues." *J Cell Biol* 217 (1): 65–77. https://doi.org/10.1083/jcb.201708092.

Melo Pereira, S., R. Ribeiro, and E. Logarinho. 2019. "Approaches towards longevity: reprogramming, senolysis, and improved mitotic competence as anti-aging therapies." *Int J Mol Sci* 20 (4). https://doi.org/10.3390/ijms20040938.

Mielczarek-Lewandowska, A., M. L. Hartman, and M. Czyz. 2020. "Inhibitors of HSP90 in melanoma." *Apoptosis* 25 (1–2): 12–28. https://doi.org/10.1007/s10495-019-01577-1.

Milanovic, M., D. N. Y. Fan, D. Belenki, J. H. M. Däbritz, Z. Zhao, Y. Yu, J. R. Dörr, L. Dimitrova, D. Lenze, I. A. Monteiro Barbosa, M. A. Mendoza-Parra, T. Kanashova, M. Metzner, K. Pardon, M. Reimann, A. Trumpp, B. Dörken, J. Zuber, H. Gronemeyer, M. Hummel, G. Dittmar, S. Lee, and C. A. Schmitt. 2018. "Senescence-associated reprogramming promotes cancer stemness." *Nature* 553 (7686): 96–100. https://doi.org/10.1038/nature25167.

Miura, Yugo, Kentaro Endo, Keiichiro Komori, and Ichiro Sekiya. 2022. "Clearance of senescent cells with ABT-263 improves biological functions of synovial mesenchymal stem cells from osteoarthritis patients." *Stem Cell Res Ther* 13 (1): 222. https://doi.org/10.1186/s13287-022-02901-4.

Moiseeva, O., X. Deschênes-Simard, E. St-Germain, S. Igelmann, G. Huot, A. E. Cadar, V. Bourdeau, M. N. Pollak, and G. Ferbeyre. 2013. "Metformin inhibits the senescence-associated secretory phenotype by interfering with IKK/NF-κB activation." *Aging Cell* 12 (3): 489–498. https://doi.org/10.1111/acel.12075.

Muñoz-Espín, D., M. Cañamero, A. Maraver, G. Gómez-López, J. Contreras, S. Murillo-Cuesta, A. Rodríguez-Baeza, I. Varela-Nieto, J. Ruberte, M. Collado, and M. Serrano. 2013. "Programmed cell senescence during mammalian embryonic development." *Cell* 155 (5): 1104–1118. https://doi.org/10.1016/j.cell.2013.10.019.

Muñoz-Espín, Daniel, and Manuel Serrano. 2014. "Cellular senescence: From physiology to pathology." *Nat Rev Mol Cell Bio* 15 (7): 482–496. https://doi.org/10.1038/nrm3823.

Mylonas, A., and A. O'Loghlen. 2022. "Cellular senescence and ageing: Mechanisms and interventions." *Front Aging* 3: 866718. https://doi.org/10.3389/fragi.2022.866718.

Nakamura, S., and T. Yoshimori. 2018. "Autophagy and longevity." *Mol Cells* 41 (1): 65–72. https://doi.org/10.14348/molcells.2018.2333.

Niedernhofer, L. J., and P. D. Robbins. 2018. "Senotherapeutics for healthy ageing." *Nat Rev Drug Discov* 17 (5): 377. https://doi.org/10.1038/nrd.2018.44.

Novakova, Z., S. Hubackova, M. Kosar, L. Janderova-Rossmeislova, J. Dobrovolna, P. Vasicova, M. Vancurova, Z. Horejsi, P. Hozak, J. Bartek, and Z. Hodny. 2010. "Cytokine expression and signaling in drug-induced cellular senescence." *Oncogene* 29 (2): 273–284. https://doi.org/10.1038/onc.2009.318.

Pal, H. C., M. Athar, C. A. Elmets, and F. Afaq. 2015. "Fisetin inhibits UVB-induced cutaneous inflammation and activation of PI3K/AKT/NFκB signaling pathways in SKH-1 hairless mice." *Photochem Photobiol* 91 (1): 225–234. https://doi.org/10.1111/php.12337.

Park, J., and D. W. Shin. 2022. "Senotherapeutics and their molecular mechanism for improving aging." *Biomol Ther (Seoul)* 30 (6): 490–500. https://doi.org/10.4062/biomolther.2022.114.

Russo, T., and M. Riessland. 2022. "Age-related midbrain inflammation and senescence in parkinson's disease." *Front Aging Neurosci* 14: 917797. https://doi.org/10.3389/fnagi.2022.917797.

Salminen, A. 2021. "Immunosuppressive network promotes immunosenescence associated with aging and chronic inflammatory conditions." *J Mol Med (Berl)* 99 (11): 1553–1569. https://doi.org/10.1007/s00109-021-02123-w.

Samaraweera, L., A. Adomako, A. Rodriguez-Gabin, and H. M. McDaid. 2017. "A novel indication for panobinostat as a senolytic drug in NSCLC and HNSCC." *Sci Rep* 7 (1): 1900. https://doi.org/10.1038/s41598-017-01964-1.

Sang, Q., X. Liu, L. Wang, L. Qi, W. Sun, W. Wang, Y. Sun, and H. Zhang. 2018. "Curcumin protects an SH-SY5Y cell model of parkinson's disease against toxic injury by regulating HSP90." *Cell Physiol Biochem* 51 (2): 681–691. https://doi.org/10.1159/000495326.

Schmitt, Clemens A., Boshi Wang, and Marco Demaria. 2022. "Senescence and cancer—role and therapeutic opportunities." *Nat Rev Clinl Oncol* 19 (10): 619–636. https://doi.org/10.1038/s41571-022-00668-4.

Shao, J., J. Liu, and S. Zuo. 2022. "Roles of epigenetics in cardiac fibroblast activation and fibrosis." *Cells* 11 (15). https://doi.org/10.3390/cells11152347.

Sharma, A. K., R. L. Roberts, R. D. Benson, Jr., J. L. Pierce, K. Yu, M. W. Hamrick, and M. E. McGee-Lawrence. 2020. "The senolytic drug navitoclax (ABT-263) causes trabecular bone loss and impaired osteoprogenitor function in aged mice." *Front Cell Dev Biol* 8: 354. https://doi.org/10.3389/fcell.2020.00354.

Si, H., and D. Liu. 2014. "Dietary antiaging phytochemicals and mechanisms associated with prolonged survival." *J Nutr Biochem* 25 (6): 581–591. https://doi.org/10.1016/j.jnutbio.2014.02.001.

Sierra, F. 2016. "The emergence of geroscience as an interdisciplinary approach to the enhancement of health span and life span." *Cold Spring Harb Perspect Med* 6 (4): a025163. https://doi.org/10.1101/cshperspect.a025163.

Soto-Gamez, A., and M. Demaria. 2017. "Therapeutic interventions for aging: The case of cellular senescence." *Drug Discov Today* 22 (5): 786–795. https://doi.org/10.1016/j.drudis.2017.01.004.

Surmachevska, N., and J. Rubio. 2023. "Senescence in osteoarthritis: Overview of mechanisms and therapeutics." *Eur J Rheumatol* 11 (Suppl 1): S3–6. https://doi.org/10.5152/eurjrheum.2023.22077.

Tang, X., P. H. Li, and H. Z. Chen. 2020. "Cardiomyocyte senescence and cellular communications within myocardial microenvironments." *Front Endocrinol (Lausanne)* 11: 280. https://doi.org/10.3389/fendo.2020.00280.

Tchkonia, T., A. K. Palmer, and J. L. Kirkland. 2021. "New horizons: Novel approaches to enhance healthspan through targeting cellular senescence and related aging mechanisms." *J Clin Endocrinol Metab* 106 (3): e1481–e1487. https://doi.org/10.1210/clinem/dgaa728.

Tilstra, J. S., C. L. Clauson, L. J. Niedernhofer, and P. D. Robbins. 2011. "NF-κB in aging and disease." *Aging Dis* 2 (6): 449–465.

Tilstra, J. S., A. R. Robinson, J. Wang, S. Q. Gregg, C. L. Clauson, D. P. Reay, L. A. Nasto, C. M. St Croix, A. Usas, N. Vo, J. Huard, P. R. Clemens, D. B. Stolz, D. C. Guttridge, S. C. Watkins, G. A. Garinis, Y. Wang, L. J. Niedernhofer, and P. D. Robbins. 2012. "NF-κB inhibition delays DNA damage-induced senescence and aging in mice." *J Clin Invest* 122 (7): 2601–2612. https://doi.org/10.1172/jci45785.

Toso, A., A. Revandkar, D. Di Mitri, I. Guccini, M. Proietti, M. Sarti, S. Pinton, J. Zhang, M. Kalathur, G. Civenni, D. Jarrossay, E. Montani, C. Marini, R. Garcia-Escudero, E. Scanziani, F. Grassi, P. P. Pandolfi, C. V. Catapano, and A. Alimonti. 2014. "Enhancing chemotherapy efficacy in Pten-deficient prostate tumors by activating the senescence-associated antitumor immunity." *Cell Rep* 9 (1): 75–89. https://doi.org/10.1016/j.celrep.2014.08.044.

Tovar, C., B. Graves, K. Packman, Z. Filipovic, B. Higgins, M. Xia, C. Tardell, R. Garrido, E. Lee, K. Kolinsky, K. H. To, M. Linn, F. Podlaski, P. Wovkulich, B. Vu, and L. T. Vassilev. 2013. "MDM2 small-molecule antagonist RG7112 activates p53 signaling and regresses human tumors in preclinical cancer models." *Cancer Res* 73 (8): 2587–2597. https://doi.org/10.1158/0008-5472.Can-12-2807.

Triana-Martínez, F., P. Picallos-Rabina, S. Da Silva-Álvarez, F. Pietrocola, S. Llanos, V. Rodilla, E. Soprano, P. Pedrosa, A. Ferreirós, M. Barradas, F. Hernández-González, M. Lalinde, N. Prats, C. Bernadó, P. González, M. Gómez, M. P. Ikonomopoulou, P. J. Fernández-Marcos, T. García-Caballero, P. Del Pino, J. Arribas, A. Vidal, M. González-Barcia, M. Serrano, M. I. Loza, E. Domínguez, and M. Collado. 2019. "Identification and characterization of cardiac glycosides as senolytic compounds." *Nat Commun* 10 (1): 4731. https://doi.org/10.1038/s41467-019-12888-x.

Valieva, Y., E. Ivanova, A. Fayzullin, A. Kurkov, and A. Igrunkova. 2022. "Senescence-associated β-galactosidase detection in pathology." *Diagnostics (Basel)* 12 (10). https://doi.org/10.3390/diagnostics12102309.

van Deursen, Jan M. 2014. "The role of senescent cells in ageing." *Nature* 509 (7501): 439–446. https://doi.org/10.1038/nature13193.

Vicente, R., A. L. Mausset-Bonnefont, C. Jorgensen, P. Louis-Plence, and J. M. Brondello. 2016. "Cellular senescence impact on immune cell fate and function." *Aging Cell* 15 (3): 400–406. https://doi.org/10.1111/acel.12455.

Wagner, K. D., and N. Wagner. 2022. "The senescence markers p16INK4A, p14ARF/p19ARF, and p21 in organ development and homeostasis." *Cells* 11 (12). https://doi.org/10.3390/cells11121966.

Wakita, Masahiro, Akiko Takahashi, Osamu Sano, Tze Mun Loo, Yoshinori Imai, Megumi Narukawa, Hidehisa Iwata, Tatsuyuki Matsudaira, Shimpei Kawamoto, Naoko Ohtani, Tamotsu Yoshimori, and Eiji Hara. 2020. "A BET family protein degrader provokes senolysis by targeting NHEJ and autophagy in senescent cells." *Nat Commun* 11 (1): 1935. https://doi.org/10.1038/s41467-020-15719-6.

Wang, Y., J. Chang, X. Liu, X. Zhang, S. Zhang, X. Zhang, D. Zhou, and G. Zheng. 2016. "Discovery of piperlongumine as a potential novel lead for the development of senolytic agents." *Aging (Albany NY)* 8 (11): 2915–2926. https://doi.org/10.18632/aging.101100.

Waugh, D. J., and C. Wilson. 2008. "The interleukin-8 pathway in cancer." *Clin Cancer Res* 14 (21): 6735–6741. https://doi.org/10.1158/1078-0432.Ccr-07-4843.

Wiley, C. D., N. Schaum, F. Alimirah, J. A. Lopez-Dominguez, A. V. Orjalo, G. Scott, P. Y. Desprez, C. Benz, A. R. Davalos, and J. Campisi. 2018. "Small-molecule MDM2 antagonists attenuate the senescence-associated secretory phenotype." *Sci Rep* 8 (1): 2410. https://doi.org/10.1038/s41598-018-20000-4.

Wissler Gerdes, E. O., Y. Zhu, T. Tchkonia, and J. L. Kirkland. 2020. "Discovery, development, and future application of senolytics: Theories and predictions." *FEBS J* 287 (12): 2418–2427. https://doi.org/10.1111/febs.15264.

Xiao, S., D. Qin, X. Hou, L. Tian, Y. Yu, R. Zhang, H. Lyu, D. Guo, X. Z. Chen, C. Zhou, and J. Tang. 2023. "Cellular senescence: A double-edged sword in cancer therapy." *Front Oncol* 13: 1189015. https://doi.org/10.3389/fonc.2023.1189015.

Xie, S., S. C. Xu, W. Deng, and Q. Tang. 2023. "Metabolic landscape in cardiac aging: Insights into molecular biology and therapeutic implications." *Signal Transduct Target Ther* 8 (1): 114. https://doi.org/10.1038/s41392-023-01378-8.

Xu, M., A. K. Palmer, H. Ding, M. M. Weivoda, T. Pirtskhalava, T. A. White, A. Sepe, K. O. Johnson, M. B. Stout, N. Giorgadze, M. D. Jensen, N. K. LeBrasseur, T. Tchkonia, and J. L. Kirkland. 2015. "Targeting senescent cells enhances adipogenesis and metabolic function in old age." *Elife* 4: e12997. https://doi.org/10.7554/eLife.12997.

Xu, M., T. Pirtskhalava, J. N. Farr, B. M. Weigand, A. K. Palmer, M. M. Weivoda, C. L. Inman, M. B. Ogrodnik, C. M. Hachfeld, D. G. Fraser, J. L. Onken, K. O. Johnson, G. C. Verzosa, L. G. P. Langhi, M. Weigl, N. Giorgadze, N. K. LeBrasseur, J. D. Miller, D. Jurk, R. J. Singh, D. B. Allison, K. Ejima, G. B. Hubbard, Y. Ikeno, H. Cubro, V. D. Garovic, X. Hou, S. J. Weroha, P. D. Robbins, L. J. Niedernhofer, S. Khosla, T. Tchkonia, and J. L. Kirkland. 2018. "Senolytics improve physical function and increase lifespan in old age." *Nat Med* 24 (8): 1246–1256. https://doi.org/10.1038/s41591-018-0092-9.

Xu, M., T. Tchkonia, H. Ding, M. Ogrodnik, E. R. Lubbers, T. Pirtskhalava, T. A. White, K. O. Johnson, M. B. Stout, V. Mezera, N. Giorgadze, M. D. Jensen, N. K. LeBrasseur, and J. L. Kirkland. 2015. "JAK inhibition alleviates the cellular senescence-associated secretory phenotype and frailty in old age." *Proc Natl Acad Sci U S A* 112 (46): E6301–6310. https://doi.org/10.1073/pnas.1515386112.

Yamazaki, Y., D. J. Baker, M. Tachibana, C. C. Liu, J. M. van Deursen, T. G. Brott, G. Bu, and T. Kanekiyo. 2016. "Vascular cell senescence contributes to blood-brain barrier breakdown." *Stroke* 47 (4): 1068–1077. https://doi.org/10.1161/strokeaha.115.010835.

Yang, Jennifer H., Annalise E. Miner, Ashley Fair, Revere Kinkel, and Jennifer S. Graves. 2024. "Senescence marker p16INK4a expression in patients with multiple sclerosis."

Mult Scler Relat Disord 84: 105498. https://www.sciencedirect.com/science/article/pii/S2211034824000774.

Yin, Hao, and J. Geoffrey Pickering. 2023. "Telomere length: Implications for atherogenesis." *Curr Atheroscler Rep* 25 (3): 95–103. https://doi.org/10.1007/s11883-023-01082-6.

Yosef, R., N. Pilpel, R. Tokarsky-Amiel, A. Biran, Y. Ovadya, S. Cohen, E. Vadai, L. Dassa, E. Shahar, R. Condiotti, I. Ben-Porath, and V. Krizhanovsky. 2016. "Directed elimination of senescent cells by inhibition of BCL-W and BCL-XL." *Nat Commun* 7: 11190. https://doi.org/10.1038/ncomms11190.

Yousefzadeh, M. J., Y. Zhu, S. J. McGowan, L. Angelini, H. Fuhrmann-Stroissnigg, M. Xu, Y. Y. Ling, K. I. Melos, T. Pirtskhalava, C. L. Inman, C. McGuckian, E. A. Wade, J. I. Kato, D. Grassi, M. Wentworth, C. E. Burd, E. A. Arriaga, W. L. Ladiges, T. Tchkonia, J. L. Kirkland, P. D. Robbins, and L. J. Niedernhofer. 2018. "Fisetin is a senotherapeutic that extends health and lifespan." *EBioMedicine* 36: 18–28. https://doi.org/10.1016/j.ebiom.2018.09.015.

Yun, S. P., Y. S. Han, J. H. Lee, S. M. Kim, and S. H. Lee. 2018. "Melatonin rescues mesenchymal stem cells from senescence induced by the uremic toxin p-cresol via inhibiting mTOR-dependent autophagy." *Biomol Ther (Seoul)* 26 (4): 389–398. https://doi.org/10.4062/biomolther.2017.071.

Zhang, C., Y. Xie, H. Chen, L. Lv, J. Yao, M. Zhang, K. Xia, X. Feng, Y. Li, X. Liang, X. Sun, C. Deng, and G. Liu. 2020. "FOXO4-DRI alleviates age-related testosterone secretion insufficiency by targeting senescent Leydig cells in aged mice." *Aging (Albany NY)* 12 (2): 1272–1284. https://doi.org/10.18632/aging.102682.

Zhang, L., L. E. Pitcher, V. Prahalad, L. J. Niedernhofer, and P. D. Robbins. 2023. "Targeting cellular senescence with senotherapeutics: Senolytics and senomorphics." *FEBS J* 290 (5): 1362–1383. https://doi.org/10.1111/febs.16350.

Zhang, L., P. Yang, J. Chen, Z. Chen, Z. Liu, G. Feng, F. Sha, Z. Li, Z. Xu, Y. Huang, X. Shi, X. Li, J. Cui, C. Zhang, P. Fan, L. Cui, Y. Shen, G. Zhou, H. Jing, and S. Ma. 2023. "CD44 connects autophagy decline and ageing in the vascular endothelium." *Nat Commun* 14 (1): 5524. https://doi.org/10.1038/s41467-023-41346-y.

Zhang, P., Y. Kishimoto, I. Grammatikakis, K. Gottimukkala, R. G. Cutler, S. Zhang, K. Abdelmohsen, V. A. Bohr, J. Misra Sen, M. Gorospe, and M. P. Mattson. 2019. "Senolytic therapy alleviates Aβ-associated oligodendrocyte progenitor cell senescence and cognitive deficits in an Alzheimer's disease model." *Nat Neurosci* 22 (5): 719–728. https://doi.org/10.1038/s41593-019-0372-9.

Zhang, Xin, Suping Zhang, Xingui Liu, Yingying Wang, Jianhui Chang, Xuan Zhang, Samuel G. Mackintosh, Alan J. Tackett, Yonghan He, Dongwen Lv, Dongwen Lv, Remi-Martin Laberge, Judith Campisi, Jianrong Wang, Guangrong Zheng, and Daohong Zhou. 2018. "Oxidation resistance 1 is a novel senolytic target." *Aging Cell* 17 (4): e12780. https://doi.org/10.1111/acel.12780.

Zhang, Yinan, Jeffrey Atkinson, Christin E. Burd, Jennifer Graves, and Benjamin M. Segal. 2023. "Biological aging in multiple sclerosis." *Mult Scler J* 29 (14): 1701–1708. https://doi.org/10.1177/13524585231204122.

Zhang, Yong, Yinhui Dong, Michael W. Melkus, Shutao Yin, Su-Ni Tang, Peixin Jiang, Kartick Pramanik, Wei Wu, Sangyub Kim, and Min Ye. 2018. "Role of P53-senescence induction in suppression of LNCaP prostate cancer growth by cardiotonic compound bufalin." *Mol Cancer Ther* 17 (11): 2341–2352. https://doi.org/10.1158/1535-7163.MCT-17-1296.

Zhang, Zhao, Ji Jing, Youqiong Ye, Zhiao Chen, Ying Jing, Shengli Li, Wei Hong, Hang Ruan, Yaoming Liu, Qingsong Hu, Jun Wang, Wenbo Li, Chunru Lin, Lixia Diao, Yubin Zhou, and Leng Han. 2020. "Characterization of the dual functional effects of heat shock proteins (HSPs) in cancer hallmarks to aid development of HSP inhibitors." *Genome Med* 12 (1): 101. https://doi.org/10.1186/s13073-020-00795-6.

Zheng, L., S. He, H. Wang, J. Li, Y. Liu, and S. Liu. 2024. "Targeting cellular senescence in aging and age-related diseases: Challenges, considerations, and the emerging role of senolytic and senomorphic therapies." *Aging Dis*. https://doi.org/10.14336/ad.2024.0206.

Zhu, Y., E. J. Doornebal, T. Pirtskhalava, N. Giorgadze, M. Wentworth, H. Fuhrmann-Stroissnigg, L. J. Niedernhofer, P. D. Robbins, T. Tchkonia, and J. L. Kirkland. 2017. "New agents that target senescent cells: The flavone, fisetin, and the BCL-X(L) inhibitors, A1331852 and A1155463." *Aging (Albany NY)* 9 (3): 955–963. https://doi.org/10.18632/aging.101202.

Zhu, Y., T. Tchkonia, H. Fuhrmann-Stroissnigg, H. M. Dai, Y. Y. Ling, M. B. Stout, T. Pirtskhalava, N. Giorgadze, K. O. Johnson, C. B. Giles, J. D. Wren, L. J. Niedernhofer, P. D. Robbins, and J. L. Kirkland. 2016. "Identification of a novel senolytic agent, navitoclax, targeting the Bcl-2 family of anti-apoptotic factors." *Aging Cell* 15 (3): 428–35. https://doi.org/10.1111/acel.12445.

Zhu, Y., T. Tchkonia, T. Pirtskhalava, A. C. Gower, H. Ding, N. Giorgadze, A. K. Palmer, Y. Ikeno, G. B. Hubbard, M. Lenburg, S. P. O'Hara, N. F. LaRusso, J. D. Miller, C. M. Roos, G. C. Verzosa, N. K. LeBrasseur, J. D. Wren, J. N. Farr, S. Khosla, M. B. Stout, S. J. McGowan, H. Fuhrmann-Stroissnigg, A. U. Gurkar, J. Zhao, D. Colangelo, A. Dorronsoro, Y. Y. Ling, A. S. Barghouthy, D. C. Navarro, T. Sano, P. D. Robbins, L. J. Niedernhofer, and J. L. Kirkland. 2015. "The Achilles' heel of senescent cells: from transcriptome to senolytic drugs." *Aging Cell* 14 (4): 644–658. https://doi.org/10.1111/acel.12344.

Chapter 6

An Emerging Approach of Senotherapeutics for the Treatment of Lung Disorders

Molecular Mechanisms and Therapeutic Potential

Anwar A. Alghamdi, Aftab Ahmad, Muhammad Afzal, Mohammad Jaffar Sadiq Mantargi, Shah Alam Khan, and Asif Husain

6.1 INTRODUCTION

Senotherapeutics targeted at senescent cells have surfaced as prospective therapeutic interventions for diverse pulmonary disorders. The irreversible cessation of the cell cycle is termed cellular senescence, which contributes to aging and associated illnesses such as chronic obstructive pulmonary disorder (COPD), idiopathic pulmonary fibrosis, and asthma. The accumulation of senescent cells triggers the release of proinflammatory cytokines, chemokines, and proteases, resulting in the senescence-associated secretory phenotype (SASP), which plays a role in the development of chronic pulmonary illnesses.

Senolytics like fenofibrate selectively induce apoptosis, making them potential therapeutic agents. Studies using INK-ATTAC mouse models have demonstrated that removing senescent cells can increase health span and delay carcinogenesis by lowering proinflammatory cytokines, which are high in case of lung disorders (Schafer et al. 2017b).

However, study of adverse drug reactions and long-term impacts are critical for avoiding off-target effects and toxicities. Their heterogenicity limits developing a universal senotherapeutics treatment, calling for a thorough characterization of senescent cells. The current treatment rarely provides improvements rather than treating the underlying causes, pressing the need for novel, effective therapy. Further, the interaction between immune cells and senescence adds more difficulties of creating tailored senotherapeutics for lung disorders. However, despite these challenges, the development of senotherapeutics in recent years has shown promising outcomes overcoming the obstacles faced by patients with chronic pulmonary disorders.

DOI: 10.1201/9781003493969-6

6.2 EPIDEMIOLOGY OF SENESCENT CELL–INDUCED LUNG DISORDERS

Research pertaining to senescent cells in pulmonary pathologies is progressively expanding, yielding considerable ramifications for comprehending and managing chronic respiratory ailments. Senescent cells, defined as those that have permanently ceased to proliferate and exhibit a proinflammatory secretory phenotype, accumulate within the pulmonary system as individuals age, thereby contributing to a spectrum of pulmonary diseases.

1. As an individual's age progresses, senescent cells accumulate in the epithelial, endothelial, fibroblastic, and immunological regions of the lung. This accumulation is particularly pronounced in patients with chronic pulmonary disorders such as COPD and IPF, which are prevalent illnesses.
2. The frequency of chronic respiratory conditions, such as COPD and interstitial lung diseases including pulmonary fibrosis and pneumonia, increases with age. Senescent cells in lung tissues are believed to significantly contribute to the rising prevalence of these illnesses. Senescent cells have been identified in the aging lung and the compromised lungs of persons with lung fibrosis and COPD, affecting bronchial and alveolar epithelial cells, along with mesenchymal and vascular cells (Bartling 2013).
3. Mechanisms and consequences: Senescent cells contribute to pulmonary illnesses by several methods, including the secretion of pro-inflammatory cytokines, chemokines, and other inflammatory mediators. The SASP can provoke persistent inflammation and tissue damage. Furthermore, oxidative stress resulting from environmental factors, such as cigarette smoke, triggers cellular senescence, hence aggravating lung injury (Bezerra et al. 2023). Cellular senescence not only diminishes lung function but also facilitates the advancement of chronic respiratory illnesses. Consequently, comprehending the processes of oxidative stress and its effects on pulmonary health is essential for formulating successful therapeutic approaches.
4. Therapeutic implications: The selective targeting of senescent cells is a viable treatment strategy for chronic lung illnesses. Senescent cells signify a prospective therapeutic strategy for lung illnesses associated with cigarette smoke exposure (Mikawa et al. 2020). Currently, senolytic or senotherapeutic agents that specifically target and eradicate senescent cells are under investigation.
5. Alongside age-related chronic pulmonary illnesses, there is growing interest in the influence of cellular senescence on the advancement of chronic lung disorders that may manifest in childhood or even during the neonatal period (Liu Z et al. 2024).

The accumulation of senescent cells in the pulmonary system substantially influences the epidemiology of chronic lung diseases, facilitating disease development through ongoing inflammation and tissue deterioration. The targeted eradication of these cells may enable the advancement of innovative treatment strategies for managing and treating these illnesses.

6.3 CLASSIFICATION OF SENESCENT CELL–INDUCED LUNG DISORDERS

Senescent cells have been associated with a plethora of pulmonary disorders, encompassing both chronic and developmental lung pathologies.

6.3.1 Chronic Disorders of the Respiratory System

- *Chronic obstructive pulmonary disease* (COPD): Individuals with COPD have demonstrated a significant rise in the incidence of senescent cells inside their pulmonary tissues.

  The elevation of senescence markers in the pneumocytes of individuals with COPD indicates that senescent pneumocytes may contribute to the pathophysiology of this condition (Bartling 2013). Furthermore, senescent cells are found to accumulate within the epithelial, endothelial, fibroblastic, and immunological compartments of the pulmonary system in these patients (Liu et al. 2022).
- *Idiopathic pulmonary fibrosis* (IPF): Similar to COPD, individuals suffering from IPF exhibit a significant accumulation of senescent cells within their lung tissues. The heightened levels of senescence markers in the pneumocytes of IPF patients suggest a potential involvement of these cells in the disease mechanism. Senescent cells in pulmonary tissue substantially contribute to the heightened incidence of pulmonary diseases, including IPF (Bartling 2013).
- *Pulmonary arterial hypertension* (PAH): In patients with PAH, there is an observed elevation in the levels of cytokines, chemokines, and other inflammatory mediators, which are closely associated with clinical outcomes. The accumulation of senescent cells within various lung compartments is recognized as a pivotal factor in the pathogenesis of this disease (Liu et al. 2022).
- *Emphysema*: The prevalence of senescent cells within the airways and lung parenchyma increases with advancing age, particularly within regions affected by age-related pulmonary diseases such as emphysema (Campisi 2016)

6.3.2 Developmental Lung Disorders: Bronchopulmonary Dysplasia

Cellular senescence has been studied in relation to the onset of pulmonary issues that often emerge during childhood or the neonatal period. Bronchopulmonary dysplasia (BPD) is a specific disorder where the implications of cellular senescence are currently under investigation (Liu et al. 2024).

Senescent cells are implicated in a diverse array of pulmonary disorders, inclusive of chronic conditions such as COPD, IPF, PAH, and emphysema, as well as developmental disorders such as BPD. Senescent cells in lung tissues greatly contribute to the etiology and progression of these disorders (Sugimoto 2024; Mikawa et al. 2020). Innovative therapeutic strategies aimed at restoring pulmonary function and improving patient outcomes may emerge from comprehending the mechanisms that govern the growth of senescent cells. Researchers seek to enhance tissue repair mechanisms and mitigate the adverse effects of these cells by targeted investigation.

6.4 PATHOPHYSIOLOGY OF SENESCENT CELL–INDUCED LUNG DISORDERS

Senescent cells are implicated in the etiology of pulmonary disorders through a multitude of mechanisms.

Cellular senescence, characterized by the SASP, is a state defined by the irreversible cessation of the cell cycle induced by many stressors. As individuals age, senescent cells accumulate in various mammalian tissues, particularly within the pulmonary system, and are especially abundant in areas impacted by age-related disorders such as emphysema and COPD (Campisi 2016).

Senescent cells facilitate the progression of pulmonary diseases through numerous approaches.

1. *Chronic inflammation*: Senescent cells secrete proinflammatory proteases, chemokines, and cytokines, which initiate chronic inflammation and facilitate tissue remodeling. The inflammatory microenvironment is essential in the pathogenesis of conditions such as COPD and IPF (Parikh et al. 2019).
2. *Fibrosis*: In pathologies such as IPF, senescent cells are instrumental in interstitial remodeling and fibrosis, which culminates in compromised pulmonary function. The detection of senescence markers within IPF lung tissues, coupled with the restoration of pulmonary health in aged murine models post-senescence cell ablation, underscores the crucial involvement of these cells in fibrosis (Schafer et al. 2017b).
3. *Dysfunction of lung epithelium and endothelium due to senescence*: Senescent cells residing in the lung epithelium, endothelium, and fibroblasts can hinder normal cellular operations, thereby contributing to the onset of chronic pulmonary disorders. For instance, senescent airway epithelial cells provoke persistent pulmonary inflammation, and diminishing their population can lead to a reduction in pulmonary inflammatory responses.
4. *Senescence spread*: Empirical evidence suggests that senescence can be transmitted from senescent cells to neighboring non-senescent cells, intensifying the accumulation of senescent cells and their harmful effects (Waters et al. 2021).

5. *Therapeutic targeting*: Senolytic drugs, which selectively target and eradicate senescent cells, have demonstrated efficacy in decelerating the advancement of pulmonary diseases. This method has been investigated as a novel therapy approach for persistent respiratory disorders (Parikh et al. 2019; Yanai et al. 2015). The development of senescent cells in the pulmonary system is pivotal in maintaining chronic inflammation, fostering fibrosis, hindering cellular function, and enabling the propagation of senescence. These mechanisms are significant factors in the development and progression of lung illnesses, such as IPF and COPD. The strategic targeting of these cells presents a promising therapeutic intervention for managing these diseases.

6.5 MANAGEMENT OF SENESCENT CELL–INDUCED LUNG DISORDERS

The management of senescent cells in pulmonary pathologies constitutes a promising area of inquiry, with various methodologies being explored to mitigate their effects on persistent lung diseases.

6.5.1 Senolytic Pharmacotherapy

A principal approach involves the application of senolytic pharmacotherapy, which specifically targets and eliminates senescent cells. Dasatinib and quercetin have been employed in clinical investigations as senolytic agents, yielding promising outcomes in ameliorating physical limitations in individuals diagnosed with IPF (de Godoy et al. 2024).

6.5.2 Targeting Senescent Alveolar Type 2 Cells

Empirical research has indicated that the ablation of senescent alveolar type 2 (AT2) cells, coupled with the administration of senolytic agents, can significantly enhance pulmonary function and alleviate manifestations of radiation-induced pulmonary fibrosis. These results imply that the strategic targeting of AT2 cell senescence may represent a viable therapeutic strategy for addressing fibrotic lung conditions (Zhou et al. 2022).

Senescent cells have become significant therapeutic targets for numerous pulmonary disorders, including IPF and COPD. The elimination of senescent cells has been shown to improve respiratory function in aged mouse models, indicating a potential therapeutic advantage in treating pulmonary disorders.

6.5.3 Mechanisms of Action and Molecular Targets

Elucidating the molecular mechanisms of action and mitochondrial dysfunctions that govern cellular senescence is imperative for the development of efficacious strategies to modify the senescent cell phenotype within the lung. This understanding can facilitate the creation of targeted therapeutic modalities for chronic pulmonary ailments associated with senescence.

Senolytics possess the capacity to ameliorate pulmonary pathology by specifically targeting senescent cells, a notion that is currently under investigation. This approach has the potential to address inflammation, hypercontractility, and remodeling/fibrosis, all of which are critical characteristics of various pulmonary diseases (Parikh et al. 2019)

In conclusion, the management of senescent cells in pulmonary diseases necessitates an integrative approach that encompasses senolytic pharmacotherapy, the targeting of distinct senescent cell populations, and a comprehensive understanding of the underlying molecular pathways. These strategies hold promise for enhancing clinical outcomes in chronic lung disorders, comprising IPF and COPD.

Figures 6.1 and 6.2 depict the role of senolytic agents, highlighting two key approaches: checkpoint inhibitors and CAR-T cell therapy. Checkpoint inhibitors,

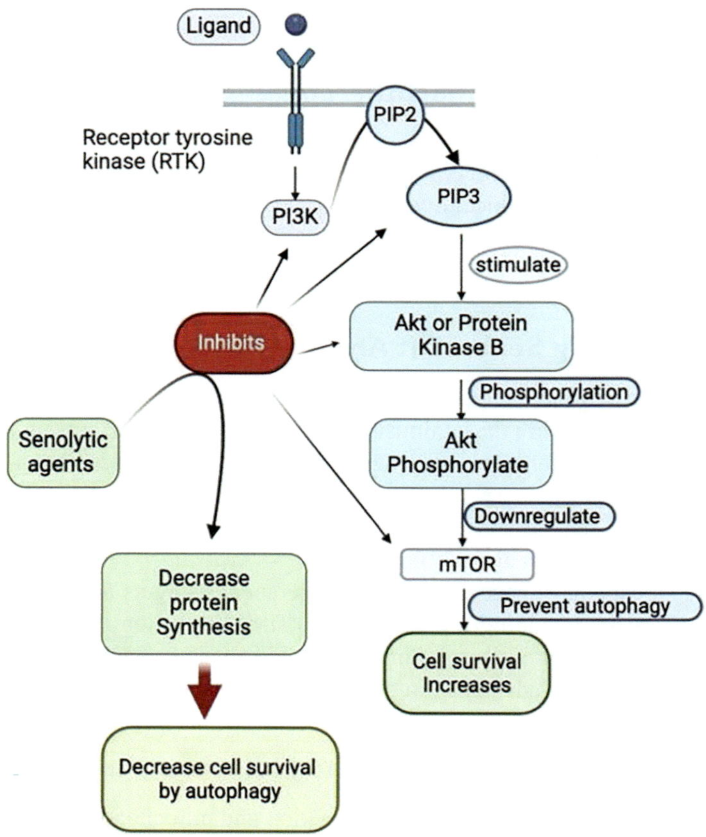

Figure 6.1 The mechanism of senolytic of the drugs and their molecular targets.

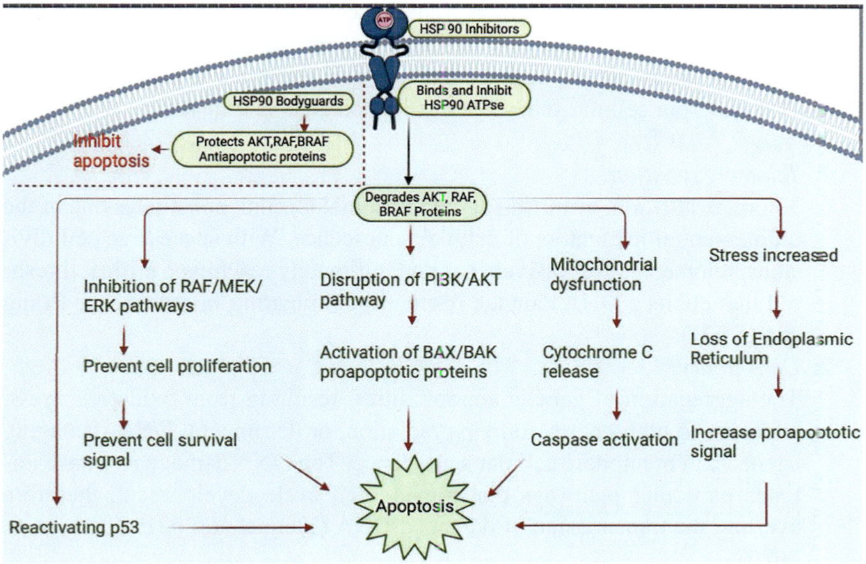

Figure 6.2 The role of senolytic agents and their pathways.

including anti-PD-1/PD-L1 antibodies, augment T-cell activity by obstructing immune-suppressive signals from senescent cells, thus enabling T cells to identify and eradicate these cells. Chimeric antigen receptor T (CAR-T) cell therapy entails the modification of T cells to recognize specific surface markers on senescent cells, leading to direct lethal effects upon contact. Both methodologies enhance immune surveillance, promoting the targeted elimination of senescent cells and alleviating inflammation linked to the SASP.

Senescent cells manifest a range of distinctive characteristics and biomarkers that are critical for their identification and analysis. These cells exhibit irreversible halt of division, modifications in metabolic processes, and resistance to apoptosis, manifesting across many organ systems in response to diverse stimuli (Song et al. 2020). Their variability in structural, functional, and tissue distribution attributes complicates their detection and characterization (Sun 2023).

Senescent cells can influence tissues and organs either beneficially or detrimentally, contingent upon the unique cell type and its metabolic environment. They have an important part in a multitude of physiological and pathological events, like embryonic progression, tissue mending, immune engagement, and hindering tumor formation. However, their accumulation within tissues as a consequence of aging has been correlated with a spectrum of age-associated declines and disorders (Munk et al. 2017; Yu et al. 2022).

Hence, the characterization and identification of senescent cells necessitate acknowledging their irreversible cessation of cell division, metabolic changes, evasion of apoptosis, inherent heterogeneity, and the requirement for many biomarkers for precise detection (Song et al. 2020; Sun 2023; Zimmermann et al.

2022; Adewoye et al. 2020). Cellular senescence represents a multifaceted biological phenomenon delineated by irreversible cell cycle arrest, which may be instigated by an array of both intrinsic and extrinsic stimuli. The principal mechanisms that underpin cellular senescence are articulated as follows:

1. *Telomere attrition:*
   Telomere attrition, occurring at chromosomal termini, constitutes one of the quintessential instigators of cellular senescence. With successive cell divisions, telomeres progressively shorten, ultimately reaching a critical threshold that elicits a DNA damage response, culminating in senescence (Yang et al. 2021).
2. *DNA injury:*
   The aggregation of genetic abnormalities, resulting from oxidative stress, exposure to high-energy ionizing radiation, or detrimental DNA-damaging agents, can precipitate cellular senescence. The DNA damage response initiates particular pathways that impede cell cycle development, therefore averting the transmission of damaged DNA (Yang et al. 2021; Zhang et al. 2020).
3. *Activation of oncogenes:*
   Aberrant activation of oncogenes can result in oncogene-induced senescence (OIS). This mechanism serves as a tumor-suppressive strategy by curtailing the proliferation of cells harboring potentially oncogenic mutations (Yang et al. 2021; Zhang et al. 2020).
4. *Mitochondrial dysfunction:*
   Mitochondrial failure can increase the production of reactive oxygen species (ROS), resulting in oxidative damage to essential macromolecules, such as DNA. Oxidative stress is a crucial element in initiating cellular senescence.
5. *Epigenetic alterations:*
   Changes in the epigenetic landscape, including adjustments in DNA methylation patterns and alterations in histone structure, can induce cellular senescence. Epigenetic changes can modulate gene expression patterns and contribute to the enduring cell cycle arrest characteristic of senescent cells (Kim et al. 2017).
6. *Additional stressors:*
   Mechanical or shear stress, infections, and metabolic perturbations can all elicit cellular senescence. These stresses activate many signaling pathways that lead to the senescence program (Zhang et al. 2020).

   In summary, cellular senescence is instigated by a multitude of mechanisms, encompassing telomere attrition, DNA damage, activation of oncogenes, mitochondrial dysfunction, epigenetic alterations, and various cellular stresses. These pathways collectively contribute to the intricate phenomenon of cellular senescence, which assumes critical roles in the processes of aging, tumor suppression, and tissue regeneration (Yang et al. 2021; Zhang et al. 2020; Kim et al. 2017).

Cellular senescence is a crucial feature of aging that comprises a self-defense mechanism of action that is activated in response to both intrinsic and external stimuli. This process is linked to the onset and progression of chronic respiratory disorders including IPF, COPD, and other inflammatory lung diseases. Chronic pulmonary diseases are a substantial public health issue, leading to severe morbidity and mortality globally (Goecke et al. 2024).

Despite advances in understanding the mechanism of actions underlying these diseases, present medications generally address symptoms rather than the underlying causes, such as cellular senescence (Goecke et al. 2024; Meng et al. 2024). Senotherapeutics provide a novel strategy for treating chronic lung disorders by targeting senescent cells that contribute to disease progression. Senolytics has the capability to eradicate senescent cells from pulmonary tissue, thereby diminishing inflammation and fibrosis—two principal pathological characteristics of chronic lung diseases (Faner et al. 2014; Gibson et al. 2017).

The senotherapeutics signify a promising avenue in the management of pulmonary diseases by addressing the fundamental mechanisms underlying cellular senescence. This innovative strategy has the potential to yield more efficacious and possibly curative interventions for chronic respiratory ailments by simultaneously addressing both the clinical manifestations and the root causes (Faner et al. 2014; Gibson et al. 2017). Senotherapeutics, which specifically focus on cellular senescence, have emerged as a credible methodology for improving pulmonary health, particularly in relation to aging and chronic respiratory conditions. The state of cellular senescence is noted for its stable halting of proliferation as cells face various physiological stresses. This scenario is marked by various phenotypic changes, including the secretion of pro-inflammatory signaling molecules, including as cytokines, immune-modulating chemokines, and tissue-degrading proteases, together known as the SASP.

With the flow of time there comes a rise in aged cells, altering the pathophysiological landscape of many age-linked health issues, which include persistent respiratory disorders including IPF, COPD, and asthma (Goecke et al. 2024; Pramanik et al. 2021) These disorders are marked by chronic inflammatory responses and compromised pulmonary function, which are further intensified by the accumulation of senescent cells (Allam et al. 2022). Studies have investigated therapies focused on senescent cells for their potential role in COPD, emphasizing the promise of senolytic and anti-aging pharmaceutical agents as new treatment possibilities (Easter et al. 2020).

Additionally, the appearance of aging cells in the lung after exposure to radiation has been associated with the development of tumors, suggesting that focusing on cellular aging might provide beneficial treatment options in cancer care. This underscores the significant relevance of senotherapeutics not only in mitigating chronic pulmonary diseases but also in addressing lung cancer, which is increasingly prevalent among the aging population (Nomori et al. 2010).

A recent report of FOXO4-DRI, a senolytic peptide designed to selectively induce apoptosis in senescent cells, represents a leading-edge progress in the field of senotherapeutics, particularly for aging-related diseases and fibrotic disorders like IPF and COPD. FOXO4 peptide inhibitors specifically target the FOXO4-p53 axis, which facilitates the evasion of apoptosis by senescent cells. Furthermore, it was also revealed that FOXO4-DRI mitigate radiation-induced pulmonary fibrosis (RIPF) by selectively targeting senescence-like fibroblasts in vivo (Meng et al. 2021). The present study has the potential to redefine the understanding of senescent cells and their impact on the treatment of respiratory disorders.

Similarly, a growing body of literature reports that pirfenidone use may be associated with reduced lung cancer risk in patients with IPF (Yoon et al. 2025). As targeting senescent cells has emerged as a promising therapeutic strategy for pulmonary fibrosis (PF), growing evidence supports the potential of several molecular agents to serve as future anti-IPF therapies. Among them, sirtuins—particularly SIRT3—have gained attention for their role in regulating mitochondrial function, oxidative stress, and cellular aging. SIRT3 activation has been shown to alleviate fibrotic changes by reducing ROS levels and improving mitochondrial integrity in alveolar epithelial cells, thereby attenuating fibroblast activation and extracellular matrix deposition in preclinical models of PF. Honokiol, a bioactive natural compound, exhibits potent antioxidant, anti-inflammatory, and anti-senescent properties. Recent studies have demonstrated that honokiol can inhibit TGF-β1–induced fibroblast-to-myofibroblast differentiation, reduce senescence markers and suppress fibrosis-related gene expression in lung tissues, suggesting its therapeutic relevance in managing pulmonary fibrosis (Pulivendala et al. 2020; Wang et al. 2024). Bone morphogenetic protein 4 (BMP4), part of the TGF-β superfamily, is another key player in lung tissue remodeling and fibrosis. Modulation of BMP4 signaling has been shown to counteract TGF-β–driven profibrotic pathways by promoting epithelial repair and inhibiting fibroblast proliferation. Experimental modulation of BMP4 has resulted in decreased collagen deposition and fibrosis markers in murine models, pointing to its utility as a therapeutic target. Together, these agents represent a growing class of senescence-modulating interventions that not only target the molecular roots of pulmonary fibrosis but also offer the promise of slowing or even reversing disease progression. Continued research into their mechanisms and clinical translation may redefine the landscape of IPF management in the coming years (Wang et al. 2024).

In summary, with their ability to focus on the core mechanisms of cellular aging, senotherapeutics hold great promise for improving pulmonary health, addressing chronic inflammatory responses, tissue harm, and disease development in the respiratory system. Enhanced research efforts and clinical trials are imperative to elucidate their efficacy and to formulate effective therapeutic strategies aimed at aging-related respiratory pathologies (Wang et al. 2024).

6.6 APPLICABILITY AND ANALYSIS OF SENOTHERAPY IN LUNG DISORDERS

Senescent cells are integral to the pathophysiology of specific pulmonary diseases. These cells manifest irreversible cell cycle arrest, metabolic dysregulation, and an enhanced resistance to apoptosis, thus potentially resulting in chronic pathologies and tissue dysfunction if their presence is excessively pronounced within tissues (Song et al. 2020).

Senescent cells have been identified in the lungs of patients exhibiting aging and respiratory pathologies, such as IPF and COPD. These cells are allocated among many lung compartments, encompassing immune cells, as well as epithelial, endothelial, and fibroblast cells. Senescent cells facilitate the progression of chronic pulmonary diseases by inciting inflammation and promoting tissue remodeling. For instance, preclinical investigations conducted on murine models have illustrated that senescent airway epithelial cells can instigate chronic pulmonary inflammation, and diminishing the population of these cells may mitigate pulmonary inflammatory responses. Moreover, the identification of senescent cells in pulmonary tissues correlates with heightened susceptibility to age-related illnesses and a decline in lung function. The accumulation of senescent cells in lung tissue has been associated with an increased prevalence of chronic respiratory illnesses, including COPD and interstitial lung diseases, as persons age (Bartling 2013). Additionally, these senescent cells possess the capacity to transmit their senescent characteristics to adjacent nonsenescent cells, thereby exacerbating the pathological condition (Waters et al. 2021).

Due to their significant role in pulmonary diseases, senescent cells are currently being assessed as viable therapeutic targets. Therapeutic techniques aimed at the elimination or regulation of these cells, referred to as senolytic or senotherapeutic drugs, are being investigated for their potential application in the treatment of chronic pulmonary illnesses.

6.7 CONCLUSION

The investigation into the implications of senotherapeutics on pulmonary conditions has revealed considerable promise for addressing the underlying etiologies of chronic respiratory pathologies. Our research indicates that the strategic targeting of senescent cells, which proliferate with advancing age and are implicated in ailments including IPF and COPD, has the potential to diminish inflammation and tissue remodeling, thereby enhancing pulmonary function. Senolytic agents, which preferentially eliminate senescent cells, along with senomorphics, which modify the SASP, have exhibited encouraging results in preclinical investigations and nascent clinical trials (Yanai et al. 2015; Parimon et al. 2021).

Nonetheless, the translational application of these therapeutic modalities is fraught with numerous challenges. The heterogeneity of senescent cells, compounded by the absence of standardized biomarkers, complicates their identification and eradication. Moreover, the potential adverse effects of senolytic agents, including unintended off-target consequences and disruption of normal tissue homeostasis, warrant meticulous consideration and further examination (Mikawa et al. 2020).

To enhance our comprehension, forthcoming investigations should prioritize the identification of specific biomarkers for senescent cells within the pulmonary system and the development of more precisely targeted senolytic therapies. It is essential to evaluate the long-term consequences of senotherapeutics and their effects on the overall health and functions of the pulmonary system. Furthermore, investigating the influence of senescent cells on developmental lung diseases, and their potential as therapeutic targets may reveal new therapy options (Liu et al. 2024).

In summary, while senotherapeutics present a promising approach for managing chronic pulmonary illnesses by targeting senescent cells, further study is crucial to overcome current limitations and fully clarify their therapeutic potential. Confronting these obstacles will promote the advancement of more efficacious and safer therapies for lung disorders linked to cellular senescence.

Addressing these challenges would facilitate the development of more effective and safer interventions for lung diseases associated with cellular senescence.

REFERENCES

Adewoye AB, Tampakis D, Follenzi A and Stolzing A. "Multiparameter flow cytometric detection and quantification of senescent cells in vitro." *Biogerontology* 2020; 21(6):773–786.

Allam VSRR, Chellappan DK, Jha NK, Shastri MD, Gupta G, Shukla SD, Singh SK, Sunkara K, Chitranshi N, Gupta V, Wich PR, MacLoughlin R, Oliver BGG, Wernersson S, Pejler G and Dua K. "Treatment of chronic airway diseases using nutraceuticals: Mechanistic insight." *Critical Reviews in Food Science and Nutrition* 2022; 62(27):7576–7590.

Bartling B. "Cellular senescence in normal and premature lung aging." *Zeitschrift für Gerontologie und Geriatrie* 2013; 46:613–622.

Bezerra FS, Lanzetti M, Nesi RT, Nagato AC, Silva CPE, Kennedy-Feitosa E, Melo AC, Cattani-Cavalieri I, Porto LC and Valenca SS. "Oxidative stress and inflammation in acute and chronic lung injuries." *Antioxidants (Basel)* 2023; 12(3):548. https://doi.org/10.3390/antiox12030548.

Campisi J. "Cellular senescence and lung function during aging." *Annals of the American Thoracic Society* 2016; 13: S402–S406.

de Godoy MC, Macedo JA and Gambero A. "Researching new drug combinations with senolytic activity using senescent human lung fibroblasts MRC-5 cell line." *Pharmaceuticals* 2024; 17(1).

Easter M, Bollenbecker S, Barnes JW and Krick S. "Targeting aging pathways in chronic obstructive pulmonary disease." *International Journal of Molecular Sciences* 2020; 21(18).

Faner R, Cruz T, López-Giraldo A and Agustí A. "Network medicine, multimorbidity and the lung in the elderly." *European Respiratory Journal* 2014; 44(3):775.

Gibson PG, Peters MJ and Wainwright CE. "Targeted therapy for chronic respiratory disease: A new paradigm." *Medical Journal of Australia* 2017; 206(3):136–140.

Goecke T, Ius F, Ruhparwar A and Martin U. "Unlocking the future: Pluripotent stem cell-based lung repair." *Cells* 2024; 13(7).

Kim C, Kang D, Lee EK and Lee J-S. "Long noncoding RNAs and RNA-binding proteins in oxidative stress, cellular senescence, and age-related diseases." *Oxidative Medicine and Cellular Longevity* 2017; 2017(1):2062384.

Liu L, Wei Y, Giunta S, He Q and Xia S. "Potential role of cellular senescence in pulmonary arterial hypertension." *Clinical and Experimental Pharmacology and Physiology* 2022; 49(10):1042–1049.

Liu Z, Zhang Y, Li D and Fu J. "Cellular senescence in chronic lung diseases from newborns to the elderly: An update literature review." *Biomedicine & Pharmacotherapy* 173 (2024):116463.

Meng J, Li Y, Wan C, Sun Y, Dai X, Huang J, Hu Y, Gao Y, Wu B, Zhang Z, Jiang K, Xu S, Lovell JF, Hu Y, Wu G, Jin H and Yang K. "Targeting senescence-like fibroblasts radiosensitizes non-small cell lung cancer and reduces radiation-induced pulmonary fibrosis." *JCI Insight* 2021; 6(23):e146334. https://doi.org/10.1172/jci.insight.146334.

Meng M, Zhang WW, Chen SF, Wang DR and Zhou CH. "Therapeutic utility of human umbilical cord-derived mesenchymal stem cells-based approaches in pulmonary diseases: Recent advancements and prospects." *World Journal of Stem Cells* 2024; 16(2):70–88.

Mikawa R, Sato T, Suzuki Y, Baskoro H, Kawaguchi K and Sugimoto M. "p19Arf exacerbates cigarette smoke-induced pulmonary dysfunction." *Biomolecules* 10(3) (2020): 462. https://doi.org/10.3390/biom10030462.

Munk R, Panda AC, Grammatikakis I, Gorospe M and Abdelmohsen K. "Chapter four—senescence-associated microRNAs." In: Galluzzi L, Vitale I, editors. *International Review of Cell and Molecular Biology*. 334: Academic Press; 2017. pp. 177–205.

Nomori H. "Treatment for elderly patients with non-small cell lung cancer." *Cancer & Chemotherapy* 2010; 37(13):2833–2837.

Parikh P, Wicher S, Khandalavala K, Pabelick CM, Britt RD and Prakash YS. "Cellular senescence in the lung across the age spectrum." *American Journal of Physiology-Lung Cellular and Molecular Physiology* 316(5) 2019:L826–L842.

Parimon T, Hohmann MS and Yao C. "Cellular senescence: Pathogenic mechanisms in lung fibrosis." *International Journal of Molecular Sciences* 2021; 22(12):6214.

Pramanik S, Mohanto S, Manne R, Rajendran RR, Deepak A, Edapully SJ, Patil T and Katari O "Nanoparticle-based drug delivery system: The magic bullet for the treatment of chronic pulmonary diseases." *Molecular Pharmaceutics* 2021; 18(10):3671–3718.

Pulivendala G, Bale S and Godugu C. "Honokiol: A polyphenol neolignan ameliorates pulmonary fibrosis by inhibiting TGF-β/Smad signaling, matrix proteins and IL-6/CD44/STAT3 axis both in vitro and in vivo." *Toxicol Appl Pharmacol* 2020; 391:114913. https://doi.org/10.1016/j.taap.2020.114913.

Schafer MJ, White TA, Iijima K, Haak AJ, Ligresti G, Atkinson EJ, Oberg AL, Birch J, Salmonowicz H, Zhu Y, Mazula DL, Brooks RW, Fuhrmann-Stroissnigg H, Pirtskhalava T, Prakash YS, Tchkonia T, Robbins PD, Aubry MC, Passos JF, Kirkland JL, Tschumperlin DJ, Kita H and LeBrasseur NK. "Cellular senescence mediates fibrotic pulmonary disease." *Nature Communications* 2017b; 8(1):14532.

Song P, An J and Zou M-H. "Immune clearance of senescent cells to combat ageing and chronic diseases." *Cells* 2020; 9(3):671.

Sugimoto M. "Targeting cellular senescence: A promising approach in respiratory diseases." *Geriatrics & Gerontology International* 2024; 24(S1):60–66.

Sun Y. "Pathophysiological implications of cellular senescence and prospects for novel anti-aging drugs." *Sheng Li Xue Bao* 2023; 75(6):847–863.

Wang J, Li K, Hao D, Li X, Zhu Y, Yu H and Chen H. "Pulmonary fibrosis: Pathogenesis and therapeutic strategies." *MedComm (2020)* 2024; 5(10):e744. https://doi.org/10.1002/mco2.744.

Waters DW, Schuliga M, Pathinayake PS, Wei L, Tan HY, Blokland KEC, Jaffar J, Westall GP, Burgess JK, Prêle CM, Mutsaers SE, Grainge CL and Knight DA. "A senescence bystander effect in human lung fibroblasts." *Biomedicines* 2021; 9(9).

Yanai H, Shteinberg A, Porat Z, Budovsky A, Braiman A, Zeische R, Fraifeld VE. "Cellular senescence-like features of lung fibroblasts derived from idiopathic pulmonary fibrosis patients." *Aging (Albany NY)* 2015; 7(9):664–672.

Yang J, Liu M, Hong D, Zeng M and Zhang X. "The paradoxical role of cellular senescence in cancer." *Frontiers in Cell and Developmental Biology* 2021; 9.

Yoon HY, Kim H, Bae Y and Song JW. "Pirfenidone and risk of lung cancer development in idiopathic pulmonary fibrosis: A nationwide population-based study." *European Respiratory Journal* 2025; 65(2):2401484. https://doi.org/10.1183/13993003.01484-2024.

Yu X, Quan J, Chen S, Yang X, Huang S, Yang G and Zhang Y. "A protocol for rapid construction of senescent cells." *Frontiers Integrative Neuroscience* 2022; 16:929788. https://doi.org/10.3389/fnint.2022.929788.

Zhang Y, Yang B, Wang J, Cheng F, Shi K, Ying L, Wang C, Xia K, Huang X, Gong Z, Yu C, Li F, Liang C and Chen Q. "Cell senescence: A nonnegligible cell state under survival stress in pathology of intervertebral disc degeneration." *Oxidative Medicine and Cellular Longevity* 2020; 2020(1):9503562.

Zhou S, Zhu J, Zhou P-K and Gu Y. "Alveolar type 2 epithelial cell senescence and radiation-induced pulmonary fibrosis." *Frontiers in Cell and Developmental Biology* 2022; 10.

Zimmermann T, Pommer M, Kluge V, Chiheb C, Muehlich S and Bosserhoff A-K. "Detection of cellular senescence in human primary melanocytes and malignant melanoma cells in vitro." *Cells* 2022; 11(9):1489.

Chapter 7

Senotherapeutics in Bone Diseases

Neha Sharma, Shreshta Jain, and Divya Vohora

7.1 INTRODUCTION

Bone has a vastly dynamic structure with a hard exterior and a functional bone marrow comprising numerous types of immune cells, stem cells, cytokines and growth factors (Morrison and Scadden 2014). However, the physiological functionality of bone, somatic cells and precursor cells deteriorates with evolving age, causing a decline in bone strength and bone density (Morrison and Scadden 2014, Massaro et al. 2023). Bone has been strongly associated with cellular senescence observed in bones and cartilage joints brought about by age-related insults such as telomere attrition and genomic instability, contributing to the progression of senile joint disorders and bone diseases (Childs et al. 2017). Senescence in bone is a cellular defence in response to stress that helps prevent acquired damage. It is necessary for tissue homeostasis and wound healing, and it also plays physiological roles during normal development. However, excessive cellular senescence reduces the bone's ability to regenerate and repair (Marie 2014, Farr and Khosla 2019). The main disorders that are caused by senescence of bone and cartilage cells are osteoarthritis, osteoporosis, and intervertebral disc disorder (Zhao et al. 2024, He et al. 2023). Osteoarthritis is a joint disorder caused by senescence in the cartilage cells affecting the subchondral bone and joints, while osteoporosis and intervertebral disc disorder are characterized by age-related loss in bone composition and degeneration in intervertebral discs, respectively. The treatment available for the above diseases is mainly symptomatic and relief oriented. Hence, there is a need for developing new strategies like senotherapeutics that directly target the bone senescent cells and help in tissue regeneration.

Senotherapeutics are agents that target the senescent cells in bone and cartilage to inhibit disease progression. They have the potential to be used clinically against various bone disorders, including osteoarthritis, osteoporosis, intervertebral disc disorders and bone fractures, as evidenced by multiple preclinical findings. The first recognized senotherapeutic in bone disorders was dasatinib, used in combination with quercetin, which promoted the bone formation process and reduced bone resorption (Zhu et al. 2015). Scientists have been vigorously employing the use of senotherapeutics as treatment against age-related bone and joint disorders.

DOI: 10.1201/9781003493969-7

Senotherapeutics attenuate bone disorders by either causing the elimination of senescent bone cells and chondrocytes by initiating apoptosis selectively or by neutralizing the secretory phenotypes, known as senescence-associated secretory phenotype (SASP), leading to reduced inflammation, thereby triggering tissue regeneration (Zhou et al. 2021). Multiple categories of senotherapeutics target bone and cartilage. The two main categories of senotherapeutics are mainly divided into senolytics and senomorphics. This chapter details the recent progress and pivotal role of senotherapeutics in the prevention and treatment of major bone and joint disorders (osteoporosis and osteoarthritis, respectively).

7.2 CELLULAR SENESCENCE AND ITS ROLE IN BONE BIOLOGY AND BONE HEALTH

Bone remodelling is a process of substitution of old bone cells with new bone-forming cells. At a cellular level, the accumulation of bone matrix, bone mineralization and remodelling is managed by three main sorts of cells, such as osteoclasts, osteoblasts and osteocytes (Yasuda et al. 1998). Osteoclast differentiation is aggravated by the release of receptor activator of nuclear factor kappa-B ligand (RANKL), which binds to the receptor present on the osteoclast surface called RANK (Boyle, Simonet, and Lacey 2003, Li et al. 2000). The osteoblasts improve the new bone formation process in contrast to osteoclasts. Wingless-related integration site (WNT) signalling is the critical pathway that regulates the differentiation of bone mesenchymal stem cells (BMSCs) into osteoblasts via the WNT/β-catenin pathway through stabilization of β-catenin, and other non-canonical WNT pathways (Corr 2008). With aging, the ability of BMSCs to differentiate into osteoblasts reduces, and adipocyte differentiation occurs. This causes increased adipogenesis. WNT signalling also decreases with age, thereby further reducing osteoblast number (Stevens et al. 2010, Rauner, Sipos, and Pietschmann 2008). Senescent cells impair bone remodelling by disturbing the bone formation process by osteoblasts and osteoblast progenitor cell function, thus promoting osteoclastogenesis. A set of stressors, like telomere shortening (replicative senescence), DNA damage, oxidative stress and genomic instability, are responsible for creating stress in the cells. The contribution of all these above factors, along with physiological and pathological processes such as remodelling, aging and traumatic injury, promotes senescence in bone (Farr and Khosla 2019). There is a very prominent feature of senescent cells called SASP, which acts as the primary contributor to the worsening of the bone, osteoblasts, cartilage cells and joints. SASP, through various mechanisms, triggers inflammatory responses in bone (Pignolo, Law, and Chandra 2021). The cell cycle arrest in senescent cells is mainly because of signalling pathways (Chandrakar, Ambatwar, and Khatik 2024), which are elaborated in section 7.6.

Bone loss is also a natural aging process in both men and women. The inflammatory disorders impact whole joints and bones. Aging can boost the ability of

Table 7.1 Cell Types in Bone Undergoing Senescence

Cell Types	*Senescence Associated Changes*	*Mechanism*
Bone marrow-derived mesenchymal stem cells (BMSCs)	Number of BMSCs is decreased, adipogenic differentiation is elevated while osteogenic differentiation is reduced, decreased sensitivity to respond to IGF-1, glucose uptake and fracture healing	Downregulation of WNT signalling, upregulation of PPAR-γ
Osteoblasts	Decreased function and proliferation; apoptosis is increased	Downregulation of RUNX2 and osterix due to increased oxidative stress and DNA damage accumulation
Osteoclasts	Their activity is increased resulting in increased bone resorption	Altered RANKL/RANK signalling, SASP-mediated inflammatory cytokine release
Osteocytes	Their number decreases due to cellular apoptosis, senescent osteocytes have reduced dendrites	Increased SASP production
Chondrocytes	Matrix degradation due to increased senescent cells in cartilage	SASP-induced secretion of MMPs and inflammatory cytokines

synovial fibroblasts, immune cells, fat cells, chondrocytes and other bone cells to release inflammatory cytokines and chemokines (Pignolo, Law, and Chandra 2021). This increase is often linked to senescent cells and oxidative stress. Alterations in articular cartilage due to aging can lead to the onset and worsening of osteoarthritis. In older articular cartilage, chondrocytes show a decline in their ability to grow and produce new material; however, they can still create pro-inflammatory substances and enzymes that break down the matrix (Harbo et al. 2013). Table 7.1 shows the various bone and cartilage cell types undergoing senescence.

7.3 BONE DISORDERS ASSOCIATED WITH AGING AND SENESCENCE

7.3.1 Osteoporosis

Aging and cellular senescence play a vital part in the loss of bone density, leading to pathologies like osteoporosis and osteopenia (Ginaldi, Mengoli, and De

Martinis 2009, ADAMS, Davies, and Sweetnam 1970). In bone remodelling, resorption by osteoclasts and formation by osteoblasts become imbalanced with aging (Sims and Vrahnas 2014). Mitochondrial dysfunction in osteoblast and osteoclast cells contributes to reactive oxygen species (ROS) that harm protein and lipids in DNA, further activating the senescence pathways like MAPK and NF-κB signalling pathways, promoting inflammation and upregulation of p16ink4 and SASP (Salminen et al. 2012, Zinovkin et al. 2014, Kim et al. 2010, Farr et al. 2016). WNT signalling drives osteoblast differentiation by stabilizing β-catenin and inducing osteogenic genes, namely, Runt-related transcription factor 2 (Runx2) and osterix (Osx); however, Wnt inhibitors such as sclerostin and Dickkopf-related protein 1 (DKK1) increase with aging, thereby suppressing osteoclastogenesis (Baron and Kneissel 2013). As a result, reduced β-catenin signalling decreases bone formation and promotes adipogenesis (Liu, Xiao, et al. 2022). Occasionally, hormonal deficiency, such as oestrogen deficiency, suppresses osteoclast activity and inflammatory cytokines, such as tumour necrosis factor (TNF)-α and interleukin-6 (IL-6), and increases RANKL/OPG ratio, thus favouring osteoclastogenesis (Jilka 1998, Wang et al. 2024)

7.3.2 Osteoarthritis

Osteoarthritis is a widely recognized age-related disease (ARD) that worsens as people get older and aging plays a major role in its development. Philipot and colleagues showed in a lab experiment that p16INK4a is sufficient to generate senescence and hence osteoarthritis in chondrocytes, which helps in the development of osteoarthritis (Philipot et al. 2014a). When chondrocytes encounter a complex network of pro-inflammatory mediator cytokines such as IL-1, IL-6, IL-8, and IL-1β, they generate matrix-remodelling enzymes known as matrix metalloproteases (MMPs), MMP1 and MMP13, that are responsible for the pathophysiology of osteoarthritis (Molnar et al. 2021). These enzymes show signs of SASP. The SASP factors, along with other pathways, activate p16, which drives cells toward senescence (Wu et al. 2022). Research conducted with mice indicates that removing p16INK4a-positive cells helped reduce age-related bone loss (Baker et al. 2011).

7.4 KEY SENESCENCE MARKERS IN BONE DISORDERS

Senescence markers are grave markers for identifying and comprehending the role of senescent cells in bone disorders. These markers promote critical pathologies including osteoporosis, osteoarthritis and impaired bone healing fractures.

7.4.1 p16INK4a (CDKN2A)

It is a tumour suppressor protein related to senescence and age-related morbidities and involved in the cell cycle's G1 phase. It is elevated in aged and senescent osteoblasts, osteocytes and bone marrow-derived mesenchymal stem cells, inducing osteoporosis. Osteoblastogenesis and bone formation are reduced by promoting cell cycle arrest by inhibiting CDK4/6, leading to senescence (Diekman et al. 2018b). p16INK4a also upregulates SASP, thereby enhancing inflammation and bone resorption (Safwan-Zaiter, Wagner, and Wagner 2022). A team of scientists measured SASP markers in vivo with rt-qPCR in B cells, T cells, myeloid cells, osteoblasts, and osteocytes in both 6-month-old and 24-month-old C57BL/6 wild-type (WT) mice. The study revealed a significant increase in p16INK4a in the osteoprogenitors, osteoblasts and osteocytes, as well as in the immune cells of the aged mice (Farr et al. 2016). These findings suggest that this marker is centralized in the pathology of osteoporosis. Besides, it is also involved in the progression of osteoarthritis by aging the chondrocytes and increasing inflammation by releasing SASP mediators (Diekman et al. 2018a, Philipot et al. 2014b)

7.4.2 p21CIP1/WAF1 (CDKN1A)

It is a cyclin-dependent kinase inhibitor regulated by p53 (Kreis, Louwen, and Yuan 2019). It accumulates in osteocytes and osteoprogenitors in response to DNA damage and is elevated in bone cells during aging. Impaired bone remodelling and reduced repair capacity are the key responses of this marker in the senescent bone cells. It regulates senescence through the induction of G1/S cell cycle arrest and enhances SASP expression, thereby influencing the bone microenvironment (Gascoyne et al. 2015, Pignolo et al. 2019). The role of this marker has been implicated in both osteoporosis and osteoarthritis. On modulating the activity of p21, cartilage regenerative capabilities increase further, as reported in both in vitro and in vivo (Molnar et al. 2021). Mesenchymal progenitor cells (MPCs) were derived from normal and osteoarthritic knee joints and were analysed for p21 at the mRNA and protein levels. The levels of p21 in osteoarthritic MPCs were higher, and chondrogenic differentiation decreased with inflammation within the tissue of the synovium (Masson et al. 2015). The marker is also related to bone loss in osteoporosis. The low levels of p21 are found to exhibit protection against osteoporosis in ovariectomized mice (Premnath et al. 2019).

7.4.3 Senescence-Associated β-Galactosidase (SA-β-Gal)

It is an aging hallmark and an enzyme that reflects the activity associated with lysosomal β-galactosidase for ascertaining the senescent cells in bone tissues (Itahana, Campisi, and Dimri 2007). SA-β-Gal activity is found to be upregulated in osteoblasts and osteocytes in aged or damaged bone and in osteoarthritic conditions (Ryu et al. 2008). Senescent cells are a significant therapeutic target in bone disorders (Wang, Huang, and He 2022).

7.4.4 SASP Factors

These include proinflammatory cytokines like IL-6, IL-8, TNF-α, MMPs, and vascular endothelial growth factor (VEGF) that are released by senescent cells, causing degradation of bone matrix and inhibition of bone formation (Lopes-Paciencia et al. 2019, Zhu et al. 2022). SASP factors promote chronic inflammation and bone resorption by recruiting immune cells. These factors are especially secreted by senescent osteoblasts, osteocytes and chondrocytes, amplifying tissue damage. They play a special role in degrading cartilage and subchondral bone, leading to osteoarthritis (Fang, Liu, and Wan 2023b, Farr and Khosla 2019). The presence of SASP factors was found to be increased in the senescence-related osteoporosis animal model (Farr et al. 2016).

7.4.5 γ-H2AX

It is a DNA marker associated with genomic instability in bone cells. It accumulates in osteoblasts and osteocytes during aging. It works on the mechanism of DNA damage via the senescence pathway through activation of p53 and p21 (Bai et al. 2020, Facchini et al. 2014). ROS and oxidative stress exposure increase the levels of this marker and cause stress-induced DNA damage. γ-H2AX is indirectly involved in causing DNA damage in osteoarthritis. The levels of --H2AX are raised in the osteoporotic mouse model (Chen et al. 2019).

7.4.6 Telomere Attrition

It is observed in osteoblasts and BMSCs during aging that limit the regenerative capacity of bone-forming cells contributes to osteoporosis (Bekaert, De Meyer, and Van Oostveldt 2005, Tang et al. 2010).

7.4.7 Reactive Oxygen Species

They are the most vital indicators of oxidative stress in osteoblasts and osteocytes, triggering senescence and bone loss in osteoporosis and osteoarthritis (Tudorachi et al. 2021). ROS works on the mechanism of DNA damage response and p53/p21 signalling pathways (Callaway and Jiang 2015). There are various senotherapeutic drugs which target ROS and manage to treat osteoporosis and osteoarthritis.

7.4.8 High-Mobility Group Box 1

It is a nonhistone nuclear protein released by macrophages that is involved in chromatin remodelling, inflammatory signalling and matrix degradation in bone diseases, including osteoarthritis and osteoporosis (Callaway and Jiang 2015, Heinola et al. 2010). In a study, an *in vitro* osteoblast model of SaOS-2 induced with high-mobility group box 1 (HMGB1) showed increased proliferation, migration and osteogenic differentiation that can propose HMGB1 as a potent bone remodelling signal (Martinotti et al. 2016). HMGB1 regulates bone marrow macrophages (BMMs) through receptor for advanced glycation end product (RAGE) and promotes osteoclastogenesis in vitro and in vivo (Zhou et al. 2008). HMGB1 is secreted by human cell lines of oral squamous cell cancer (OSCC) and promotes bone destruction via osteoclastogenesis by upregulating the expression of nuclear factor kappa B (NF-κB) ligand in osteoblasts and osteocytes (Sakamoto et al. 2020).

7.5 SENOTHERAPEUTIC STRATEGIES FOR BONE DISORDERS

There are three main strategies for combating regenerating aging cells in the bone: (1) pharmacological methods using senotherapeutics; (2) non-pharmacological methods involving biologics and biomaterials; and (3) lifestyle changes. The pharmacological methods utilize different drug treatments aimed at destroying or discarding growing senescent cells. Non-pharmacological methods employ materials, including biologics such as platelet-rich plasma (PRP), which have shown the ability to fight aging and senescence in older cells and ARDs (Lawrence et al. 2024a). Finally, the lifestyle approach focuses on various dietary changes, intermittent fasting or incorporating more antioxidants in the daily diet to help reduce oxidative stress that leads to senescence, along with regular exercise to improve the cellular health of bone and joints naturally (Militello et al. 2024). Here we focus on the pharmacological senotherapeutic strategies for bone disorders as given below:

- Senolytics (e.g., dasatinib, quercetin, navitoclax)
- Senomorphics (e.g., rapamycin, metformin, resveratrol)
- Stem cell therapy
- Senescence pathway inhibitors (JAK/STAT inhibitors).

7.5.1 Senolytics

Senescent cells are eradicated by this subclass of senotherapeutics thereby alleviating several age-related disorders such as senile osteoporosis and osteoarthritis without affecting the normal cells (Lawrence et al. 2024b). The selective removal of aging cells is the recognized mechanism of senolytics, which is helpful in halting disease progression in osteoarthritis and other ARDs (Farr et al. 2017, Hou et al. 2018). The senolytics treat osteoarthritis and osteoporosis by acting mechanistically on senescent cells through various pathways.

7.5.1.1 Dasatinib and Quercetin

Dasatinib (Sprycel) is a well-known senolytic drug discovered and developed by Bristol-Myers Squibb that was approved by the US Food and Drug Administration in 2006 for treating chronic and acute leukaemia. Quercetin is a natural flavonoid, first isolated in 1936 by Albert Szent- Gyorgyi (Formica and Regelson 1995). The dasatinib and quercetin combination is the first generation of senolytic treatment for bone disorders. There are various preclinical studies in vivo and in vitro that provide sufficient evidence for their role in attenuating bone-related disorders. As evidenced in a study intervention, dasatinib inhibited the bone resorption effects and exhibited bone anabolic effects on osteoblasts, primary human bone marrow mesenchymal stem cells (hMSCs), hMSC-TERT and the MG-63 cell lines. This study showed the potential use of dasatinib in bone diseases such as osteoporosis, osteolytic bone metastasis and myeloma bone diseases (Garcia-Gomez et al. 2012).

Since then, there have been many research studies performed on dasatinib and quercetin combination specifically. The combination has been used in various in vitro studies on mouse mesenchymal stem cells (MSCs), human mesenchymal stem cells–telomerase reverse transcriptase (hMSC-TERT) and the MG-63 cell lines, senescent osteocyte, osteoclast cells, aged BMSCs in mice and bone marrow, and the effects were found to be significantly productive in elimination of osteoporosis by inhibiting osteoclastogenesis. (Casado-Díaz et al. 2016, Farr et al. 2017; Zhang et al. 2020). The combination helps reduce senescent biomarkers like p16INK4a and p21 gene expression in many cases. The bone resorption process is also reduced on administration of treatment (Chandra et al. 2020).

Besides this, osteogenic potential under osteoarthritic conditions in cartilage is also alleviated (Zhang et al. 2020, Maurer et al. 2025). In addition, SASP factors (IL-6, CXCL1) were also found to be reduced in human osteoarthritic chondrocytes (Maurer et al. 2025). The dasatinib and quercetin combination was found to help treat human degenerative lumbar facet joints. Facet joint cartilage degeneration is associated with chondrocyte cellular senescence in both humans and mice. Treatment with dasatinib significantly reduces senescence in chondrocytes thereby reducing degeneration of facet joints (Zhao et al. 2025). A long-term treatment with dasatinib and quercetin ameliorated age-dependent intervertebral disc degeneration in mice by decreasing SASP markers (Novais et al. 2021). Summarizing the in vitro, in vivo and clinical studies as shown in Tables 7.2, 7.3 and 7.4, it is clearly evident that dasatinib and quercetin are effective against senescence and thereby in bone and joint diseases.

7.5.1.2 Navitoclax (Bcl2 Inhibitor)

It is a novel chemotherapeutic drug also known as ABT-263 and one of the highly investigated target treatments in preclinical studies. It is a Bcl-2 pathway inhibitor responsible for apoptosis in senescent cells (Tse et al. 2008, Wilson et al. 2010). These studies thus target various elements of the senescent bone cells via anti-apoptotic pathways. In a study, navitoclax's therapeutic effect was evaluated on post-traumatic osteoarthritis in a destabilization of the medial meniscus (DMM) rat model in which it reduced inflammation, attenuated the osteoarthritic condition by selectively eliminating senescent chondrocyte cells in the cartilage tissue,

Table 7.2 Senolytics and Senomorphics in Osteoarthritis: Evidence from Preclinical Studies

S.No.	*Senotherapeutic Agent*	*Model*	*Major Findings*
1	Dasatinib + quercetin (Zhang et al., 2020)	Senescent rat BMSCs	Chondrogenic gene expression for COL2A1, ACAN and SOX9 was increased
2	Dasatinib + quercetin (Maurer et al., 2025)	Human osteoarthritic chondrocytes	SASP factors (IL-6, CXCL1) were reduced
3	Navitoclax (Yang et al., 2020)	Post-traumatic osteoarthritis in DMM rat model, osteoarthritis chondrocyte pellet culture	Reduced inflammation, by selectively eliminating senescent chondrocyte cells in the cartilage tissue, supported the aggregation of cartilage matrix in osteoarthritis chondrocyte pellet culture and promoted chondrogenic phenotype
4	Navitoclax (Miura et al., 2022)	Synovial MSCs from osteoarthritis patients	Selective elimination of senescent cells, lower expression of SASP factors (MMP-13 and IL-6) and senescence markers (p16 and p21)
5	UBX0101 (Jeon et al., 2017)	C57BL/6 mice model of osteoarthritis	Reduced senescent cell markers, matrix metalloproteinases and suppressed inflammation, improving the cartilage health
6	Fenofibrate (Nogueira-Recalde et al., 2019)	Human chondrocytes with IL-6–induced senescence	Reported reduction in senescent cells and inflammation, reversing damage in senescent osteoarthritis cells, lowering the PPARα levels
7	Fisetin (Zheng et al., 2017)	In vitro: primary human chondrocytes In vivo: 10-week-old C57BL/6 male osteoarthritis mice models induced by destabilization of the medial meniscus (DMM)	Decreased inflammatory mediators
8	Berberine (Li et al., 2022)	In vivo: AMPKα1 KO mice and congenic WT mice with C57BL/6/129 In vitro: human and mouse articular chondrocytes	Attenuated structural changes and pain in joint

(*Continued*)

Table 7.2 (Continued) Senolytics and Senomorphics in Osteoarthritis: Evidence from Preclinical Studies

S.No.	*Senotherapeutic Agent*	*Model*	*Major Findings*
9	Spermidine (Ou et al., 2024)	In vivo: 10-week-old male C57BL/6 mice In vitro: human primary chondrocytes and bone marrow–derived macrophages (BMDMs)	Inhibited p65/NF-κB signalling in macrophages; in vivo, it protected articular cartilage
10	Panobinostat (Wen et al., 2021)	In vivo: murine osteoarthritis model	Cartilage, synovium and subchondral bone were protected by reducing MMPs and inflammatory mediators
11	Rapamycin (Bao et al., 2020)	Wistar rats	Reduced IL-1 and inhibited NF-kB
12	Resveratrol (Luo et al., 2019)	IL-1β–induced human chondrocytes in vitro	Lowered matrix metalloproteinases like MMP-3 and MMP-9
13	Resveratrol (Yang, Sun, and Zhang, 2022)	In vivo: MIA-induced Sprague Dawley rats	Decreased inflammatory mediators IL-1β, MMP-13
14	Resveratrol (Su et al., 2020)	In vitro: H_2O_2 induced porcine chondrocytes	Anti-inflammatory effects by decreasing TNF-α, IL-1β, MMP-1 and MMP-13
15	Resveratrol (Wei et al., 2018)	In vivo: MIA-induced knee osteoarthritis in Wistar rats	Activated HO-1/Nrf2 signalling pathways
16	Resveratrol (Xu et al., 2019)	In vivo: high-fat diet–induced osteoarthritis in C57BL/6 mice In vitro: IL-1β–induced SW1353 cells	Suppressed TLR4 signalling pathway

Table 7.3 Senolytics and Senomorphics in Osteoporosis: Evidence from Preclinical Studies

S.No.	*Senotherapeutic Agent*	*Model*	*Major Findings*
1	Dasatinib (Garcia-Gomez et al., 2012)	In vitro: primary human bone marrow mesenchymal stem cells (hMSCs), hMSC-TERT and the MG-63 cell lines	Inhibition of bone resorption and attenuation of osteoporosis, osteolytic bone metastasis, myeloma bone disease
2	Dasatinib + quercetin (Farr et al., 2017)	Bone marrow	Selectively cleared senescent osteocyte, osteoclasts cells and by suppressing the activity of bone resorption; the combination attenuated the trabecular microarchitecture at spine and femur
3	Dasatinib + quercetin (Chandra et al., 2020)	In vivo: FRT-induced osteoporosis in C57BL/6 mice	Decreasing the number of senescent osteoblasts and suppression of senescent markers p16INK4a and p21 gene expression
4	Dasatinib + quercetin (Zhou et al., 2021)	In vivo: Old mice In vitro: B6MSCs from old mice	Osteoblast formation and improved osteogenic potential
5	Dasatinib + quercetin and bone morphogenetic protein 2 (BMP2) (Wang et al., 2023b)	Mesenchymal stem cells	Rejuvenation of osteoporotic bone
6	Navitoclax (Su et al., 2023)	UHMWPE particle-induced osteolysis in 8-week-old male C57bL/6j mice	Inhibited the activation of osteoclasts and rejuvenated the UHMWPE particle–induced osteolysis
7	Navitoclax (Yang et al., 2024)	In vitro: bone marrow-derived mesenchymal stem cells from young and aged mice In vivo: 1,25(OH)2D-insufficient (Cyp27b1+-) mice	Induced apoptosis in senescent bone marrow-derived mesenchymal stem cells cells by downregulating bcl2, corrected bone loss by increasing bone density, bone volume, trabecular number and trabecular thickness
8	Fisetin (Molagoda et al., 2021)	In vitro: mouse preosteoblast MC3T3-E1 cells In vivo: zebrafish larvae	Inhibits osteoclastogenesis and promotes osteoblastogenesis GSK-3β phosphorylation at Ser9 and consequent β-catenin activation
9	Fisetin (Xu et al., 2021)	Osteoporosis model ovariectomized (OVX) Sprague Dawley rats	Augmented the bone density and bone mineral content

(*Continued*)

Table 7.3 (Continued) Senolytics and Senomorphics in Osteoporosis: Evidence from Preclinical Studies

S.No.	*Senotherapeutic Agent*	*Model*	*Major Findings*
10	Fisetin (Feng, Shu, and Zhao, 2022)	In silico: docking study of fisetin and alendronate on the vitamin D and oestrogen (α and β) receptors was conducted In vitro: SaOS-2 osteosarcoma cells (osteoblast like human) In vivo: ovariectomy-induced osteoporosis in rats	Increased levels of bone mineral density (BMD), bone mineral content (BMC), and biochemical parameters like stiffness, energy and maximum load
11	Piperlongumine (Luo et al., 2024)	In vitro: primary human chondrocytes In vivo: 10-week-old C57BL/6 osteoarthritis models induced by destabilization of the medial meniscus (DMM)	Protected ovariectomy-induced osteoporosis by inhibiting osteoclastogenesis via suppression of p38
12	Piperlongumine (Liu, Diao, et al., 2022)	In vivo: titanium (Ti) particle–induced calvarial osteolysis model In vitro: bone marrow–derived macrophage (BMM) cells of mouse human osteoblasts (hFOB 1.19)	By suppressing RANKL-induced signalling pathways, reduced the osteoclastic marker genes' mRNA expressions
13	Curcumin (Hatefi et al., 2018)	Osteoporosis in patients with spinal cord injuries	Bone mineral density of lumbar, femoral neck and total hip significantly decreased in control group and increased in curcumin group at the end of the study
14	Berberine (Jin et al., 2017)	In vivo: BALB/c-nu/nu mice, male, 5–6 weeks old weighing 18–20 g In vitro: human Saos-2 and MG-63 cell lines	Apoptosis in senescent cells and reduced inflammation
15	Rapamycin (Martin et al., 2021)	In vivo: young and adult mice	Decreased bone mineral content and bone mineral density
16	Resveratrol (Wei et al., 2023)	In vivo: ovariectomy-induced osteoporosis in Wistar rats	Inhibited bcl2 and bcl1 pathway, promoted autophagy and reduced oxidative stress
17	Metformin (Ruan et al., 2023)	Women patients	Accelerated fracture healing by expanding type H vessel, increased bone mineral density

Table 7.4 Senolytics in Clinical Trials

S.No.	*Senolytic*	*Study Title*	*Study Design and Status*	*Reference*	*Results*
1	Dasatinib + quercetin, fisetin	Targeting cellular senescence with senolytics to improve skeletal health in older humans	Phase 2, randomized, open-label, current	NCT04313634	Change in bone turnover markers, bone mineral density and SASP mediators
2	Fisetin	Use of senolytic and anti-fibrotic agents to improve the beneficial effect of bone marrow-derived mesenchymal stem cells for osteoarthritis	Phase 1/2, randomized, double-blind, active-control, current	NCT04815902	Results have not yet published as the trial is ongoing
3	Fisetin	Senolytic drugs attenuate osteoarthritis-related articular cartilage degeneration: a clinical trial	Phase 1/2, randomized, double-blind, placebo-controlled, current	NCT04210986	Completed in 2023; results not yet posted
4	Fisetin	Targeting senescence to reduce osteoarthritis pain and cartilage breakdown	Phase 1/2, randomized, double-blind, placebo-controlled, current	NCT04770064	Completed in 2023; results not yet posted
5	UBX0101	Safety and tolerability and long-term follow-up studies of patients with osteoarthritis of the knee treated with UBX0101 or placebo	Phase 2, randomized, double-blind, placebo-controlled, competed but it failed to achieve primary endpoint	NCT03513016 AND NCT04349956	Ongoing
6	UBX0101	A study to assess the safety and efficacy of a single or repeat doses of UBX0101 in patients with osteoarthritis of the knee	Current	NCT04229225 AND NCT04129944	Results not disclosed from phase 1 study; in phase 2 trial, UBX0101 not effective in alleviating osteoarthritis
7	Dasatinib + quercetin + fisetin	To determine if senolytic drugs reduce senescent cell burden and reduce bone resorption markers/increase bone formation markers in elderly women	Phase 2, single-center, 20-week, open-label, randomized controlled trial	NCT04313634	Change in C-terminal telopeptide of type I collagen (CTX), change in plasma senescence-associated secretory phenotype (SASP)

encouraged the aggregation of cartilage matrix in osteoarthritis chondrocyte pellet culture and promoted chondrogenic phenotype (Yang et al. 2020). In another study (Miura et al. 2022), navitoclax acts as a potential disease-modifying drug in osteoarthritis and osteoporosis in synovial mesenchymal cells from osteoarthritic patients. The basic mechanisms involved included selective elimination of senescent cells as evidenced by the lower expression of SASP factors (MMP-13 and IL-6) and crucial senescence markers (p16 and p21) and inhibition of the activation of osteoclasts. In a study in an ultra-high molecular weight polyethylene (UHMWPE)-induced mouse calvarial (cranial) osteolysis model, navitoclax reduced the inflammatory microenvironment, inhibiting osteoclast formation and alleviating bone loss (Su et al. 2023). ABT263 cleared senescent skeletal cells selectively, which shows its therapeutic characteristic in BMSCs caused by vitamin D insufficiency. It acts by improving osteoblast activity, decreasing the activity of osteoclasts, and improving overall bone health (Yang et al. 2024). On the contrary, navitoclax is also reported to cause trabecular bone loss and impair osteoprogenitor function in old mice thereby showing negative effects on bone (Sharma et al. 2020) Other bcl-2 inhibitors include ABT-737, effective in osteoporosis, A1331852, effective in cartilage and bone aging alleviation, A1155463, effective in both osteoarthritis and osteoporosis and UBX1325, a future senolytic therapy in bone disorders. They commonly cause apoptosis in senescent bone cells (Souers et al. 2013, Tao et al. 2014, Croce and Reed 2016).

7.5.1.3 UBX0101 and PPARα Agonist

Additional senolytic substances under investigation in bone disorders are p53 activators such as UBX0101 and fenofibrate, PPARα agonist (Pawge and Khatik 2021) (Nogueira-Recalde et al. 2019). UBX0101 is a small senolytic molecule developed by Unity Biotechnology. In a preclinical study, it reduced senescent cell markers and MMPs, suppressed inflammation, and improved cartilage health in a C57BL/6 mouse model of osteoarthritis by modulating the MDM2-p53 pathway (Chin et al. 2023). A phase 1 clinical trial demonstrated the safety and tolerability of intra-articular UBX0101 in patients with moderate-to-severe osteoarthritis of the knee, but a phase 2 study reported that at higher doses, it failed to meet the primary endpoint of pain reduction compared to placebo. In a Phase 2, randomized, double-blind, placebo-controlled trial, a single injection of UBX0101 targeting senescent synoviocytes showed improvement in patients, but it was not significant compared to placebo (Lane et al. 2021). Despite its failure, the concept of modulating the MDM2-p53 pathway remains promising and ongoing research in senolytics may yield more refined molecules with better efficacy (Jeon et al. 2017).

One study on fenofibrate reported a reduction in senescent cells and inflammation, reversing damage in senescent osteoarthritis cells, and lowering of PPARα levels, suggesting fibrate drugs as potential targets for osteoarthritis (Nogueira-Recalde et al. 2019). Cell proliferation, differentiation and apoptosis are regulated by mitogen-activated protein kinase (MAPK) in bone development. Another attractive target is p38/MAPK. p38/MAPK comes under the sub-family of MAPK pathway and gets activated in response to stress markers including oxidative stress, environmental stress, heat and osmotic shock. Interestingly, p38/MAPK inhibitors have the potential to attenuate inflammation in rheumatoid arthritis and their senescence-related role is confirmed in chondrogenesis (Gaur et al. 2022, Ganguly et al. 2023). Drugs such as SB203580, UR-13756 and BIRB-796 have been newly synthesized, which inhibit the p38/MAPK pathway by triggering cell cycle arrest and inducing senescence in them. p38/MAPK inhibitors have been shown to block SASP secretion in senescent osteoblast cells (Li, Dai, et al. 2022). SB2023580 suppresses p16 signalling and SA-β-Gal activity, through which cell cycle arrest is well mediated (Dimitriou et al. 2011). It also downregulates RANK/RANKL (Chen et al. 2015). In an in vivo study using human fibroblasts, R-13756 and BIRB-796 are other novel second-generation p38 inhibitors that showed higher specificity (Alimbetov et al. 2016).

7.5.1.4 Fisetin

It is a natural flavonoid and senolytic compound found in various fruits and vegetables such as strawberries, apples and grapes. It is known for its antioxidant, anti-inflammatory and anti-carcinogenic properties (Arai et al. 2000). It also downregulates anti-apoptotic proteins, including Bcl-2, which is particularly effective in reducing the secretion of the SASP. It works by two mechanisms: (1) by inhibiting the mammalian target of rapamycin (mTOR) signalling pathway, thereby delaying cellular senescence in bone and cartilage cells; and (2) by activating nuclear factor erythroid 2–related factor 2 (Nrf2) signalling, a master regulator of antioxidant signalling pathways that enhances the cell's antioxidant defences by controlling redox balance, detoxification and inflammation.

A study on osteoblast physiology was reported by Fisetin treatment in vivo and in vitro. The study proved that fisetin stimulated proliferation and differentiation of rat preosteoblasts in vitro by upregulating the transcriptional activity of the key transcription factor Runx2, which also leads to expression of crucial structural and functional genes involved in the formation of mineralized bone matrix (Léotoing et al. 2014). Fisetin improved bone and joint health through its dual actions in producing senolytic and anti-inflammatory effects, and acted as a more naturally prominent senolytic alternative for chronic bone disorders. In preclinical studies of osteoporosis and osteoarthritis, fisetin has been shown to reduce senescence markers and improve bone density and cartilage health (Zheng et al. 2017). Clinical trials are assessing it for its senolytic effects in various age-related conditions, specifically for bone disorders (NCT04210986).

In a Zmpste24−/− Progeria mouse model that exhibits multiple established hallmarks of aging and senescence, including musculoskeletal deterioration, fisetin attenuated bone degeneration. Fisetin significantly increased runt-related transcription factor 2 (RUNX2), ALP, collagen type I alpha, osterix, osteocalcin and bone morphogenetic protein expression. Fisetin inhibited anti-osteoblastic genes, while fisetin-induced osteogenic effects were activated via phosphorylation of glycogen synthase kinase-3β at Ser 9 (Molagoda et al. 2021). Oral administration of fisetin in ovariectomized rats for 16 weeks produced better protection against osteoporosis via augmenting bone density and bone mineral content (Xu et al. 2021).

A systematic review on fisetin on bone and cartilage defines various strategies that demonstrate how beneficial fisetin is for osteoarthritis and osteoporosis (Yamaura et al. 2022). It has also shown an anti-osteoporotic effect on ovariectomy-induced osteoporosis in silico, in vitro and in vivo, where it has been shown to be a useful senolytic phytoconstituent for postmenopausal prevention and treatment (Feng, Shu, and Zhao 2022).

7.5.1.5 Piperlongumine

It is a potential natural alkaloid and senolytic derived from the fruits of the long pepper plant (*Piper longum*) (Yadav, Krishnan, and Vohora 2020). Recently, it has gained more attention from scientists as a potential senotherapeutic agent due to its multidimensional property to selectively induce apoptosis in senescent cells, through oxidation resistance 1 (OXR1) receptor modulation (Zhang et al. 2018) and anti-inflammatory action, making it a promising candidate for targeting aging and ARDs, including bone disorders (Thatikonda et al. 2020). Mechanistically, it works by increasing intracellular ROS levels in target bone cells by inhibiting glutathione-S-transferase pi 1 (GSTP1), a critical enzyme in ROS detoxification (Harshbarger et al. 2017). The build-up of ROS induces oxidative stress, particularly in senescent cells, causing apoptosis (Chen et al. 2016). Piperlongumine inhibits osteoclastogenesis via suppression of signalling pathways p38 and c-Jun N-terminal kinase (JNK) in the ovariectomy-induced osteoporosis model (Luo et al. 2024). This study shows its usage in osteoporotic fractures. Piperlongumine also inhibits osteolysis induced by titanium particles-induced osteolysis in bone, osteoclast formation and signalling pathways induced by RANKL in vivo, which could help treat osteoclast-related diseases, including periprosthetic osteolysis (Liu, Diao, et al. 2022). In vitro and in silico studies done on Wharton's jelly mesenchymal stem cells (WJMSCs) treated with piperlongumine identified the significant osteogenic effects in mesenchymal cells and mechanisms of alleviating cartilage destruction and joint inflammation (Sanap et al. 2021; Jo et al. 2024).

7.5.1.6 Natural Compounds with Senolytic Properties

Spermidine and curcumin have already been evaluated in at least 129 clinical trials for various conditions like acute kidney injury, cancer, lymphocytic leukaemia, cardiovascular abnormalities, chronic kidney disease and cystic fibrosis. Curcumin is reported to promote osteogenic differentiation by modifying the Wnt/β-catenin signalling (Yamaguchi et al. 2012). Besides this, it also improved the apoptosis induced by oxidative stress in senescent osteoblasts (Inchingolo et al. 2022). Various in vitro studies also show that curcumin modulates senescence-related pathways to inhibit osteoclast formation and differentiation via promoting autophagic activity (Ke et al. 2020).

In a recent randomized controlled trial, postmenopausal women with osteoporosis and osteopenia were administered curcumin orally in a dose of 80 mg daily along with *Nigella sativa* oil. It was found that there was no significant increase in bone mineral density and overall quality of life score; however, a significant increase was observed in femoral neck bone mineral density and lumbar spine bone mineral density. In patients with osteoarthritis, curcumin was compared to a placebo in treating osteoarthritic pain and was recommended as a traditional therapy for treating osteoarthritis pain (Van Ameyde and Hodgden 2022).

Berberine is an isoquinoline alkaloid that is known for preventing various diseases, including musculoskeletal disorders. Berberine is reported to suppress the proliferation of osteosarcoma cells by targeting multiple signalling pathways, including Wnt/β-catenin, AMP-activated protein kinase (AMPK), PI3K/Akt, NF-κB, Hedgehog, RANK/RANKL/OPG and oxidative stress signalling (Xu et al. 2010, Zhang, Ma, and Zhang 2021, Jin et al. 2017). Berberine was studied in post-traumatic osteoarthritis, which showed positive effects by reducing joint structural change and pain (Zhang, Ma, and Zhang 2021).

Spermidine is an anti-aging natural substance. It ameliorated articular cartilage degeneration and osteophyte in animal models of osteoarthritis through apoptosis and anti-inflammatory effects (Ou et al. 2024).

7.5.1.7 HSP90 Inhibitors

They are heat shock protein 90 molecular chaperones that help in proper folding, stabilization and cell cycle regulation. Significantly high levels of pro-survival proteins are expressed in senescent cells present in the bone microenvironment (e.g., osteoblasts, osteocytes, osteoclast precursors), which are stabilized by HSP90 by stabilizing their survival rate. Hence, the HSP90 inhibitors induce apoptosis in these kinds of cells, reducing SASP-mediated inflammation and bone matrix degradation. Geldanamycin (the first discovered HSP90 inhibitor), tanespimycin (17 AAG), alvespimycin (17-DMAG) are examples of HSP90 inhibitors (Siebelt et al. 2013a, Siebelt et al. 2013b).

The senolytics in various phases of clinical trials for bone diseases are shown in Table 7.4.

7.5.2 Senomorphics in Bone Disorders

These treatments focus on influencing the processes and elements linked to senescent cells without destroying the aging cells themselves. Senomorphics are commonly referred to as SASP inhibitors. These substances aim to make aging cells behave like younger ones by controlling their inflammation and age-related signalling pathways (Lagoumtzi and Chondrogianni 2021a) (Lagoumtzi and Chondrogianni 2021b). Some of the most well-known senomorphics studied in bone disorders include rapamycin, resveratrol, metformin, NF-κB, JAK/STAT, and p38MAPK inhibitors (Moiseeva et al. 2013).

7.5.2.1 *Rapamycin*

Rapamycin, also known as sirolimus, is an mTOR inhibitor that has been found to reduce IL-1 expression by inhibiting NF-kB. Rapamycin decreases the pro-inflammatory actions of IL-18 and shows a promising chondroprotective effect in rats (Bao et al. 2020). The effects of rapamycin treatment on bone accrual mass, architecture, and indices of bone turnover were examined in a healthy adult mouse model. In a research study, the results of intraperitoneal injection of rapamycin reduced femur bone mineral content, bone mineral density, and bone volume in comparison to mice treated with a vehicle. This data showed that the negative impact of rapamycin should also be taken into account (Martin et al. 2021). Rapamycin has shown positive results in inhibiting osteoclastogenesis in vitro by upregulating nuclear factor erythroid-2–related factor, glutamate-cysteine ligase catalytic subunit (Nrf2/GCLC) signalling pathway, and suppressing the intracellular redox reactions (Feng et al. 2023). Everolimus and temsirolimus are the analogues of rapamycin (Lin et al. 2022). Everolimus in combination with exemestane has shown bone protection in postmenopausal women (Gnant et al. 2013) while temsirolimus has shown protection in patients with bone metastases. It is yet to be explored for aging bone (Huelsmann et al. 2015).

7.5.2.2 *Resveratrol*

It is a plant-based antioxidant that originates in organic fruits like grapes and red wine and that activates the SIRT-1 pathway. In an in vitro study on IL-1β–induced human chondrocytes, resveratrol combined with curcumin lowered MMP-3 and MMP-9 by suppressing the NF-κB signalling pathway (Luo et al. 2019). In an in vivo study involving monoiodoacetate (MIA)-induced Sprague Dawley rats, oral administration of resveratrol 5–10 mg/kg/day for 2 weeks reduced levels of IL-1, IL-6, TNF-α and MMP-13 and inhibited the COX-2/iNOS signalling pathway (Yang, Sun, and Zhang 2022). Recently, studies have shown the effect of resveratrol on knee osteoarthritis in preclinical and clinical studies. An in vitro study on H_2O_2-induced porcine chondrocytes showed anti-inflammatory effects by decreasing IL-1β, TNF-α, MMP-1 and MMP-13 levels (Su et al. 2020). In MIA-induced knee osteoarthritis, resveratrol showed potential in reducing symptoms through activating the HO-1/Nrf2 signalling pathways (Wei et al. 2018). Resveratrol may also work by suppressing the TLR4 signalling pathway to reduce the incidence of osteoarthritis, as observed in IL-1β–induced SW1353 cells and high-fat diet–induced osteoarthritis in C57BL/6J mice (Xu et al. 2019). From the above studies, it is clear that resveratrol has shown potential for chondroprotective effects. There are few clinical studies of resveratrol on osteoarthritis. In a randomized, double blind study of 110 patients, resveratrol (500 mg/day) along with meloxicam (15 mg/day) significantly improved joint function as compared to placebo (Hussain et al. 2018). In addition to this, it was found to reduce inflammatory cytokines in osteoarthritis patients after 90 days of treatment. Additionally, patients' conditions significantly improved after receiving a dose of 500 mg/day for 90 days. In a double blind study of healthy postmenopausal women, resveratrol supplementation improved knee pain (Wong, Evans, and Howe 2017).

Resveratrol is also useful in maintaining conditions caused due to osteoporosis. There are several studies done to test the effects. In osteoporotic rats induced via ovariectomy, resveratrol activated autophagy by inhibiting Bcl-1/Bcl-2 complex in AMPK/JNK1-dependent pathway, eventually regulating osteocytes' function (Wei et al. 2023). A randomized clinical study done on post-menopausal women reported that regular supplementation improved bone mineral density. In age-related bone loss models, it increased cortical bone and increased trabecular bone in old animals. In oestrogen-deficiency induced bone loss, resveratrol showed increased femur epiphysis, increased femur calcium, and increased femur neck bone mineral density (Wong et al. 2020).

7.5.2.3 *Metformin*

Metformin is a diabetic medication and a widely known senomorphic (Acar et al. 2021) that has a potential role in mitigating osteoarthritis as well as osteoporosis and fracture risks through its anti-inflammatory and anti-aging properties. Some studies have shown that metformin has shown potential osteogenic effects, which are crucial for bone formation, especially in type 2 diabetes patients (Wang et al. 2020, Loh, Kadirvelu, and Pamidi 2022). It works through the AMPK pathway to induce osteogenesis. Other anti-osteoporotic effects include accelerated fracture healing and improved bone metabolism by lowering markers of bone turnover and raising bone mineral density, particularly in women (Ruan et al. 2023). These studies are mentioned in Table 7.3.

Along with anti-osteoporotic effects, metformin has proven to be a better candidate in preclinical studies in osteoarthritis as well. A 4-month administration of metformin in non-diabetic osteoarthritis patients showed significant beneficial effects (Alimoradi et al. 2023). In combination with celecoxib, metformin reduced cartilage damage in the obese osteoarthritis population, reduced pain and modulated autophagy to protect the cartilage (Aiad et al. 2024). Metformin has previously been associated with increased bone mineral density as recorded from the population of China (Sun, Liu, et al. 2022). It also has beneficial effects in ovariectomized-induced bone loss; however, the underlying mechanism is still vague.

7.5.3 Stem Cell Therapy

This therapy provides insights into rejuvenating the aged bone cells and promoting new bone formation by self-renewal and differentiation into multiple tissues such as bone and cartilage (Iaquinta et al. 2019). Rejuvenating bone marrow-derived mesenchymal stem cells, their derived vesicles as senolytic drugs, show promise in reducing inflammation to combat osteoarthritis (Rizzo et al. 2023). Allogeneic and autologous BM-MSCs, autologous adipose-derived mesenchymal stem cells (AD-MSCs) have been used in humans for studying anti-ostearthritic potential, where these MSCs protected the joint, subchondral bone and cartilage regeneration occurred without causing any adverse effects (Kim et al. 2014, Davatchi et al. 2011, Jo et al. 2014).

In a recent study of microarray analysis, MSCs from patients having primary osteoporosis had a different transcriptome than the control MSCs of non-osteoporotic patients. RUNX2, LRP5 and COL1A1 were enhanced in osteoporotic MSCs (Benisch et al. 2012). The types of mesenchymal cells used in various studies to regenerate bone were autologous enriched bone marrow MSCs for repairing osteoporotic bone defects and xenogeneic human umbilical cord blood–derived mesenchymal stem cells (hUCB-MSCs) (Hong et al. 2018, Jones et al. 2014). They are useful in disc degeneration, as evidenced by a finding in a porcine model where a reduction in inflammatory markers was seen, and BMP2 was elevated (Omlor et al. 2018).

7.5.4 JAK/STAT Inhibitors

Another very popular anti-aging compound is JAK/STAT inhibitors, widely applied in mitigating myeloproliferative diseases. They have been proclaimed to mitigate senescence-related bone loss in mice, attributing to their capability to halt SASP secretions, thereby acting as senomorphics (Godoi et al. 2023, Komagamine et al. 2023). The JAK/STAT pathway is a potential therapeutic target for osteolytic diseases as it regulates the increase in bone mass to boost osteoblast activity (Yari et al. 2023). Tofacitinib, baricitinib and upadacitinib are examples of JAK/STAT signalling pathway inhibitors useful in mitigating inflammation-driven aging and chronic diseases (Hu, Liu, and Zhang 2022, Angelini et al. 2020). Generally, they work by suppressing osteoclastogenesis and promoting osteoblastogenesis in osteoporosis, reducing joint erosion, and ameliorating periarticular osteopenia (bone thinning around joints) and bone loss (Yari et al. 2023, Komagamine et al. 2023).

7.6 SENESCENCE PATHWAYS AND MOLECULAR CROSSTALK IN BONE REMODELLING

SASP factors are produced within the bone microenvironment by the senescent BMSCs, which are detrimental to bone health (Fang, Liu, and Wan 2023a). Senolytics eliminate these senescent cells while senomorphics inhibit the SASPs. The key targets are described in the following sections.

7.6.1 RANK/RANKL/OPG Pathway (Osteoclast Regulation)

RANK is a receptor expressed on osteoclasts and other cells. RANKL is a protein that binds to the RANK receptor (Boyce and Xing 2007). This interaction is useful in bone resorption by promoting osteoclast differentiation, their activation and survival (Kiechl et al. 2006). Osteoprotegerin (OPG) is a protein that blocks RANKL and RANK interaction, preventing activation of osteoclasts (Boyce and Xing 2007). The mechanism behind this pathway drives bone resorption due to increased RANKL and decreased OPG levels, thereby enhancing osteoclast activity (De Leon-Oliva et al. 2023). RANKL binds to the RANK receptor on osteoclast precursors, which further activates NF-κB, c-Fos signalling and OPG, a decoy receptor for RANKL, thereby inhibiting osteoclastogenesis (Silva and Branco 2011).

Senotherapeutics interact with the RANK/RANKL/OPG pathway, influencing bone health and disease progression (Kim et al. 2020, Pignolo, Law, and Chandra 2021). Senolytic ABT-263 was administered to aged mice for 5 days to check the effect on RANKL expression, and it revealed reduced bone loss due to decreased RANKL expression (Kim et al. 2020). Dasatinib and quercetin target this pathway by reducing RANKL-induced osteoclastogenesis. Resveratrol (He et al. 2010) and metformin (Mai et al. 2011) follow this pathway.

7.6.2 JAK/STAT Pathway

It is a Janus kinase-signal transducer and activator of transcription signalling pathway that induces gene expression and cellular processes in the chondrocytes, osteoblasts and osteoclasts, involved in inflammation and ARDs (Sanpaolo et al. 2020). SASP mediators such as IL-6, IL-4 and TNF-α activate this pathway by binding to its receptors. This in turn triggers JAKs, resulting in the stimulation of STAT (Damerau et al. 2020). These proteins stimulate osteoclasts, chondrocytes and osteoblasts (Sims 2020).

The JAK pathway is activated in aging, which is responsible for causing bone disorders. Hence, collectively senotherapeutics like ruxolitinib (JAK1/2 inhibitor) and tofacitinib (JAK1/3 inhibitor) target this pathway (Xu, Tchkonia, and Kirkland 2016) (Xu et al. 2015). Metformin and rapamycin indirectly affect the JAK-STAT pathway in terms of oxidative stress and promoting stem cell function, respectively (Xu, Tchkonia, and Kirkland 2016).

7.6.3 p53-p21 Pathway

The p16INK4a/Rb pathway (cell cycle regulators)-p53 is a tumour-suppressor protein acting in response to cellular stress caused during aging, and p21 is a cyclin-dependent kinase inhibitor and a target gene of p52 (Mijit et al. 2020). These are activated during cellular stress in bone. p21, which is also called CIP1 and WAF1, a protein made from CDKN1A gene. It may cause cells to stop dividing through both p53-dependent and p53-independent ways (Xu et al. 2020). Englund and colleagues showed that p21 plays a part in causing cells to age through DNA damage response (DDR) as well as inflammatory pathways in specially modified mice, where p21 is overproduced in their skeletal muscles. The increase of p21 in aging cells was linked to tissue scarring, decreased skeletal muscle size and lower physical abilities. Research studies have also shown that the loss of p53 in mouse BMSC affects bone remodelling and might also affect cancer-related bone changes by negatively regulating OPG (Engeland 2022, Chen et al. 2022). p16INK4a/Rb is a protein associated with aging, osteoarthritis and osteoporosis (Khosla, Farr, and Monroe 2022, Saul et al. 2024).

Drugs targeting senescent osteoclasts selectively eliminate p16INK4a-positive cells (Baker et al. 2011). Senolytic drugs like fisetin target and eliminate p16INK4a-positive cells (Yousefzadeh et al. 2018).

7.6.4 Growth Promotion Pathways: mTOR and SIRT-1

7.6.4.1 mTOR

It is a nutrient-sensing signalling cascade that plays an important role as a negative regulator of autophagy and the regulation of growth and metabolism of cells (Wang et al. 2023a). It gets activated through a series of actions involving PI3K kinase and protein kinase B (Akt kinase) which leads to the inhibition of autophagy promoting cell growth, cell differentiation and cell survival (Chen and Long 2018). mTOR forms two main protein complexes similar in structure but differ in function: mTORC1, which helps control cell growth and metabolism which is essential for normal cartilage, and mTORC2, which manages cell proliferation and survival and skeletal development. Pal and colleagues found a link between the increased levels of mTOR and the progress of the disease using a mouse model for osteoarthritis (Pal et al. 2015). By removing mTOR at the genetic level, they were able to reduce osteoarthritis development by boosting autophagy (Saxton and Sabatini 2017). Luo and his team showed that fixing the autophagy block in chondrocytes in the osteoarthritis mouse model, cartilage damage was reduced by the PI3K/AKT/mTOR pathway. (Luo et al. 2019). When mTOR signalling is dysregulated, it inhibits BMSC proliferation and differentiation resulting in bone loss and osteoporosis (Chen and Long 2018).

Hence, senomorphics like mTOR inhibitors (e.g., rapamycin) showed beneficial effects in osteoporosis by inhibiting mTOR (Chen and Long 2018, Wu et al. 2019).

7.6.4.2 SIRTs

SIRTs, or sirtuins, are a category of proteins dependent on nicotinamide adenine dinucleotide (NAD+) to mechanistically promote longevity of senescent cells and stabilize them in ARDs. SIRTs can regulate mitochondrial homeostasis in chondrocytes for their survival (Liu et al. 2023). There are seven members in this family, named SIRT1 through SIRT7, which are present in the nucleus, regulating and managing the expression of specific genes. SIRT-1 is especially important for keeping cartilage healthy because it helps chondrocyte cells to survive and support the stability of the extracellular matrix (ECM) in the cellular environment by maintaining homeostasis (Lu et al. 2022). It has been linked to longer life and aging.

Research shows that activating SIRT-1 can help protect against osteoarthritis by improving the health of certain bones and preventing chondrocyte death. SIRT-1 participates in several pathways that includes NF-κB, AMPK, mTOR, p53 and family of transcription factors (FoxOs) which are involved in inflammation, creating new mitochondria, breaking down waste in cells, managing energy use, and dealing with oxidative stress. Many clinical studies have found SIRT1 in treating bone disorders like osteoporosis and osteonecrosis (Chen et al. 2021, Domazetovic et al. 2017). SIRT3, an essential mitochondrial metabolic regulatory enzyme, has been reported to reduce oxidative stress in rodent BMSCs by reducing the generation of ROS (Sun, Wu, et al. 2022) and regulating AGEs-induced BMSCs senescence and senile osteoporosis (Guo, Jia, et al. 2021). SIRT3 has the potential to target different types of osteoporosis. SIRT3 enhances the osteogenic potential and osteoblastic activity of bone marrow-derived mesenchymal stem cells. It is found to play a role in different types of osteoporosis, including postmenopausal osteoporosis, diabetic osteoporosis, glucocorticoid-induced osteoporosis, and senescence-related osteoporosis (Pan et al. 2024, Hu and Wang 2022).

7.6.5 DNA Damage Induced by Reactive Oxygen Species and the Role of Type I Interferon and the STING Pathway

The cyclic GMP–AMP synthase–stimulator of interferon genes (cGAS-STING) pathway is a host's innate immune response to pathogenic DNA, mild and continuous aging and mechanical stress. Inflammation leads to a peak rise in ROS, which successively causes oxidative stress and DNA damage to osteoblasts and chondrocytes, impairing their proliferation and differentiation (Domazetovic et al. 2017). It is a newly discovered pathway playing a role in both osteoporosis and osteoarthritis. Type H vessels are recently discovered blood vessels that play a role in angiogenesis and osteogenesis, helping in bone formation, which provide bone tissue with vital nutrition, oxygen and growth factors (Wang et al. 2017). They are surrounded by osteoprogenitors expressing osterix, which contributes to the process of bone formation (Nakashima et al. 2002). Therefore, the STING pathway directly affects the osteoblasts and osteoclasts, followed by the angiogenesis process of Type H vessels during aging and stress (Wang et al. 2017, Huang et al. 2018).

Oxidative stress causes DNA damage in older cells and is associated with various diseases affecting nearly every organ. When damaged cells release mitochondrial

DNA, the innate immune system gets activated. Cyclic GMP–AMP synthase (cGAS) is a fundamental component of this immune response and the STING signalling pathway, or the interferon gene stimulator (Hu et al. 2021). The escaped DNA is then recognized by the cGAS enzyme, which stimulates the production of cyclic GMP-AMP. This cGAMP then adheres to STING, and initiates the STING pathway, thereby activating different downstream targets, including TANK-binding kinase 1 (TBK1), a key regulator of NF-κB signalling, interferon regulatory factor 3 (IRF-3), which drives inflammation, and IκB kinase (IKK), which influences osteoclastogenesis (Zhou et al. 2023). As a result, the production of type 1 interferons begins. The STING pathway modulates NF-κB signalling in chondrocytes, which are associated with SASP and aging (Guo, Chen, et al. 2021b).

The cGAS–cGAMP–STING pathway is proposed to be a crucial connection between DNA damage, cellular aging, cancer and inflammatory mediators (Guo, Chen, et al. 2021b). The expression of STING increases in osteoarthritis and further deteriorating articular cartilage in humans. Further, according to available literature, STING expression is increased in the DMM model, which accelerates the malfunctioning of the ECM by increasing the levels of enzymes that degrade the matrix, specifically ADAMTS5 and MMP13, which are a segment of the SASP (Yang, Zhao, and Pang 2024).

STING pathway activation is linked to processes such as cellular aging and apoptosis in IL-1β–treated chondrocytes, which is directly linked to osteoarthritis. Research by Guo and colleagues showed that reducing STING using a lentivirus in a mouse model of osteoarthritis improves issues related to cell aging, apoptosis and ECM imbalance in chondrocytes through regulating the NF-κB pathway (Guo, Chen, et al. 2021a). Because of their significant purpose in swelling and tenderness and in raising SASP factors, these enzymes are becoming a promising choice for therapies directed at treating cellular senescence-related osteoarthritis and osteoporosis.

7.6.6 Seno-Inflammation

The term denotes a dysregulated response towards immunity that indicates chronic inflammation. Seno-inflammation is a "steady-state age-related inflammation" as first proposed by Chung and coworkers, where it was described as a process that aggravates chronic diseases in the skeletal system. Combining age and age-related inflammation introduces the concept of inflammaging (Chung et al. 2019). Inflammation produced by the senescent chondrocytes and osteoblasts triggers NF-κB signalling and hence, inflammation. Chemokines, interleukins, adhesion molecules and C-reactive protein are upregulated in this process, prompting immune system instigation (Liu et al. 2017). Aging in humans has been linked with dysregulated macrophage activity.

Macrophage activity in senescent cells is linked to changes in the Toll-like receptor (TLR) signalling pathway, interferon-gamma (IFN)-γ activity, and NF-κB signalling. In vitro and in vivo, proteoglycan-4 (PRG-4/lubricin) regulates TLR signalling and the inflammatory response (Iqbal et al. 2016). In the synovial fluid of human osteoarthritic joints, PRG-4 adheres to TLR2 and reduces TLR4 activity, which is considered to be a potential anti-inflammatory therapeutic effect (Alquraini et al. 2015). The other remedial biomarkers related to bone that are also being explored in restoring seno-inflammation are senescence-associated secretomes and growth factors. Growth hormones such as pegvisomant are considered dynamic therapeutic agents as they inhibit the growth hormone/insulin-like growth factor-1 (IGF1) axis and inflammation (Chesnokova et al. 2024). The cells lowered inflammatory stress, which was measured using markers IL-1β and SA-β-Gal.

7.7 CONCLUSION

The senotherapeutic agents are widely investigated in cancer and myelofibrative diseases and are now also showing progress in bone disorders that affect the older population. Various research studies, as discussed, show the potential of senotherapeutics for treating and preventing the progression of bone disorders associated with aging, particularly osteoporosis and osteoarthritis. Their mechanistic actions that improve bone deterioration are worth proving their application clinically to improve health span and extend longevity, specifically in elderly people. Senolytics like navitoclax and dasatinib + quercetin that selectively kill senescent cells have shown strong preclinical efficacy. Although these drugs progressed to early-phase clinical trials, their toxicity concerns still exist. Senomorphics such as metformin and rapamycin are backed by more clinical evidence, although they are mostly in the experimental stage for bone and joint disorders. Simultaneously, stem cell therapy holds promise in preserving bone and cartilage, regulating the inflammatory microenvironment. Combination of senotherapeutics with stem cell therapy may enhance regenerative outcomes. However, more rigorous preclinical and clinical studies are necessary to establish the role of senotherapeutics in the treatment of bone disorders.

7.8 ACKNOWLEDGEMENT

We acknowledge the support of the Department of Science and Technology (DST), Government of India and Hamdard National Foundation (HNF) for the fellowship to NS.

REFERENCES

Acar, M. B., Ş Ayaz-Güner, Z. Gunaydin, M. Karakukcu, G. Peluso, G. Di Bernardo, S. Özcan, and U. Galderisi. 2021. "Proteomic and biological analysis of the effects of metformin senomorphics on the mesenchymal stromal cells." *Frontiers in Bioengineering and Biotechnology* 9:730813. https://doi.org/10.3389/fbioe.2021.730813.

Adams, Peter, G. T. Davies, and P. Sweetnam. 1970. "Osteoporosis and the effects of ageing on bone mass in elderly men and women1." *QJM: An International Journal of Medicine* 39 (4):601–616.

Aiad, Amany Abd Elaal, Sahar Mohamed El-Haggar, Amal Mohamed El-Barbary, and Dalia Refat El-Afify. 2024. "Metformin as adjuvant therapy in obese knee osteoarthritis patients." *Inflammopharmacology* 32 (4):2349–2359.

Alimbetov, Dauren, Terence Davis, Amy J. C. Brook, Lynne S. Cox, Richard G. A. Faragher, Talgat Nurgozhin, Zhaxybay Zhumadilov, and David Kipling. 2016. "Suppression of the senescence-associated secretory phenotype (SASP) in human fibroblasts using small molecule inhibitors of p38 MAP kinase and MK2." *Biogerontology* 17:305–315.

Alimoradi, Nahid, Mohammad Tahami, Negar Firouzabadi, Elham Haem, and Amin Ramezani. 2023. "Metformin attenuates symptoms of osteoarthritis: Role of genetic diversity of Bcl2 and CXCL16 in osteoarthritis." *Arthritis Research & Therapy* 25 (1):35. https://doi.org/10.1186/s13075-023-03025-7.

Alquraini, Ali, Steven Garguilo, Gerard D'Souza, Ling X. Zhang, Tannin A. Schmidt, Gregory D. Jay, and Khaled A. Elsaid. 2015. "The interaction of lubricin/proteoglycan 4 (PRG4) with toll-like receptors 2 and 4: An anti-inflammatory role of PRG4 in synovial fluid." *Arthritis Research & Therapy* 17:1–12.

Angelini, J., R. Talotta, R. Roncato, G. Fornasier, G. Barbiero, L. Dal Cin, S. Brancati, and F. Scaglione. 2020. "JAK-inhibitors for the treatment of rheumatoid arthritis: A focus on the present and an outlook on the future." *Biomolecules* 10 (7). https://doi.org/10.3390/biom10071002.

Arai, Yusuke, Shaw Watanabe, Mitsuru Kimira, Kayoko Shimoi, Rika Mochizuki, and Naohide Kinae. 2000. "Dietary intakes of flavonols, flavones and isoflavones by Japanese women and the inverse correlation between quercetin intake and plasma LDL cholesterol concentration." *The Journal of Nutrition* 130 (9):2243–2250.

Bai, Jiangtao, Yuyang Wang, Jianping Wang, Jianglong Zhai, Feilong He, and Guoying Zhu. 2020. "Irradiation-induced senescence of bone marrow mesenchymal stem cells aggravates osteogenic differentiation dysfunction via paracrine signaling." *American Journal of Physiology-Cell Physiology* 318 (5):C1005–C1017.

Baker, D. J., T. Wijshake, T. Tchkonia, N. K. LeBrasseur, B. G. Childs, B. van de Sluis, J. L. Kirkland, and J. M. van Deursen. 2011. "Clearance of p16Ink4a-positive senescent cells delays ageing-associated disorders." *Nature* 479 (7372):232–236. https://doi.org/10.1038/nature10600.

Bao, Jiapeng, Zhonggai Chen, Langhai Xu, Lidong Wu, and Yan Xiong. 2020. "Rapamycin protects chondrocytes against IL-18-induced apoptosis and ameliorates rat osteoarthritis." *Aging (Albany NY)* 12 (6):5152.

Baron, Roland, and Michaela Kneissel. 2013. "WNT signaling in bone homeostasis and disease: From human mutations to treatments." *Nature Medicine* 19 (2):179–192. https://doi.org/10.1038/nm.3074.

Bekaert, Sofie, Tim De Meyer, and Patrick Van Oostveldt. 2005. "Telomere attrition as ageing biomarker." *Anticancer Research* 25 (4):3011–3021.

Benisch, Peggy, Tatjana Schilling, Ludger Klein-Hitpass, Sönke P. Frey, Lothar Seefried, Nadja Raaijmakers, Melanie Krug, Martina Regensburger, Sabine Zeck, and Thorsten Schinke. 2012. "The transcriptional profile of mesenchymal stem cell populations in primary osteoporosis is distinct and shows overexpression of osteogenic inhibitors." *PLoS ONE* 7 (9):e45142. https://doi.org/10.1371/journal.pone.0045142.

Boyce, Brendan F., and Lianping Xing. 2007. "Biology of RANK, RANKL, and osteoprotegerin." *Arthritis Research & Therapy* 9 (1):S1. https://doi.org/10.1186/ar2165.

Boyle, William J., W. Scott Simonet, and David L. Lacey. 2003. "Osteoclast differentiation and activation." *Nature* 423 (6937):337–342.

Callaway, Danielle A., and Jean X. Jiang. 2015. "Reactive oxygen species and oxidative stress in osteoclastogenesis, skeletal aging and bone diseases." *Journal of Bone and Mineral Metabolism* 33:359–370.

Casado-Díaz, Antonio, Jaouad Anter, Gabriel Dorado, and José Manuel Quesada-Gómez. 2016. "Effects of quercetin, a natural phenolic compound, in the differentiation of human mesenchymal stem cells (MSC) into adipocytes and osteoblasts." *The Journal of Nutritional Biochemistry* 32:151–162. https://doi.org/10.1016/j.jnutbio.2016.03.005.

Chandra, Abhishek, Anthony B. Lagnado, Joshua N. Farr, David G. Monroe, Sean Park, Christine Hachfeld, Tamar Tchkonia, James L. Kirkland, Sundeep Khosla, and João F. Passos. 2020. "Targeted reduction of senescent cell burden alleviates focal radiotherapy-related bone loss." *Journal of Bone and Mineral Research* 35 (6):1119–1131.

Chandrakar, Lokesh, Ramesh Ambatwar, and Gopal L. Khatik. 2024. "Cellular senescence and senolytic agents: Recent updates on their role and applications." *Current Topics in Medicinal Chemistry* 24 (2):157–178.

Chen, D., Y. Li, F. Guo, Z. Lu, C. Hei, P. Li, and Q. Jin. 2015. "Protective effect of p38 MAPK inhibitor on wear debris-induced inflammatory osteolysis through downregulating RANK/RANKL in a mouse model." *Genetics Molecular Research* 14 (1):40–52. https://doi.org/10.4238/2015.January.15.6.

Chen, Jianquan, and Fanxin Long. 2018. "mTOR signaling in skeletal development and disease." *Bone Research* 6 (1):1. https://doi.org/10.1038/s41413-017-0004-5.

Chen, L., G. Wang, Q. Wang, Q. Liu, Q. Sun, and L. Chen. 2019. "N-acetylcysteine prevents orchiectomy-induced osteoporosis by inhibiting oxidative stress and osteocyte senescence." *American Journal of Translational Research* 11 (7):4337–4347.

Chen, S. Y., G. H. Liu, W. Y. Chao, C. S. Shi, C. Y. Lin, Y. P. Lim, C. H. Lu, P. Y. Lai, H. R. Chen, and Y. R. Lee. 2016. "Piperlongumine suppresses proliferation of human oral squamous cell carcinoma through cell cycle arrest, apoptosis and senescence." *International Journal of Molecular Sciences* 17 (4). https://doi.org/10.3390/ijms17040616.

Chen, Ye, Feng Zhou, Hanghang Liu, Jiaxuan Li, Huiling Che, Jiaqi Shen, and En Luo. 2021. "SIRT1, a promising regulator of bone homeostasis." *Life Sciences* 269:119041. https://doi.org/10.1016/j.lfs.2021.119041.

Chen, Yi-Peng, Xin-Yu Wang, Yong-Li Ma, Wen Wen, Xin-Hua Fang, Min Wu, Shi-Jie Dai, and Jun-Fei He. 2022. "p53/p21 inhibits osteoarthritis progression by regulating chondrocyte pyroptosis." *Journal of Biomedical Nanotechnology* 18 (12):2721–2729.

Chesnokova, Vera, Svetlana Zonis, Tugce Apaydin, Robert Barrett, and Shlomo Melmed. 2024. "Non-pituitary growth hormone enables colon cell senescence evasion." *Aging Cell*:e14193.

Childs, Bennett G., Martina Gluscevic, Darren J. Baker, Remi-Martin Laberge, Dan Marquess, Jamie Dananberg, and Jan M. Van Deursen. 2017. "Senescent cells: An emerging target for diseases of ageing." *Nature Reviews Drug Discovery* 16 (10):718–735.

Chin, A. F., J. Han, C. C. Clement, Y. Choi, H. Zhang, M. Browne, O. H. Jeon, and J. H. Elisseeff. 2023. "Senolytic treatment reduces oxidative protein stress in an aging male murine model of post-traumatic osteoarthritis." *Aging Cell* 22 (11):e13979. https://doi.org/10.1111/acel.13979.

Chung, Hae Young, Dae Hyun Kim, Eun Kyeong Lee, Ki Wung Chung, Sangwoon Chung, Bonggi Lee, Arnold Y. Seo, Jae Heun Chung, Young Suk Jung, and Eunok Im. 2019. "Redefining chronic inflammation in aging and age-related diseases: Proposal of the senoinflammation concept." *Aging and Disease* 10 (2):367.

Corr, Maripat. 2008. "Wnt–β-catenin signaling in the pathogenesis of osteoarthritis." *Nature Clinical Practice Rheumatology* 4 (10):550–556. https://doi.org/10.1038/ncprheum0904.

Croce, C. M., and J. C. Reed. 2016. "Finally, an apoptosis-targeting therapeutic for cancer." *Cancer Research* 76 (20):5914–5920. https://doi.org/10.1158/0008-5472.Can-16-1248.

Damerau, A., T. Gaber, S. Ohrndorf, and P. Hoff. 2020. "JAK/STAT activation: A general mechanism for bone development, homeostasis, and regeneration." *International Journal of Molecular Sciences* 21 (23). https://doi.org/10.3390/ijms21239004.

Davatchi, Fereydoun, Bahar Sadeghi Abdollahi, Mandana Mohyeddin, Farhad Shahram, and Behrooz Nikbin. 2011. "Mesenchymal stem cell therapy for knee osteoarthritis. Preliminary report of four patients." *International Journal of Rheumatic Diseases* 14 (2):211–215.

De Leon-Oliva, D., S. Barrena-Blázquez, L. Jiménez-Álvarez, O. Fraile-Martinez, C. García-Montero, L. López-González, D. Torres-Carranza, L. M. García-Puente, S. T. Carranza, MÁ Álvarez-Mon, M. Álvarez-Mon, R. Diaz, and M. A. Ortega. 2023. "The RANK-RANKL-OPG system: A multifaceted regulator of homeostasis, immunity, and cancer." *Medicina (Kaunas)* 59 (10). https://doi.org/10.3390/medicina59101752.

Diekman, B. O., G. A. Sessions, J. A. Collins, A. K. Knecht, S. L. Strum, N. K. Mitin, C. S. Carlson, R. F. Loeser, and N. E. Sharpless. 2018a. "Expression of p16(INK)(4a) is a biomarker of chondrocyte aging but does not cause osteoarthritis." *Aging Cell* 17 (4):e12771. https://doi.org/10.1111/acel.12771.

Diekman, Brian O., Garrett A. Sessions, John A. Collins, Anne K. Knecht, Susan L. Strum, Natalia K. Mitin, Cathy S. Carlson, Richard F. Loeser, and Norman E. Sharpless. 2018b. "Expression of p16 INK 4a is a biomarker of chondrocyte aging but does not cause osteoarthritis." *Aging Cell* 17 (4):e12771.

Dimitriou, Rozalia, Elena Jones, Dennis McGonagle, and Peter V. Giannoudis. 2011. "Bone regeneration: Current concepts and future directions." *BMC Medicine* 9:1–10.

Domazetovic, V., G. Marcucci, T. Iantomasi, M. L. Brandi, and M. T. Vincenzini. 2017. "Oxidative stress in bone remodeling: Role of antioxidants." *Clinical Cases in Mineral & Bone Metabolism* 14 (2):209–216. https://doi.org/10.11138/ccmbm/2017.14.1.209.

Engeland, Kurt. 2022. "Cell cycle regulation: p53-p21-RB signaling." *Cell Death & Differentiation* 29 (5):946–960. https://doi.org/10.1038/s41418-022-00988-z.

Facchini, Annalisa, Silvia Cetrullo, Stefania D'Adamo, Serena Guidotti, Manuela Minguzzi, Andrea Facchini, Rosa Maria Borzì, and Flavio Flamigni. 2014. "Hydroxytyrosol prevents increase of osteoarthritis markers in human chondrocytes treated with hydrogen peroxide or growth-related oncogene α." *PLoS One* 9 (10):e109724.

Fang, C. L., B. Liu, and M. Wan. 2023a. "'Bone-SASP' in skeletal aging." *Calcified Tissue International* 113 (1):68–82. https://doi.org/10.1007/s00223-023-01100-4.

Fang, Ching-Lien, Bin Liu, and Mei Wan. 2023b. "'Bone-SASP' in skeletal aging." *Calcified Tissue International* 113 (1):68–82.

Farr, Joshua N., Daniel G. Fraser, Haitao Wang, Katharina Jaehn, Mikolaj B. Ogrodnik, Megan M. Weivoda, Matthew T. Drake, Tamara Tchkonia, Nathan K. LeBrasseur, and James L. Kirkland. 2016. "Identification of senescent cells in the bone microenvironment." *Journal of Bone and Mineral Research* 31 (11):1920–1929.

Farr, Joshua N., and Sundeep Khosla. 2019. "Cellular senescence in bone." *Bone* 121:121–133.

Farr, Joshua N., Ming Xu, Megan M. Weivoda, David G. Monroe, Daniel G. Fraser, Jennifer L. Onken, Brittany A. Negley, Jad G. Sfeir, Mikolaj B. Ogrodnik, and Christine M. Hachfeld. 2017. "Targeting cellular senescence prevents age-related bone loss in mice." *Nature Medicine* 23 (9):1072–1079.

Farr, Joshua N., Ming Xu, Megan M. Weivoda, David G. Monroe, Daniel G. Fraser, Jennifer L. Onken, Brittany A. Negley, Jad G. Sfeir, Mikolaj B. Ogrodnik, Christine M. Hachfeld, Nathan K. LeBrasseur, Matthew T. Drake, Robert J. Pignolo, Tamar Pirtskhalava, Tamara Tchkonia, Merry Jo Oursler, James L. Kirkland, and Sundeep Khosla. 2017. "Targeting cellular senescence prevents age-related bone loss in mice." *Nature Medicine* 23 (9):1072–1079. https://doi.org/10.1038/nm.4385.

Feng, Chong, Yan Liu, Bao-Yi Zhang, Hao Zhang, Fa-Yu Shan, Tian-Qi Li, Zhi-Ning Zhao, Zi-Rou Wang, Qiong-Lin Li, and Lan-Lan Liang. 2023. "Rapamycin inhibits osteoclastogenesis and prevents LPS-induced alveolar bone loss via an increase in autophagy flux and the suppression of oxidative stress." *ACS Omega* 8 (23):20739–20754.

Feng, P., S. Shu, and F. Zhao. 2022. "Anti-osteoporosis effect of fisetin against ovariectomy induced osteoporosis in rats: In silico, in vitro and in vivo Activity." *Journal of Oleo Science* 71 (1):105–118. https://doi.org/10.5650/jos.ess21252.

Formica, J. V., and W. Regelson. 1995. "Review of the biology of quercetin and related bioflavonoids." *Food and Chemical Toxicology* 33 (12):1061–1080. https://doi.org/10.1016/0278-6915(95)00077-1.

Ganguly, Payal, Tom Macleod, Chi Wong, Mark Harland, and Dennis McGonagle. 2023. "Revisiting p38 Mitogen-Activated Protein Kinases (MAPK) in inflammatory arthritis: A narrative of the emergence of MAPK-Activated Protein kinase inhibitors (MK2i)." *Pharmaceuticals* 16 (9):1286.

Garcia-Gomez, Antonio, Enrique M. Ocio, Edvan Crusoe, Carlos Santamaria, Pilar Hernández-Campo, Juan F. Blanco, Fermin M. Sanchez-Guijo, Teresa Hernández-Iglesias, Jesús G. Briñón, and Rosa M. Fisac-Herrero. 2012. "Dasatinib as a bone-modifying agent: anabolic and anti-resorptive effects." *PloS One* 7 (4):e34914.

Gascoyne, Duncan M., Hayley Spearman, Linden Lyne, Rathi Puliyadi, Marta Perez-Alcantara, Les Coulton, Simon E. Fisher, Peter I. Croucher, and Alison H. Banham. 2015. "The forkhead transcription factor FOXP2 is required for regulation of p21WAF1/CIP1 in 143B osteosarcoma cell growth arrest." *PloS One* 10 (6):e0128513.

Gaur, Rajula, Kofi A. Mensah, Jason Stricker, Mary Adams, Anastasia Parton, Dorota Cedzik, Jamie Connarn, Michael Thomas, Gerald Horan, and Peter Schafer. 2022. "CC-99677, a novel, oral, selective covalent MK2 inhibitor, sustainably reduces pro-inflammatory cytokine production." *Arthritis Research & Therapy* 24 (1):199.

Ginaldi, Lia, Lucia P. Mengoli, and Massimo De Martinis. 2009. "Osteoporosis, inflammation and ageing." *Handbook on Immunosenescence: Basic Understanding and Clinical Applications*:1329–1352.

Gnant, M., J. Baselga, H. S. Rugo, S. Noguchi, H. A. Burris, M. Piccart, G. N. Hortobagyi, J. Eakle, H. Mukai, H. Iwata, M. Geberth, L. L. Hart, P. Hadji, M. El-Hashimy, S. Rao, T. Taran, T. Sahmoud, D. Lebwohl, M. Campone, and K. I. Pritchard. 2013. "Effect of everolimus on bone marker levels and progressive disease in bone in BOLERO-2." *Journal of the National Cancer Institute* 105 (9):654–663. https://doi.org/10.1093/jnci/djt026.

Godoi, M. A., A. C. Camilli, K. G. A. Gonzales, V. B. Costa, E. Papathanasiou, F. R. M. Leite, and M. R. Guimarães-Stabili. 2023. "JAK/STAT as a potential therapeutic target for osteolytic diseases." *International Journal of Molecular Sciences* 24 (12). https://doi.org/10.3390/ijms241210290.

Guo, Q., X. Chen, J. Chen, G. Zheng, C. Xie, H. Wu, Z. Miao, Y. Lin, X. Wang, W. Gao, X. Zheng, Z. Pan, Y. Zhou, Y. Wu, and X. Zhang. 2021a. "STING promotes senescence, apoptosis, and extracellular matrix degradation in osteoarthritis via the NF-κB signaling pathway." *Cell Death & Disease* 12 (1):13. https://doi.org/10.1038/s41419-020-03341-9.

Guo, Qiang, Ximiao Chen, Jiaoxiang Chen, Gang Zheng, Chenglong Xie, Hongqiang Wu, Zhimin Miao, Yan Lin, Xiangyang Wang, Weiyang Gao, Xiangtao Zheng, Zongyou Pan, Yifei Zhou, Yaosen Wu, and Xiaolei Zhang. 2021b. "STING promotes senescence, apoptosis, and extracellular matrix degradation in osteoarthritis via the NF-κB signaling pathway." *Cell Death & Disease* 12 (1):13. https://doi.org/10.1038/s41419-020-03341-9.

Guo, Y., X. Jia, Y. Cui, Y. Song, S. Wang, Y. Geng, R. Li, W. Gao, and D. Fu. 2021. "Sirt3-mediated mitophagy regulates AGEs-induced BMSCs senescence and senile osteoporosis." *Redox Biology* 41:101915. https://doi.org/10.1016/j.redox.2021.101915.

Harbo, M., J. M. Delaisse, P. Kjaersgaard-Andersen, F. B. Soerensen, S. Koelvraa, and L. Bendix. 2013. "The relationship between ultra-short telomeres, aging of articular cartilage and the development of human hip osteoarthritis." *Mechanisms of Ageing and Development* 134 (9):367–372. https://doi.org/10.1016/j.mad.2013.07.002.

Harshbarger, W., S. Gondi, S. B. Ficarro, J. Hunter, D. Udayakumar, D. Gurbani, W. D. Singer, Y. Liu, L. Li, J. A. Marto, and K. D. Westover. 2017. "Structural and biochemical analyses reveal the mechanism of glutathione S-transferase Pi 1 inhibition by the anti-cancer compound piperlongumine." *Journal of Biological Chemistry* 292 (1):112–120. https://doi.org/10.1074/jbc.M116.750299.

Hatefi, Masoud, Mohammad Reza Hafezi Ahmadi, Asghar Rahmani, Masoud Moghadas Dastjerdi, and Khairollah Asadollahi. 2018. "Effects of curcumin on bone loss and biochemical markers of bone turnover in patients with spinal cord injury." *World Neurosurgery* 114:e785–e791.

He, X., G. Andersson, U. Lindgren, and Y. Li. 2010. "Resveratrol prevents RANKL-induced osteoclast differentiation of murine osteoclast progenitor RAW 264.7 cells through inhibition of ROS production." *Biochemical and Biophysical Research Communications* 401 (3):356–362. https://doi.org/10.1016/j.bbrc.2010.09.053.

He, Xu, Wei Hu, Yuanshu Zhang, Mimi Chen, Yicheng Ding, Huilin Yang, Fan He, Qiaoli Gu, and Qin Shi. 2023. "Cellular senescence in skeletal disease: Mechanisms and treatment." *Cellular & Molecular Biology Letters* 28 (1):88. https://doi.org/10.1186/s11658-023-00501-5.

Heinola, T., V. P. Kouri, P. Clarijs, H. Ciferska, A. Sukura, J. Salo, and Y. T. Konttinen. 2010. "High mobility group box-1 (HMGB-1) in osteoarthritic cartilage." *Clinical & Experimental Rheumatology* 28 (4):511.

Hong, Boohwi, Sunyeul Lee, Nara Shin, Youngkwon Ko, DongWoon Kim, Jun Lee, and Wonhyung Lee. 2018. "Bone regeneration with umbilical cord blood mesenchymal stem cells in femoral defects of ovariectomized rats." *Osteoporosis and Sarcopenia* 4 (3):95–101.

Hou, Angyang, Peng Chen, He Tang, Haoye Meng, Xiaoqing Cheng, Yu Wang, Yuming Zhang, and Jiang Peng. 2018. "Cellular senescence in osteoarthritis and anti-aging strategies." *Mechanisms of Ageing and Development* 175:83–87.

Hu, L., R. Liu, and L. Zhang. 2022. "Advance in bone destruction participated by JAK/STAT in rheumatoid arthritis and therapeutic effect of JAK/STAT inhibitors." *International Immunopharmacology* 111:109095. https://doi.org/10.1016/j.intimp.2022.109095.

Hu, S., and S. Wang. 2022. "The role of SIRT3 in the osteoporosis." *Frontiers in Endocrinology (Lausanne)* 13:893678. https://doi.org/10.3389/fendo.2022.893678.

Hu, T., M. Pan, Y. Yin, C. Wang, Y. Cui, and Q. Wang. 2021. "The regulatory network of cyclic GMP-AMP synthase-stimulator of interferon genes pathway in viral evasion." *Frontier Microbiology* 12:790714. https://doi.org/10.3389/fmicb.2021.790714.

Huang, J., H. Yin, S. S. Rao, P. L. Xie, X. Cao, T. Rao, S. Y. Liu, Z. X. Wang, J. Cao, Y. Hu, Y. Zhang, J. Luo, Y. J. Tan, Z. Z. Liu, B. Wu, X. K. Hu, T. H. Chen, C. Y. Chen, and H. Xie. 2018. "Harmine enhances type H vessel formation and prevents bone loss in ovariectomized mice." *Theranostics* 8 (9):2435–2446. https://doi.org/10.7150/thno.22144.

Huelsmann, Lorel, D. Nathan W. Kim, Raquibul Hannan, Lori M. Watumull, and James Brugarolas. 2015. "Selective efficacy of temsirolimus on bone metastases in chromophobe renal cell carcinoma." *Clinical Genitourinary Cancer* 13 (4):e321–e323. https://doi.org/10.1016/j.clgc.2014.12.007.

Hussain, S. A., B. H. Marouf, Z. S. Ali, and R. S. Ahmmad. 2018. "Efficacy and safety of co-administration of resveratrol with meloxicam in patients with knee osteoarthritis: A pilot interventional study." *Clinical Interventions Aging* 13:1621–1630. https://doi.org/10.2147/cia.S172758.

Iaquinta, Maria Rosa, Elisa Mazzoni, Ilaria Bononi, John Charles Rotondo, Chiara Mazziotta, Monica Montesi, Simone Sprio, Anna Tampieri, Mauro Tognon, and Fernanda Martini. 2019. "Adult stem cells for bone regeneration and repair." *Frontiers in Cell and Developmental Biology* 7:268.

Inchingolo, Alessio Danilo, Angelo Michele Inchingolo, Giuseppina Malcangi, Pasquale Avantario, Daniela Azzollini, Silvio Buongiorno, Fabio Viapiano, Merigrazia Campanelli, Anna Maria Ciocia, and Nicole De Leonardis. 2022. "Effects of resveratrol, curcumin and quercetin supplementation on bone metabolism—a systematic review." *Nutrients* 14 (17):3519.

Iqbal, S. M., C. Leonard, S. C. Regmi, D. De Rantere, P. Tailor, G. Ren, H. Ishida, C. Y. Hsu, S. Abubacker, and D. S. J. Pang. 2016. "Lubricin/proteoglycan 4 binds to and regulates the activity of toll-like receptors in vitro." *Scientific Reports* 6 (1):18910.

Itahana, Koji, Judith Campisi, and Goberdhan P. Dimri. 2007. "Methods to detect biomarkers of cellular senescence: the senescence-associated β-galactosidase assay." *Biological Aging: Methods and Protocols*:21–31.

Jeon, Ok Hee, Chaekyu Kim, Remi-Martin Laberge, Marco Demaria, Sona Rathod, Alain P. Vasserot, Jae Wook Chung, Do Hun Kim, Yan Poon, and Nathaniel David. 2017. "Local clearance of senescent cells attenuates the development of post-traumatic osteoarthritis and creates a pro-regenerative environment." *Nature Medicine* 23 (6):775–781.

Jilka, R. L. 1998. "Cytokines, bone remodeling, and estrogen deficiency: A 1998 update." *Bone* 23 (2):75–81. https://doi.org/10.1016/S8756-3282(98)00077-5.

Jin, H., X. Jin, B. Cao, and W. Wang. 2017. "Berberine affects osteosarcoma via downregulating the caspase-1/IL-1β signaling axis." *Oncology Reports* 37 (2):729–736. https://doi.org/10.3892/or.2016.5327.

Jo, Chris Hyunchul, Young Gil Lee, Won Hyoung Shin, Hyang Kim, Jee Won Chai, Eui Cheol Jeong, Ji Eun Kim, Hackjoon Shim, Ji Sun Shin, and Il Seob Shin. 2014. 'Intra-articular injection of mesenchymal stem cells for the treatment of osteoarthritis of the knee: A proof-of-concept clinical trial." *Stem Cells* 32 (5):1254–1266.

Jo, Hee Geun, Chae Yun Baek, Donghwan Kim, Sangjin Kim, Yewon Han, Chanlim Park, Ho Sueb Song, and Donghun Lee. 2024. "Network analysis, in vivo, and in vitro experiments identified the mechanisms by which Piper longum L.[Piperaceae] alleviates cartilage destruction, joint inflammation, and arthritic pain." *Frontiers in Pharmacology* 14:1282943.

Jones, Gemma N., Dafni Moschidou, Hassan Abdulrazzak, Bhalraj Singh Kalirai, Maximilien Vanleene, Suchaya Osatis, Sandra J Shefelbine, Nicole J Horwood, Massimo Marenzana, and Paolo De Coppi. 2014. "Potential of human fetal chorionic stem cells for the treatment of osteogenesis imperfecta." *Stem Cells and Development* 23 (3):262–276.

Ke, Dianshan, Yu Wang, Yunlong Yu, Yongxuan Wang, Wang Zheng, Xiaomin Fu, Junyong Han, Guoyou Zhang, and Jie Xu. 2020. "Curcumin-activated autophagy plays a negative role in its anti-osteoclastogenic effect." *Molecular and Cellular Endocrinology* 500:110637.

Khosla, Sundeep, Joshua N. Farr, and David G. Monroe. 2022. "Cellular senescence and the skeleton: Pathophysiology and therapeutic implications." *The Journal of Clinical Investigation* 132 (3).

Kiechl, Stefan, Philipp Werner, Michael Knoflach, Martin Furtner, Johann Willeit, and Georg Schett. 2006. "The osteoprotegerin/RANK/RANKL system: A bone key to vascular disease." *Expert Review of Cardiovascular Therapy* 4 (6):801–811.

Kim, H. N., J. Xiong, R. S. MacLeod, S. Iyer, Y. Fujiwara, K. M. Cawley, L. Han, Y. He, J. D. Thostenson, E. Ferreira, R. L. Jilka, D. Zhou, M. Almeida, and C. A. O'Brien. 2020. "Osteocyte RANKL is required for cortical bone loss with age and is induced by senescence." *JCI Insight* 5 (19). https://doi.org/10.1172/jci.insight.138815.

Kim, Ji Eun, Sang Mok Lee, Soo Hyun Kim, Phil Tatman, Albert O. Gee, Deok-Ho Kim, Kyung Eun Lee, Youngmee Jung, and Sang Jun Kim. 2014. "Effect of self-assembled peptide–mesenchymal stem cell complex on the progression of osteoarthritis in a rat model." *International Journal of Nanomedicine* 9 (sup1):141–157.

Kim, Mi Kyung, Sang Woon Chung, Dae Hyun Kim, Ji Min Kim, Eun Kyeong Lee, Ji Young Kim, Young Mi Ha, Yun Hee Kim, Jae-Kyung No, and Hye Sun Chung. 2010. "Modulation of age-related NF-κB activation by dietary zingerone via MAPK pathway." *Experimental Gerontology* 45 (6):419–426.

Komagamine, Masatsugu, Noriko Komatsu, Rui Ling, Kazuo Okamoto, Shi Tianshu, Kotaro Matsuda, Tsutomu Takeuchi, Yuko Kaneko, and Hiroshi Takayanagi. 2023. "Effect of JAK inhibitors on the three forms of bone damage in autoimmune arthritis: Joint erosion, periarticular osteopenia, and systemic bone loss." *Inflammation and Regeneration* 43 (1):44. https://doi.org/10.1186/s41232-023-00293-3.

Kreis, Nina-Naomi, Frank Louwen, and Juping Yuan. 2019. "The multifaceted p21 (Cip1/Waf1/CDKN1A) in cell differentiation, migration and cancer therapy." *Cancers* 11 (9):1220.

Lagoumtzi, S. M., and N. Chondrogianni. 2021a. "Senolytics and senomorphics: Natural and synthetic therapeutics in the treatment of aging and chronic diseases." *Free Radical Biology and Medicine* 171:169–190. https://doi.org/10.1016/j.freeradbiomed.2021.05.003.

Lagoumtzi, Sofia M., and Niki Chondrogianni. 2021b. "Senolytics and senomorphics: Natural and synthetic therapeutics in the treatment of aging and chronic diseases." *Free Radical Biology and Medicine* 171:169–190. https://doi.org/10.1016/j.freeradbiomed.2021.05.003.

Lane, N., B. Hsu, J. Visich, B. Xie, A. Khan, and J. Dananberg. 2021. "A phase 2, randomized, double-blind, placebo-controlled study of senolytic molecule UBX0101 in the treatment of painful knee osteoarthritis." *Osteoarthritis and Cartilage* 29:S52–S53.

Lawrence, M., A. Goyal, S. Pathak, and P. Ganguly. 2024a. "Cellular senescence and inflammaging in the bone: Pathways, genetics, anti-aging strategies and interventions." *International Journal of Molecular Sciences* 25 (13). https://doi.org/10.3390/ijms25137411.

Lawrence, Merin, Abhishek Goyal, Shelly Pathak, and Payal Ganguly. 2024b. "Cellular senescence and inflammaging in the bone: Pathways, genetics, anti-aging strategies and interventions." *International Journal of Molecular Sciences* 25 (13):7411.

Léotoing, Laurent, Marie-Jeanne Davicco, Patrice Lebecque, Yohann Wittrant, and Véronique Coxam. 2014. "The flavonoid fisetin promotes osteoblasts differentiation through Runx2 transcriptional activity." *Molecular Nutrition & Food Research* 58 (6):1239–1248.

Li, Ji, Ildiko Sarosi, Xiao-Qiang Yan, Sean Morony, Casey Capparelli, Hong-Lin Tan, Susan McCabe, Robin Elliott, Sheila Scully, and Gwyneth Van. 2000. "RANK is the intrinsic hematopoietic cell surface receptor that controls osteoclastogenesis and regulation of bone mass and calcium metabolism." *Proceedings of the National Academy of Sciences* 97 (4):1566–1571.

Li, Jun, Yun Wang, Di Chen, and Ru Liu-Bryan. 2022. "Oral administration of berberine limits post-traumatic osteoarthritis development and associated pain via AMP-activated protein kinase (AMPK) in mice." *Osteoarthritis and Cartilage* 30 (1):160–171.

Li, Z., A. Dai, M. Yang, S. Chen, Z. Deng, and L. Li. 2022. "p38MAPK signaling pathway in osteoarthritis: Pathological and therapeutic aspects." *Journal of Inflammation Research* 15:723–734. https://doi.org/10.2147/jir.S348491.

Lin, Hong, Felipe Salech, Anthony Lim, Sara Vogrin, and Gustavo Duque. 2022. "The effect of rapamycin and its analogues on age-related musculoskeletal diseases: A systematic review." *Aging Clinical and Experimental Research* 34 (10):2317–2333.

Liu, Jiaqi, Qing Xiao, Jiani Xiao, Chenxi Niu, Yuanyuan Li, Xiaojun Zhang, Zhengwei Zhou, Guang Shu, and Gang Yin. 2022. "Wnt/β-catenin signalling: Function, biological mechanisms, and therapeutic opportunities." *Signal Transduction and Targeted Therapy* 7 (1):3. https://doi.org/10.1038/s41392-021-00762-6.

Liu, Ting, Lingyun Zhang, Donghyun Joo, and Shao-Cong Sun. 2017. "NF-κB signaling in inflammation." *Signal Transduction and Targeted Therapy* 2 (1):1–9.

Liu, Xuan, Li Diao, Yudie Zhang, Xue Yang, Junnan Zhou, Yuhang Mao, Xiaotian Shi, Fuli Zhao, and Mei Liu. 2022. "Piperlongumine inhibits titanium particles-induced osteolysis, osteoclast formation, and RANKL-induced signaling pathways." *International Journal of Molecular Sciences* 23 (5):2868.

Liu, Y., Z. Zhang, C. Liu, and H. Zhang. 2023. "Sirtuins in osteoarthritis: Current understanding." *Frontier Immunology* 14:1140653. https://doi.org/10.3389/fimmu.2023.1140653.

Loh, Darren Kin Wai, Amudha Kadirvelu, and Narendra Pamidi. 2022. "Effects of metformin on bone mineral density and adiposity-associated pathways in animal models with type 2 diabetes mellitus: A systematic review." *Journal of Clinical Medicine* 11 (14):4193.

Lopes-Paciencia, Stéphane, Emmanuelle Saint-Germain, Marie-Camille Rowell, Ana Fernández Ruiz, Paloma Kalegari, and Gerardo Ferbeyre. 2019. "The senescence-associated secretory phenotype and its regulation." *Cytokine* 117:15–22.

Lu, Qunshan, Peilai Liu, Zhuang Miao, Desu Luo, Songlin Li, and Mei Lu. 2022. "SIRT1 restoration enhances chondrocyte autophagy in osteoarthritis through PTEN-mediated EGFR ubiquitination." *Cell Death Discovery* 8 (1):203. https://doi.org/10.1038/s41420-022-00896-8.

Luo, Na, Lei Zhang, Chunmei Xiu, Xi Luo, Siyuan Hu, Kaizhong Ji, Qingbai Liu, and Jianquan Chen. 2024. "Piperlongumine, a Piper longum-derived amide alkaloid, protects mice from ovariectomy-induced osteoporosis by inhibiting osteoclastogenesis via suppression of p38 and JNK signaling." *Food & Function* 15 (4):2154–2169.

Luo, P., F. Gao, D. Niu, X. Sun, Q. Song, C. Guo, Y. Liang, and W. Sun. 2019. "The role of autophagy in chondrocyte metabolism and osteoarthritis: A comprehensive research review." *Biomed Research International* 2019:5171602. https://doi.org/10.1155/2019/5171602.

Mai, Q. G., Z. M. Zhang, S. Xu, M. Lu, R. P. Zhou, L. Zhao, C. H. Jia, Z. H. Wen, D. D. Jin, and X. C. Bai. 2011. "Metformin stimulates osteoprotegerin and reduces RANKL expression in osteoblasts and ovariectomized rats." *Journal of Cellular Biochemistry* 112 (10):2902–9. https://doi.org/10.1002/jcb.23206.

Marie, Pierre J. 2014. "Bone cell senescence: Mechanisms and perspectives." *Journal of Bone and Mineral Research* 29 (6):1311–1321.

Martin, Stephen A., Ruben T. Riordan, Rong Wang, Zhen Yu, Allan M. Aguirre-Burk, Carmen P. Wong, Dawn A. Olson, Adam J. Branscum, Russell T. Turner, Urszula T. Iwaniec, and Viviana I. Perez. 2021. "Rapamycin impairs bone accrual in young adult mice independent of Nrf2." *Experimental Gerontology* 154:111516. https://doi.org/10.1016/j.exger.2021.111516.

Martinotti, S., M. Patrone, M. Manfredi, F. Gosetti, M. Pedrazzi, E. Marengo, and E. Ranzato. 2016. "HMGB1 osteo-modulatory action on osteosarcoma SaOS-2 cell line: An integrated study from biochemical and -omics approaches." *Journal of Cellular Biochem*ical 117 (11):2559–2569. https://doi.org/10.1002/jcb.25549.

Massaro, Fulvio, Florent Corrillon, Basile Stamatopoulos, Nathan Dubois, Achille Ruer, Nathalie Meuleman, Dominique Bron, and Laurence Lagneaux. 2023. "Age-related changes in human bone marrow mesenchymal stromal cells: Morphology, gene expression profile, immunomodulatory activity and miRNA expression." *Frontiers in Immunology* 14:1267550.

Masson, A. O., R. Hess, K. O'Brien, K. L. Bertram, P. Tailor, E. Irvine, G. Ren, and R. J. Krawetz. 2015. "Increased levels of p21((CIP1/WAF1)) correlate with decreased chondrogenic differentiation potential in synovial membrane progenitor cells." *Mechanisms of Ageing and Development* 149:31–40. https://doi.org/10.1016/j.mad.2015.05.005.

Maurer, S., V. Kirsch, L. Ruths, R. E. Brenner, and J. Riegger. 2025. "Senolytic therapy combining Dasatinib and Quercetin restores the chondrogenic phenotype of human osteoarthritic chondrocytes by the release of pro-anabolic mediators." *Aging Cell* 24 (1):e14361. https://doi.org/10.1111/acel.14361.

Mijit, M., V. Caracciolo, A. Melillo, F. Amicarelli, and A. Giordano. 2020. "Role of p53 in the regulation of cellular senescence." *Biomolecules* 10 (3). https://doi.org/10.3390/biom10030420.

Militello, R., S. Luti, T. Gamberi, A. Pellegrino, A. Modesti, and P. A. Modesti. 2024. "Physical activity and oxidative stress in aging." *Antioxidants (Basel)* 13 (5). https://doi.org/10.3390/antiox13050557.

Miura, Yugo, Kentaro Endo, Keiichiro Komori, and Ichiro Sekiya. 2022. "Clearance of senescent cells with ABT-263 improves biological functions of synovial mesenchymal stem cells from osteoarthritis patients." *Stem Cell Research & Therapy* 13 (1):222. https://doi.org/10.1186/s13287-022-02901-4.

Moiseeva, Olga, Xavier Deschênes-Simard, Emmanuelle St-Germain, Sebastian Igelmann, Geneviève Huot, Alexandra E. Cadar, Véronique Bourdeau, Michael N. Pollak, and Gerardo Ferbeyre. 2013. "Metformin inhibits the senescence-associated secretory phenotype by interfering with IKK/NF-κ B activation." *Aging Cell* 12 (3):489–498.

Molagoda, Ilandarage Menu Neelaka, Chang-Hee Kang, Mi-Hwa Lee, Yung Hyun Choi, Chang-Min Lee, Seungheon Lee, and Gi-Young Kim. 2021. "Fisetin promotes osteoblast differentiation and osteogenesis through GSK-3β phosphorylation at Ser9 and consequent β-catenin activation, inhibiting osteoporosis." *Biochemical Pharmacology* 192:114676. https://doi.org/10.1016/j.bcp.2021.114676.

Molnar, V., V. Matišić, I. Kodvanj, R. Bjelica, Ž Jeleč, D. Hudetz, E. Rod, F. Čukelj, T. Vrdoljak, D. Vidović, M. Starešinić, S. Sabalić, B. Dobričić, T. Petrović, D. Antičević, I. Borić, R. Košir, U. P. Zmrzljak, and D. Primorac. 2021. "Cytokines and chemokines involved in osteoarthritis pathogenesis." *International Journal of Molecular Sciences* 22 (17). https://doi.org/10.3390/ijms22179208.

Morrison, Sean J., and David T. Scadden. 2014. "The bone marrow niche for haematopoietic stem cells." *Nature* 505 (7483):327–334.

Nakashima, Kazuhisa, Xin Zhou, Gary Kunkel, Zhaoping Zhang, Jian Min Deng, Richard R. Behringer, and Benoit de Crombrugghe. 2002. "The novel zinc finger-containing transcription factor osterix is required for osteoblast differentiation and bone formation." *Cell* 108 (1):17–29. https://doi.org/10.1016/S0092-8674(01)00622-5.

Nogueira-Recalde, Uxía, Irene Lorenzo-Gómez, Francisco J. Blanco, María I. Loza, Diego Grassi, Valery Shirinsky, Ivan Shirinsky, Martin Lotz, Paul D. Robbins, and Eduardo Domínguez. 2019. "Fibrates as drugs with senolytic and autophagic activity for osteoarthritis therapy." *EBioMedicine* 45:588–605.

Novais, Emanuel J., Victoria A. Tran, Shira N. Johnston, Kayla R. Darris, Alex J. Roupas, Garrett A. Sessions, Irving M. Shapiro, Brian O. Diekman, and Makarand V. Risbud. 2021. "Long-term treatment with senolytic drugs Dasatinib and Quercetin ameliorates age-dependent intervertebral disc degeneration in mice." *Nature Communications* 12 (1):5213. https://doi.org/10.1038/s41467-021-25453-2.

Omlor, G. W., S. Lorenz, A. G. Nerlich, T. Guehring, and W. Richter. 2018. "Disc cell therapy with bone-marrow-derived autologous mesenchymal stromal cells in a large porcine disc degeneration model." *European Spine Journal* 27:2639–2649.

Ou, Qianhua, Su'an Tang, Jianwei Zhu, Song Xue, Hong Huang, Yang Zhao, Yu Cai, Cuixi Wu, Jianmao Chen, Guangfeng Ruan, and Changhai Ding. 2024. "Spermidine ameliorates osteoarthritis via altering macrophage polarization." *Biochimica et Biophysica Acta (BBA)—Molecular Basis of Disease* 1870 (4):167083. https://doi.org/10.1016/j.bbadis.2024.167083.

Pal, B., H. Endisha, Y. Zhang, and M. Kapoor. 2015. "mTOR: A potential therapeutic target in osteoarthritis?" *Drugs R D* 15 (1):27–36. https://doi.org/10.1007/s40268-015-0082-z.

Pan, B., C. Chen, Y. Zhao, J. Cai, S. Fu, and J. Liu. 2024. "SIRT3: A potential target of different types of osteoporosis." *Cell Biochemistry and Biophysics* 82 (2):489–500. https://doi.org/10.1007/s12013-024-01254-4.

Pawge, Girija, and Gopal L. Khatik. 2021. "p53 regulated senescence mechanism and role of its modulators in age-related disorders." *Biochemical Pharmacology* 190:114651.

Philipot, D., D. Guérit, D. Platano, P. Chuchana, E. Olivotto, F. Espinoza, A. Dorandeu, Y. M. Pers, J. Piette, R. M. Borzi, C. Jorgensen, D. Noel, and J. M. Brondello. 2014a. "p16INK4a and its regulator miR-24 link senescence and chondrocyte terminal differentiation-associated matrix remodeling in osteoarthritis." *Arthritis Research & Therapy* 16 (1):R58. https://doi.org/10.1186/ar4494.

Philipot, Didier, David Guérit, Daniela Platano, Paul Chuchana, Eleonora Olivotto, Francisco Espinoza, Anne Dorandeu, Yves-Marie Pers, Jacques Piette, Rosa Maria Borzi, Christian Jorgensen, Danièle Noel, and Jean-Marc Brondello. 2014b. "p16INK4a and its regulator miR-24 link senescence and chondrocyte terminal differentiation-associated matrix remodeling in osteoarthritis." *Arthritis Research & Therapy* 16 (1):R58. https://doi.org/10.1186/ar4494.

Pignolo, Robert J., Susan F. Law, and Abhishek Chandra. 2021. "Bone aging, cellular senescence, and osteoporosis." *Journal of Bone and Mineral Research Plus* 5 (4):e10488.

Pignolo, Robert J., Rebekah M. Samsonraj, Susan F. Law, Haitao Wang, and Abhishek Chandra. 2019. "Targeting cell senescence for the treatment of age-related bone loss." *Current Osteoporosis Reports* 17:70–85.

Premnath, P., L. Ferrie, D. Louie, S. Boyd, and R. Krawetz. 2019. "Absence of p21(WAF1/CIP1/SDI1) protects against osteopenia and minimizes bone loss after ovariectomy in a mouse model." *PLoS One* 14 (4):e0215018. https://doi.org/10.1371/journal.pone.0215018.

Rauner, Martina, Wolfgang Sipos, and Peter Pietschmann. 2008. "Age-dependent Wnt gene expression in bone and during the course of osteoblast differentiation." *Age* 30:273–282.

Rizzo, Michael G., Thomas M. Best, Johnny Huard, Marc Philippon, Francis Hornicek, Zhenfeng Duan, Anthony J. Griswold, Lee D. Kaplan, Joshua M. Hare, and Dimitrios Kouroupis. 2023. "Therapeutic perspectives for inflammation and senescence in osteoarthritis using mesenchymal stem cells, mesenchymal stem cell-derived extracellular vesicles and senolytic agents." *Cells* 12 (10):1421.

Ruan, Zhe, Hao Yin, Teng-Fei Wan, Zhi-Rou Lin, Shu-Shan Zhao, Hai-Tao Long, Cheng Long, Zhao-Hui Li, Yu-Qi Liu, Hao Luo, Liang Cheng, Can Chen, Min Zeng, Zhang-Yuan Lin, Rui-Bo Zhao, Chun-Yuan Chen, Zhen-Xing Wang, Zheng-Zhao Liu, Jia Cao, Yi-Yi Wang, Ling Jin, Yi-Wei Liu, Guo-Qiang Zhu, Jing-Tao Zou, Jiang-Shan Gong, Yi Luo, Yin Hu, Yong Zhu, and Hui Xie. 2023. "Metformin accelerates bone fracture healing by promoting type H vessel formation through inhibition of YAP1/TAZ expression." *Bone Research* 11 (1):45. https://doi.org/10.1038/s41413-023-00279-4.

Ryu, Eunsook, Su Hong, Jaeku Kang, Junghoon Woo, Jungjun Park, Jongho Lee, and Jeong-Sun Seo. 2008. "Identification of senescence-associated genes in human bone marrow mesenchymal stem cells." *Biochemical and Biophysical Research Communications* 371 (3):431–436.

Safwan-Zaiter, Hasan, Nicole Wagner, and Kay-Dietrich Wagner. 2022. "P16INK4A—more than a senescence marker." *Life* 12 (9):1332.

Sakamoto, Yumi, Tatsuo Okui, Toshiyuki Yoneda, Shoji Ryumon, Tomoya Nakamura, Hotaka Kawai, Yuki Kunisada, Soichiro Ibaragi, Masanori Masui, Kisho Ono, Kyoichi Obata, Tsuyoshi Shimo, and Akira Sasaki. 2020. "High-mobility group box 1 induces bone destruction associated with advanced oral squamous cancer via RAGE and TLR4." *Biochemical and Biophysical Research Communications* 531 (3):422–430. https://doi.org/10.1016/j.bbrc.2020.07.120.

Salminen, Antero, Johanna Ojala, Kai Kaarniranta, and Anu Kauppinen. 2012. "Mitochondrial dysfunction and oxidative stress activate inflammasomes: Impact on the aging process and age-related diseases." *Cellular and Molecular Life Sciences* 69:2999–3013.

Sanap, Avinash, Kalpana Joshi, Tejas Shah, Girish Tillu, and Ramesh Bhonde. 2021. "Preconditioning of mesenchymal stem cells with piper longum L. augments osteogenic differentiation." *Journal of Ethnopharmacology* 273:113999.

Sanpaolo, E. R., C. Rotondo, D. Cici, A. Corrado, and F. P. Cantatore. 2020. "JAK/STAT pathway and molecular mechanism in bone remodeling." *Molecular Biology Reports* 47 (11):9087–9096. https://doi.org/10.1007/s11033-020-05910-9.

Saul, Dominik, Madison L. Doolittle, Jennifer L. Rowsey, Mitchell N. Froemming, Robyn L. Kosinsky, Stephanie J. Vos, Ming Ruan, Nathan K. LeBrasseur, Abhishek Chandra, and Robert J. Pignolo. 2024. "Osteochondroprogenitor cells and neutrophils expressing p21 and senescence markers modulate fracture repair." *The Journal of Clinical Investigation* 134 (12).

Saxton, R. A., and D. M. Sabatini. 2017. "mTOR signaling in growth, metabolism, and disease." *Cell* 168 (6):960–976. https://doi.org/10.1016/j.cell.2017.02.004.

Sharma, Anuj K., Rachel L. Roberts, Reginald D. Benson Jr, Jessica L. Pierce, Kanglun Yu, Mark W. Hamrick, and Meghan E. McGee-Lawrence. 2020. "The senolytic drug navitoclax (ABT-263) causes trabecular bone loss and impaired osteoprogenitor function in aged mice." *Frontiers in Cell and Developmental Biology* 8:354.

Siebelt, M., H. Jahr, H. C. Groen, M. Sandker, J. H. Waarsing, N. Kops, C. Müller, W. van Eden, M. de Jong, and H. Weinans. 2013a. "Hsp90 inhibition protects against biomechanically induced osteoarthritis in rats." *Arthritis and Rheumatism* 65 (8):2102–2112. https://doi.org/10.1002/art.38000.

Siebelt, Michiel, Holger Jahr, Harald C. Groen, Marjan Sandker, Jan H. Waarsing, Nicole Kops, Cristina Müller, Willem van Eden, Marion de Jong, and Harrie H. Weinans. 2013b. "Hsp90 inhibition protects against biomechanically induced osteoarthritis in rats." *Arthritis and Rheumatism* 65 8:2102–2112.

Silva, I., and Jaime C. Branco. 2011. "Rank/Rankl/opg: Literature review." *Acta Reumatologica Portuguesa* 36 (3).

Sims, Natalie A. 2020. "The JAK1/STAT3/SOCS3 axis in bone development, physiology, and pathology." *Experimental & Molecular Medicine* 52 (8):1185–1197. https://doi.org/10.1038/s12276-020-0445-6.

Sims, Natalie A., and Christina Vrahnas. 2014. "Regulation of cortical and trabecular bone mass by communication between osteoblasts, osteocytes and osteoclasts." *Archives of Biochemistry and Biophysics* 561:22–28.

Souers, Andrew J., Joel D. Leverson, Erwin R. Boghaert, Scott L. Ackler, Nathaniel D. Catron, Jun Chen, Brian D. Dayton, Hong Ding, Sari H. Enschede, and Wayne J. Fairbrother. 2013. "ABT-199, a potent and selective BCL-2 inhibitor, achieves antitumor activity while sparing platelets." *Nature Medicine* 19 (2):202–208.

Stevens, Jennifer R., Gustavo A. Miranda-Carboni, Meredith A. Singer, Sean M. Brugger, Karen M. Lyons, and Timothy F. Lane. 2010. "Wnt10b deficiency results in age-dependent loss of bone mass and progressive reduction of mesenchymal progenitor cells." *Journal of Bone and Mineral Research* 25 (10):2138–2147.

Su, Chen-Ying, Yongxiang Luo, Chi-Hau Fang, and Hsu-Wei Fang. 2020. "The effects of antioxidant supplements on the inflammatory gene expression of osteoarthritis-like chondrocytes." *Applied Sciences* 11 (1):239.

Su, Weiping, Yihe Hu, Xiaolei Fan, and Jie Xie. 2023. "Clearance of senescent cells by navitoclax (ABT263) rejuvenates UHMWPE-induced osteolysis." *International Immunopharmacology* 115:109694. https://doi.org/10.1016/j.intimp.2023.109694.

Sun, JunWei, Qi Liu, Huan He, Lanlan Jiang, Kok Onn Lee, Dongmei Li, and Jianhua Ma. 2022. "Metformin treatment is associated with an increase in bone mineral density in type 2 diabetes mellitus patients in China: A retrospective single center study." *Diabetes & Metabolism* 48 (5):101350. https://doi.org/10.1016/j.diabet.2022.101350.

Tang, N. L. S., J. Woo, E. W. C. Suen, C. D. Liao, J. C. S. Leung, and P. C. Leung. 2010. "The effect of telomere length, a marker of biological aging, on bone mineral density in elderly population." *Osteoporosis International* 21:89–97.

Tao, Zhi-Fu, Lisa Hasvold, Le Wang, Xilu Wang, Andrew M. Petros, Chang H. Park, Erwin R. Boghaert, Nathaniel D. Catron, Jun Chen, and Peter M. Colman. 2014. "Discovery of a potent and selective BCL-XL inhibitor with in vivo activity." *ACS Medicinal Chemistry Letters* 5 (10):1088–1093.

Thatikonda, Sowjanya, Venkatesh Pooladanda, Dilep Kumar Sigalapalli, and Chandraiah Godugu. 2020. "Piperlongumine regulates epigenetic modulation and alleviates psoriasis-like skin inflammation via inhibition of hyperproliferation and inflammation." *Cell Death & Disease* 11 (1):21. https://doi.org/10.1038/s41419-019-2212-y.

Tse, C., A. R. Shoemaker, J. Adickes, M. G. Anderson, J. Chen, S. Jin, E. F. Johnson, K. C. Marsh, M. J. Mitten, P. Nimmer, L. Roberts, S. K. Tahir, Y. Xiao, X. Yang, H. Zhang, S. Fesik, S. H. Rosenberg, and S. W. Elmore. 2008. "ABT-263: A potent and orally bioavailable Bcl-2 family inhibitor." *Cancer Research* 68 (9):3421–3428. https://doi.org/10.1158/0008-5472.Can-07-5836.

Tudorachi, Nicoleta Bianca, Eugenia Eftimie Totu, Adrian Fifere, Valeriu Ardeleanu, Veronica Mocanu, Cornelia Mircea, Ibrahim Isildak, Katarina Smilkov, and Elena Mihaela Cărăuşu. 2021. "The implication of reactive oxygen species and antioxidants in knee osteoarthritis." *Antioxidants* 10 (6):985.

Van Ameyde, M., and J. Hodgden. 2022. "In patients with osteoarthritis, is curcumin, compared to placebo, effective in reducing pain?" *Journal of the Oklahoma State Medical Association* 115 (1):28–30.

Wang, L., F. Zhou, P. Zhang, H. Wang, Z. Qu, P. Jia, Z. Yao, G. Shen, G. Li, G. Zhao, J. Li, Y. Mao, Z. Xie, W. Xu, Y. Xu, and Y. Xu. 2017. "Human type H vessels are a sensitive biomarker of bone mass." *Cell Death & Disease* 8 (5):e2760. https://doi.org/10.1038/cddis.2017.36.

Wang, L. X., G. Y. Wang, N. Su, J. Ma, and Y. K. Li. 2020. "Effects of different doses of metformin on bone mineral density and bone metabolism in elderly male patients with type 2 diabetes mellitus." *World Journal of Clinical Cases* 8 (18):4010–4016. https://doi.org/10.12998/wjcc.v8.i18.4010.

Wang, S., J. Wang, S. Wang, R. Tao, J. Yi, M. Chen, and Z. Zhao. 2023a. "mTOR signaling pathway in bone diseases associated with hyperglycemia." *International Journal of Molecular Sciences* 24 (11). https://doi.org/10.3390/ijms24119198.

Wang, T., S. Huang, and C. He. 2022. "Senescent cells: A therapeutic target for osteoporosis." *Cell Proliferation* 55 (12):e13323. https://doi.org/10.1111/cpr.13323.

Wang, Xiaohao, Zechao Qu, Songchuan Zhao, Lei luo, and Liang Yan. 2024. "Wnt/β-catenin signaling pathway: Proteins' roles in osteoporosis and cancer diseases and the regulatory effects of natural compounds on osteoporosis." *Molecular Medicine* 30 (1):193. https://doi.org/10.1186/s10020-024-00957-x.

Wang, Y., L. Che, X. Chen, Z. He, D. Song, Y. Yuan, and C. Liu. 2023b. "Repurpose dasatinib and quercetin: Targeting senescent cells ameliorates postmenopausal osteoporosis and rejuvenates bone regeneration." *Bioactive Materials* 25:13–28. https://doi.org/10.1016/j.bioactmat.2023.01.009.

Wei, L., S. Chai, C. Yue, H. Zhang, J. Li, and N. Qin. 2023. "Resveratrol protects osteocytes against oxidative stress in ovariectomized rats through AMPK/JNK1-dependent pathway leading to promotion of autophagy and inhibition of apoptosis." *Cell Death Discovery* 9 (1):16. https://doi.org/10.1038/s41420-023-01331-2.

Wei, Yulong, Jie Jia, Xin Jin, Wei Tong, and Hongtao Tian. 2018. "Resveratrol ameliorates inflammatory damage and protects against osteoarthritis in a rat model of osteoarthritis." *Molecular Medicine Reports* 17 (1):1493–1498.

Wen, Z. H., J. S. Huang, Y. Y. Lin, Z. K. Yao, Y. C. Lai, W. F. Chen, H. T. Liu, S. C. Lin, Y. C. Tsai, T. C. Tsai, and Y. H. Jean. 2021. "Chondroprotective effects of a histone deacetylase inhibitor, panobinostat, on pain behavior and cartilage degradation in anterior cruciate ligament transection-induced experimental osteoarthritic rats." *International Journal of Molecular Sciences* 22 (14). https://doi.org/10.3390/ijms22147290.

Wilson, Wyndham H., Owen A. O'Connor, Myron S. Czuczman, Ann S. LaCasce, John F. Gerecitano, John P. Leonard, Anil Tulpule, Kieron Dunleavy, Hao Xiong, and Yi-Lin Chiu. 2010. "Navitoclax, a targeted high-affinity inhibitor of BCL-2, in lymphoid malignancies: A phase 1 dose-escalation study of safety, pharmacokinetics, pharmacodynamics, and antitumour activity." *The Lancet Oncology* 11 (12):1149–1159.

Wong, R. H., J. J. Thaung Zaw, C. J. Xian, and P. R. Howe. 2020. "Regular supplementation with resveratrol improves bone mineral density in postmenopausal women: A randomized, placebo-controlled trial." *Journal of Bone Mineral Research* 35 (11):2121–2131. https://doi.org/10.1002/jbmr.4115.

Wong, R. H. X., H. M. Evans, and P. R. C. Howe. 2017. "Resveratrol supplementation reduces pain experience by postmenopausal women." *Menopause* 24 (8):916–922. https://doi.org/10.1097/gme.0000000000000861.

Wu, Chong-Jie, Ri-Xu Liu, Song-Wei Huan, Wang Tang, Yu-Kai Zeng, Jun-Cheng Zhang, Jie Yang, Zhen-Yan Li, Ying Zhou, Zhen-Gang Zha, Huan-Tian Zhang, and Ning Liu. 2022. "Senescent skeletal cells cross-talk with synovial cells plays a key role in the pathogenesis of osteoarthritis." *Arthritis Research & Therapy* 24 (1):59. https://doi.org/10.1186/s13075-022-02747-4.

Wu, Jiadong, Aifei Wang, Xiao Wang, Guangfei Li, Peng Jia, Guangsi Shen, Bin Chen, Ye Yuan, Hui Zhang, Fan Yang, and Youjia Xu. 2019. "Rapamycin improves bone mass in high-turnover osteoporosis with iron accumulation through positive effects on osteogenesis and angiogenesis." *Bone* 121:16–28. https://doi.org/10.1016/j.bone.2018.12.019.

Xu, Cong, Fei Liu, Yu Yang, Feng Yuan, Bo Zhou, and Yadong Liu. 2021. "Antiosteoporotic effect of fisetin in an estrogen deficient model of osteoporosis." *Pharmacognosy Magazine* 17 (75).

Xu, D., W. Yang, C. Zhou, Y. Liu, and B. Xu. 2010. "Preventive effects of berberine on glucocorticoid-induced osteoporosis in rats." *Planta Medica* 76 (16):1809–1813. https://doi.org/10.1055/s-0030-1250040.

Xu, M., T. Tchkonia, and J. L. Kirkland. 2016. "Perspective: Targeting the JAK/STAT pathway to fight age-related dysfunction." *Pharmacological Research* 111:152–154. https://doi.org/10.1016/j.phrs.2016.05.015.

Xu, Mao, Meng Feng, Hang Peng, Zhuang Qian, Liting Zhao, and Shufang Wu. 2020. "Epigenetic regulation of chondrocyte hypertrophy and apoptosis through Sirt1/P53/P21 pathway in surgery-induced osteoarthritis." *Biochemical and Biophysical Research Communications* 528 (1):179–185.

Xu, Ming, Tamara Tchkonia, Husheng Ding, Mikolaj Ogrodnik, Ellen R. Lubbers, Tamar Pirtskhalava, Thomas A. White, Kurt O. Johnson, Michael B. Stout, Vojtech Mezera, Nino Giorgadze, Michael D. Jensen, Nathan K. LeBrasseur, and James L. Kirkland. 2015. "JAK inhibition alleviates the cellular senescence-associated secretory phenotype and frailty in old age." *Proceedings of the National Academy of Sciences* 112 (46):E6301–E6310. https://doi.org/10.1073/pnas.1515386112.

Xu, X., X. Liu, Y. Yang, J. He, H. Gu, M. Jiang, Y. Huang, X. Liu, and L. Liu. 2019. "Resveratrol inhibits the development of obesity-related osteoarthritis via the TLR4 and

PI3K/Akt signaling pathways." *Connective Tissue Research* 60 (6):571–582. https://doi.org/10.1080/03008207.2019.1601187.

Yadav, V., A. Krishnan, and D. Vohora. 2020. "A systematic review on Piper longum L.: Bridging traditional knowledge and pharmacological evidence for future translational research." *Journal of Ethnopharmacology* 247:112255. https://doi.org/10.1016/j.jep.2019.112255.

Yamaguchi, Masayoshi, Terry W. Moore, Aiming Sun, James P. Snyder, and Mamoru Shoji. 2012. "Novel curcumin analogue UBS109 potently stimulates osteoblastogenesis and suppresses osteoclastogenesis: Involvement in Smad activation and NF-κB inhibition." *Integrative Biology* 4 (8):905–913.

Yamaura, Kohei, Anna Laura Nelson, Haruki Nishimura, Joan C. Rutledge, Sudheer K. Ravuri, Chelsea Bahney, Marc J. Philippon, and Johnny Huard. 2022. "The effects of fisetin on bone and cartilage: A systematic review." *Pharmacological Research* 185:106504. https://doi.org/10.1016/j.phrs.2022.106504.

Yang, Cuicui, Wanxin Qiao, Qi Xue, David Goltzman, Dengshun Miao, and Zhan Dong. 2024. "The senolytic agent ABT263 ameliorates osteoporosis caused by active vitamin D insufficiency through selective clearance of senescent skeletal cells." *Journal of Orthopaedic Translation* 49:107–118. https://doi.org/10.1016/j.jot.2024.08.012.

Yang, H., C. Chen, H. Chen, X. Duan, J. Li, Y. Zhou, W. Zeng, and L. Yang. 2020. "Navitoclax (ABT263) reduces inflammation and promotes chondrogenic phenotype by clearing senescent osteoarthritic chondrocytes in osteoarthritis." *Aging (Albany NY)* 12 (13):12750–12770. https://doi.org/10.18632/aging.103177.

Yang, S., M. Sun, and X. Zhang. 2022. "Protective effect of resveratrol on knee osteoarthritis and its molecular mechanisms: A recent review in preclinical and clinical trials." *Frontiers Pharmacology* 13:921003. https://doi.org/10.3389/fphar.2022.921003.

Yang, X., L. Zhao, and Y. Pang. 2024. "cGAS-STING pathway in pathogenesis and treatment of osteoarthritis and rheumatoid arthritis." *Frontiers Immunology* 15:1384372. https://doi.org/10.3389/fimmu.2024.1384372.

Yari, Shinya, Junichi Kikuta, Hotaka Shigyo, Yu Miyamoto, Daisuke Okuzaki, Yuki Furusawa, Masafumi Minoshima, Kazuya Kikuchi, and Masaru Ishii. 2023. "JAK inhibition ameliorates bone destruction by simultaneously targeting mature osteoclasts and their precursors." *Inflammation and Regeneration* 43 (1):18. https://doi.org/10.1186/s41232-023-00268-4.

Yasuda, Hisataka, Nobuyuki Shima, Nobuaki Nakagawa, Shin-Ichi Mochizuki, Kazuki Yano, Nobuaki Fujise, Yasushi Sato, Masaaki Goto, Kyoji Yamaguchi, and Masayoshi Kuriyama. 1998. "Identity of osteoclastogenesis inhibitory factor (OCIF) and osteoprotegerin (OPG): A mechanism by which OPG/OCIF inhibits osteoclastogenesis in vitro." *Endocrinology* 139 (3):1329–1337.

Yousefzadeh, M. J., Y. Zhu, S. J. McGowan, L. Angelini, H. Fuhrmann-Stroissnigg, M. Xu, Y. Y. Ling, K. I. Melos, T. Pirtskhalava, C. L. Inman, C. McGuckian, E. A. Wade, J. I. Kato, D. Grassi, M. Wentworth, C. E. Burd, E. A. Arriaga, W. L. Ladiges, T. Tchkonia, J. L. Kirkland, P. D. Robbins, and L. J. Niedernhofer. 2018. "Fisetin is a senotherapeutic that extends health and lifespan." *EBioMedicine* 36:18–28. https://doi.org/10.1016/j.ebiom.2018.09.015.

Zhang, D., K. Yu, J. Yang, S. Xie, J. Yang, and L. Tan. 2020. "Senolytic controls bone marrow mesenchymal stem cells fate improving bone formation." *American Journal of Translational Research* 12 (6):3078–3088.

Zhang, Xin, Suping Zhang, Xingui Liu, Yingying Wang, Jianhui Chang, Xuan Zhang, Samuel G. Mackintosh, Alan J. Tackett, Yonghan He, and Dongwen Lv. 2018. "Oxidation resistance 1 is a novel senolytic target." *Aging Cell* 17 (4):e12780.

Zhang, Y., J. Ma, and W. Zhang. 2021. "Berberine for bone regeneration: Therapeutic potential and molecular mechanisms." *Journal of Ethnopharmacology* 277:114249. https://doi.org/10.1016/j.jep.2021.114249.

Zhao, Jinyun, Lifu Zheng, Guoyu Dai, Yi Sun, Rundong He, Zhide Liu, Yuxin Jin, Tianding Wu, Jianzhong Hu, Yong Cao, and Chunyue Duan. 2025. "Senolytics cocktail dasatinib and quercetin alleviate chondrocyte senescence and facet joint osteoarthritis in mice." *The Spine Journal* 25 (1):184–198. https://doi.org/10.1016/j.spinee.2024.09.017

Zhao, Z., Y. Wang, Z. Wang, F. Zhang, Z. Ding, and T. Fan. 2024. "Senescence in intervertebral disc degeneration: A comprehensive analysis based on bioinformatic strategies." *Immunity, Inflammation and Disease* 12 (11):e70072. https://doi.org/10.1002/iid3.70072.

Zheng, Wenhao, Zhenhua Feng, Shengban You, Hui Zhang, Zhenyu Tao, Quan Wang, Hua Chen, and Yaosen Wu. 2017. "Fisetin inhibits IL-1β-induced inflammatory response in human osteoarthritis chondrocytes through activating SIRT1 and attenuates the progression of osteoarthritis in mice." *International Immunopharmacology* 45:135–147.

Zhou, J., Z. Zhuang, J. Li, and Z. Feng. 2023. "Significance of the cGAS-STING pathway in health and disease." *International Journal of Molecular Sciences* 24 (17). https://doi.org/10.3390/ijms241713316.

Zhou, Yueying, Xiaonan Xin, Lichao Wang, Binsheng Wang, Li Chen, Ousheng Liu, David W. Rowe, and Ming Xu. 2021. "Senolytics improve bone forming potential of bone marrow mesenchymal stem cells from aged mice." *NPJ Regenerative Medicine* 6 (1):34. https://doi.org/10.1038/s41536-021-00145-z.

Zhou, Z., J. Y. Han, C. X. Xi, J. X. Xie, X. Feng, C. Y. Wang, L. Mei, and W. C. Xiong. 2008. "HMGB1 regulates RANKL-induced osteoclastogenesis in a manner dependent on RAGE." *Journal of Bone and Mineral Research* 23 (7):1084–1096. https://doi.org/10.1359/jbmr.080234.

Zhu, Runjiu, Haoyang Wan, Hong Yang, Mingrui Song, Yu Chai, and Bin Yu. 2022. "The role of senescence-associated secretory phenotype in bone loss." *Frontiers in Cell and Developmental Biology* 10:841612.

Zhu, Y. I., Tamara Tchkonia, Tamar Pirtskhalava, Adam C. Gower, Husheng Ding, Nino Giorgadze, Allyson K. Palmer, Yuji Ikeno, Gene B. Hubbard, and Marc Lenburg. 2015. "The Achilles' heel of senescent cells: From transcriptome to senolytic drugs." *Aging Cell* 14 (4):644–658.

Zinovkin, Roman A., Valeria P. Romaschenko, Ivan I. Galkin, Vlada V. Zakharova, Olga Yu Pletjushkina, Boris V. Chernyak, and Ekaterina N. Popova. 2014. "Role of mitochondrial reactive oxygen species in age-related inflammatory activation of endothelium." *Aging (Albany NY)* 6 (8):661.

Chapter 8

Senotherapeutics and Diabetes

Aleeta Maria Jolly, Mintu Mathew, Mohit Agarwal, Anjana Krishna, and Jaya Thomas

8.1 DIABETES AND CELLULAR SENESCENCE

Diabetes mellitus (DM) is considered a fast-growing chronic illness affecting about 537 million individuals globally as per International Diabetes Federation reports of 2021 (Hossain, Al-Mamun, and Islam 2024). DM is broadly divided into two groups: type 1 and type 2 diabetes. DM persistently elevates high blood sugar levels either due to impairment in insulin secretion or due to insulin resistance elevation. Pancreatic β-cells dysfunction will reduce insulin secretion subsequently, and insulin resistance occurs due to the impairment in response of peripheral tissues such as the liver, muscles, and fat to insulin signaling (Galicia-Garcia et al. 2020). Cellular senescence is significant in the pathophysiology of diabetes directly attributed to senescence-associated secretory phenotype (SASP)-mediated tissue destruction, adipose tissue, and pancreatic β-cell dysfunction (Aguayo-Mazzucato 2020; Narasimhan et al. 2021). Obesity and aging can accelerate hyperglycemia and insulin resistance through the accumulation of dysfunctional adipose tissue thereby decline in the mass and proliferation of β-cells, which emphasizes the relevance of metabolic changes and tissue damage in diabetes (Iwasaki, Abarca, and Aguayo-Mazzucato 2023; Murakami, Inagaki, and Kondoh 2022).

8.2 PATHOPHYSIOLOGY OF CELLULAR SENESCENCE IN DIABETES

The recent advancement in aging research emphasizes the involvement of senescent cells for age-related disorders including diabetes as well as the scope of senotherapeutics. Even though the pathology of cellular senescence is not completely revealed, the influence of aging on insulin secretion is known (McHugh and Gil 2018). Acute senescence has a favorable role in repair of tissue by secreting factors involved in tissue remodeling and activating the body's immunity to resist the modeling; in contrast, chronic senescence can worsen age-related complications

 DOI: 10.1201/9781003493969-8

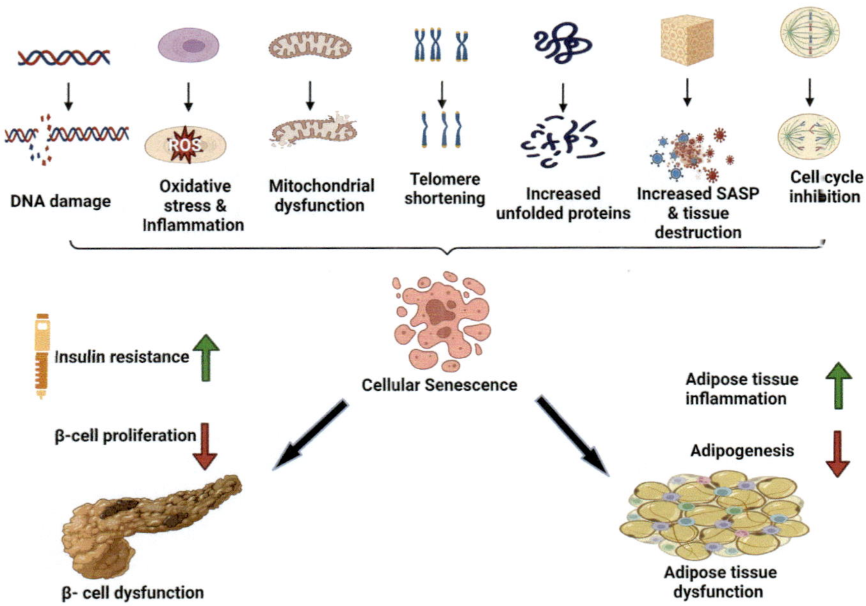

Figure 8.1 Pathophysiology of cellular senescence in diabetes.

(Narasimhan et al. 2021). The pathophysiology of senescence of cells in diabetes is represented in Figure 8.1.

Multiple factors contribute to the senescence of cells of β-cells, including:

- Cell cycle inhibitors
- SASP
- Inflammatory mediators
- Unfolded proteins
- DNA damage
- Oxidative stress and metabolic stress.

8.2.1 Cellular Senescence of β-cells of Pancreas on Aging

Reports suggest that aging can adversely affect insulin secretion by reducing pancreatic β-cell mass (BCM) or β-cell proliferation or simultaneously reducing peripheral tissue sensitivity to insulin. The direct influence of aging with the reduced ability of β-cell proliferation according to metabolic needs is evident in rodent models and humans (Aguayo-Mazzucato 2020). The age-associated functional decline in human β-cells was reported consistently in several evaluation tests such as static and perfusion systems to assess the glucose-stimulated insulin secretion, euglycemic insulin clamp oral and intravenous glucose tolerance tests (Narasimhan et al. 2021; Murakami, Inagaki, and Kondoh 2022). Chronic elderly diabetic patient's report testing positive for autoantibodies to islet proteins while some report auto-reactive T-cells (Narasimhan et al. 2021).

As age progresses there will be upregulation of cell cycle inhibitors such as wild-type activating fragment-1 (WAF1) or cyclin-dependent kinase (CDK) inhibitory protein-1 p21CIP (p21) and P16 inhibitors of CDK inhibitors 4 (p16INK4a) (p16), p15INK4b (p15), p19ARF affecting the decreased immune clearance and increased induction subsequently increasing the accumulation of senescent β-cells which have reduced activity with elevated baseline insulin (Iwasaki, Abarca, and Aguayo-Mazzucato 2023; Narasimhan et al. 2021; Murakami, Inagaki, and Kondoh 2022).

SASP, including inflammatory interleukins, growth factors, proinflammatory cytokines, chemokines, extracellular matrix-degrading enzymes, and proteases, are secreted by the senescent cells, increasing the injury to the pancreatic β-cells, and to clear the senescent β-cells SASPs mobilize the immunity locally (Narasimhan et al. 2021; Murakami, Inagaki, and Kondoh 2022; Iwasaki, Abarca, and Aguayo-Mazzucato 2023). Moreover, several factors and mechanisms such as the P16INK4A and P21WAF1/CIP1 pathways, NF-κB pathway, the p38/mitogen-activated protein kinase (MAPK) pathway, mammalian TORC1 (mTOR), transcription factors including GATA4 and C/EBPβ, cyclic GMP-AMP synthase (cGAS)-stimulator of interferon gene (STING) pathways, and the Janus kinase/signal transducer and activator of transcription 3 (JAK/STAT3) pathway regulate SASPs (Iwasaki, Abarca, and Aguayo-Mazzucato 2023; Murakami, Inagaki, and Kondoh 2022).

Senescent cells prevent the replication and mutagenesis of damaged genes with the tumor suppression mechanism; similarly, they are resistant to cell death due to the upregulation of factors in anti-apoptotic pathways (SCAP), such as p53/p21/serpines, phosphoinositide 3-kinase (PI3K)/AKT, B-cell lymphoma 2 (BCL-2)/BCL-XL, dependence receptors/tyrosine kinases, and hypoxia-inducible factor 1α (HIF-1α) (Iwasaki, Abarca, and Aguayo-Mazzucato 2023; Murakami, Inagaki, and Kondoh 2022).

Due to the involvement of free fatty acids (FFA), the β-cells start to produce and secrete the inflammatory cytokines such as interleukin (IL) [IL-1β, IL-6, IL-8] and chemokines such as CCL2 and CXCL1, which especially IL-1β enhances the stimulation of resident immune cells. This response is mediated by the toll-like receptor 4 (TLR4)-MyD88 pathway, thereby activating the proinflammatory transcription factor nuclear factor kappa B (NF-κB) pathway. Downregulation of TLR4 or Myd88 expression weaken the production and secretion of IL-1β, thereby helping to restore insulin production (Narasimhan et al. 2021; Eguchi and Nagai 2017).

All senescent β-cells experience DNA damage stimulating the DNA damage response (DDR) signaling mechanism. During the break of double-stranded DNA, DDR initiates and the MRE11/RAD50/NBS1 complex identifies the broken DNA end and incorporates the ataxia-telangiectasia mutated (ATM) kinase to the

DNA repair site. ATM helps in signal transduction, promoting DNA repair by activating several effector proteins, and it phosphorylates p53 and transcriptionally activates genes that mediate the senescence. Increased telomere-associated foci (TAF) and histone H2AX phosphorylation that help in forming foci expressing γ-H2AX present at the DNA repair site (Iwasaki, Abarca, and Aguayo-Mazzucato 2023; Murakami, Inagaki, and Kondoh 2022).

The senescent β-cells appear to be enlarged and flattened cell bodies with a change in nuclear structure and vimentin filament rearrangement, and also exhibit a frequent variation in the composition of plasma membrane due to the upregulation of caveolin-1 (Murakami, Inagaki, and Kondoh 2022; Narasimhan et al. 2021). Lack of nuclear lamina structural protein lamin B1 and other nuclear alterations, like the loss of constitutive heterochromatin condensation and formation of cytoplasmic chromatin fragments rich in epigenetic markers linked to damage in DNA, are brought on by the degradation of nuclear integrity as a result of decreased lamin B1 (Iwasaki, Abarca, and Aguayo-Mazzucato 2023). Senescent cells exhibit high lysosomal protein content due to the demand in high protein of SASP increase mTOR activity and at pH 6 stimulates lysosomal senescence-associated β-galactosidase (Aguayo-Mazzucato 2020; Iwasaki, Abarca, and Aguayo-Mazzucato 2023; Narasimhan et al. 2021).

Several preclinical studies prove that aging and obesity can increase the incidence of β-cell senescence especially in mice on a diet rich in high fat foods and observed a proportional increase in BMI and T2DM. The studies involving RNA sequencing comparison with the non-senescent (SA-β-Gal$^-$) and senescent (SA-β-Gal$^+$) β-cells help to understand the crucial involvement of specific genes in the pathophysiology of type 2 DM. The results showcase the downregulation of β-cell identity markers such as Neurod1, Ins1, Nkx6.1, MafA, and Pdx1, and the upregulation of genes such as LDHA, catalase, aging-specific markers such as IGF1R, BAMBI, increased SASPs (TNFα, IL1α, CCL2, IL6), senescence markers *p16Ink4a* and *p21Cip1* along with elevating activity of SA-β-Gal in the islet of obese mice indicates that metabolic stress can accelerate insulin resistance and senescence of β-cells (Aguayo-Mazzucato 2020; Iwasaki, Abarca, and Aguayo-Mazzucato 2023; Murakami, Inagaki, and Kondoh 2022).

The senescent cells exhibit specific transcriptional changes upon aging that directly alter the proliferation and function of pancreatic β-cells, especially insulin secretion by reducing the gene expression in cellular depolarization (voltage-gated Ca^{2+}, chloride, cation, sodium channels, ATP-dependent K^+ channel) glycolysis (*GCK*), incretin signal pathway genes (*GLP1R, GCGR*) and insulin granule components (Iwasaki, Abarca, and Aguayo-Mazzucato 2023; Narasimhan et al. 2021; Murakami, Inagaki, and Kondoh 2022).

Several studies prove the impact of oxidative stress and metabolic stress on β-cells senescence and insulin resistance stating that glucotoxicity (chronic hyperglycemia) and lipotoxicity (hyperlipidemia) can lead to dysfunction in β-cell by increasing synthesis of reactive oxygen species, stress in endoplasmic reticulum (ER), and mitochondrial dysfunction. Multiple factors such as mutation, infection lack of chaperones, and ROS can exacerbate the ER stress, resulting in the accumulation of proteins and stimulating the unfolded response in protein leading to decreased synthesis of protein, and also the export of enlarged proteins and misfolded proteins (Narasimhan et al. 2021). Hyperglycemia exacerbates insulin exocytosis and oxidative stress in β-cells, leading to dysfunction of telomerase and shorter telomere length in β-cells. Studies suggest that lifestyle modifications by including a lower calorie diet and incorporating physical exercise can help to partially reverse telomere shortening (Murakami, Inagaki, and Kondoh 2022). As age progresses, the changes in the mitochondrial activity and secretion of hormones such as glucagon-like peptide 1 and glucose-dependent insulinotropic polypeptide will directly influence secretion of insulin. Moreover, heterogeneity of age-dependent changes in insulin resistance is evident in the majority of type 2 DM (Aguayo-Mazzucato 2020).

8.2.2 Cellular Senescence of Adipose Tissue

Adipose tissue is the vital and the largest endocrine organ that regulates lipid and glucose homeostasis and helps to maintain immunity during fluctuating nutritional conditions and aging (Choe et al. 2016). Several preclinical and clinical studies report that during obesity and diabetes, there will be an increased accumulation of macrophages in the islets due to the polarization and infiltration of macrophages from the anti-inflammatory (M2) profile to the proinflammatory (M1) profile (Narasimhan et al. 2021).

The functioning of adipose tissue purely relies on calorie uptake, age, physical activity, and health conditions. Adipose tissue is of two types: brown adipose tissue (BAT) and white adipose tissue (WAT), which stores the excess energy by digesting triglycerides into FFA and glycerol and is utilized during nutritional insufficiency. In contrast, BAT utilizes the mitochondrial uncoupling process where chemical energy is generated by transforming the FFA into heat (Chait and den Hartigh 2020; Narasimhan et al. 2021). In obese patients, an increase in the visceral WAT is observed more than the subcutaneous WAT, which increases the risk of type 2 DM and cardiovascular complications. As age progresses, there is a gradual increase in fat mass due to the hypertrophy of adipocytes and excess cell counts concurrent decline in adipogenesis (Narasimhan et al. 2021; Murakami, Inagaki, and Kondoh 2022). Increased telomere shortening and oxidative stress activate p38 mitogen-activated protein kinases and overexpression of $p16^{Ink4}$, $p21^{Cip1}$, and p53 resulting in the senescence of adipose tissue leading to impaired lipid metabolism, irregular adipocytokine synthesis, and insulin resistance (Narasimhan et al. 2021).

The excess amount of lipid exerts stress on the adipocytes leading to the enlargement and initiating inflammatory response by the activating the HIF1α-NF-kB pathway; simultaneously macrophages for the cyclic ADP ribose hydrolase are elevated concerning the increase in the adipocyte senescence. It results in the accumulation of FFA and stimulates the inflammatory process, thereby secreting TNF-α, IL-8, IL-6, Il-1β, MCP-1, and CX3CL1, as well as SASPs (Narasimhan et al. 2021; Murakami, Inagaki, and Kondoh 2022). Aging, metabolic stress, and inflammatory changes in the adipose tissue will exacerbate the senescence of adipocytes and insulin resistance (Narasimhan et al. 2021). Dysfunction of these adipocytes will result in the buildup of FFA and lipid intermediates such as ceramides and diacylglycerol in the non-adipose tissues, which in turn activates the serine/threonine kinases leading to the impaired signaling of insulin due to the phosphorylation of insulin receptor substrates (Narasimhan et al. 2021).

8.3 BIOMARKERS OF CELLULAR SENESCENCE

As multiple mechanisms are involved in senescence, senescent cells have several distinct markers. The major indicators of senescent cells are their morphological alteration, such as increase in size (Li et al. 2023). Based on the difference in the cell traits, these markers are divided into cell cycle arrest factors, DNA damage or nuclear reorganization factors (P53BP1, TAF, γH2AX, lamin B1, telomere-related DNA damage foci), SASP factors (interleukins, TNFα, proteases, serpine 1, CCL3–5, monocyte chemoattractant protein-1) lysosomal compartment changes factors (lipofuscin, SA-β-gal activity, SA-α-fucosidase), and inflammatory markers (Iwasaki, Abarca, and Aguayo-Mazzucato 2023). To evaluate the impact of therapy and diabetes status of senescent cells, it is required to look at a variety of biomarkers as none of them is completely sensitive or specific (Roger, Tomas, and Gire 2021).

8.4 SENOTHERAPEUTICS AND DIABETES MELLITUS

Unfavorable senescent cells have resistance towards apoptosis. DM is caused by insulin resistance, dysfunction of pancreatic β-cells and adipose tissue due to secretion of SASP factors synthesized by senescent cells (Narasimhan et al. 2021). An environment with oxidative stress is produced by the activation of NF-kB, which is triggered by elevated amounts of proinflammatory cytokines such as IL-6 and IL−8. The development of senescent pancreatic β-cells, which secrete insulin, can result from oxidative stress in conjunction with inflammation and persistent hyperglycemia (Palmer et al. 2015). The buildup of aged endothelial cells in blood arteries aggravates vascular problems such as atherosclerosis, which is a prevalent problem in people with type 2 DM. Senescent cells in adipose tissue exacerbate insulin resistance by secreting cytokines that promote inflammation. Enhanced insulin sensitivity and elevated β-cell activity are necessary for better glucose management. Diabetes and its associated conditions may advance more slowly if senescent cells are targeted. Senescent cells were shown to have a major impact on the development of diabetes, especially in its complications

(Palmer et al. 2019). A class of drugs known as senotherapeutics focuses on treating cellular senescence, a state where cells stop dividing and progressively accumulate, contribute to aging and age-related disorders (Cha, Aguayo-Mazzucato, and Thompson 2023).

They are broadly classified into three categories: senolytics, senomorphics, and senescence-targeting immunotherapeutics (Palmer et al. 2015). Senolytics are the target signaling pathways which are activated in senescent cells and kill chronically the senescent cells. Certain examples include BCL-2 family inhibitors and HSP90 (Palmer et al. 2019). Agents used under these categories' incudes dasatinib, quercetin, navitoclax, tanespimycin, and fisetin. Senomorphics are those agents which transform characteristics of senescent cell into those of young cells by interfering with senescence-associated pathways, Certain examples of this class include metformin and ruxolitinib (Aguayo-Mazzucato et al. 2019). The other category is senescence-targeting immunotherapeutics, which includes targeting senescent cells to improve the function of the immune system. Examples of this class are NK cells and CDB T cells. Various other natural agents are discovered for senotherapeutics, which includes fisetin, a yellow compound found in various plants such as onions, strawberries, and apples. Apart from this, other substances such as quercetin, resveratrol, and curcumin are also used as senotherapeutic agents (Cha, Aguayo-Mazzucato, and Thompson 2023). Senotherapeutics may slow the development of diabetes-related problems like retinopathy, nephropathy, and cardiovascular disease by reducing the inflammation associated with aging (Murakami, Inagaki, and Kondoh 2022; Kruczkowska et al. 2024).

8.4.1 Dasatinib and Quercetin

Dasatinib and quercetin are potent drugs of senotherapeutics, especially due to their unique senolytic qualities. Senotherapy with dasatinib and quercetin reduces insulin resistance by terminating the senescent cells in WAT (Murakami, Inagaki, and Kondoh 2022)

Dasatinib is classified as a tyrosine kinase inhibitor. Senescent cells are targeted by dasatinib, which was initially created and approved for the treatment of particular types of leukemia. Dasatinib has been proven to prolong health span and enhance physical activity in preclinical models by reducing the number of senescent cells which shows enhanced insulin sensitivity and lowered inflammatory markers that are linked to senescent cells (Murakami, Inagaki, and Kondoh 2022; Iwasaki, Abarca, and Aguayo-Mazzucato 2023). This results in the cells going through an apoptotic process as shown in Figure 8.2. Salaami et al. conducted a clinical study among the diabetic population and found that patients treated with dasatinib for 1 year had reduced glucose levels and HbA1C levels in comparison with the patients treated with imatinib (Salaami et al. 2021).

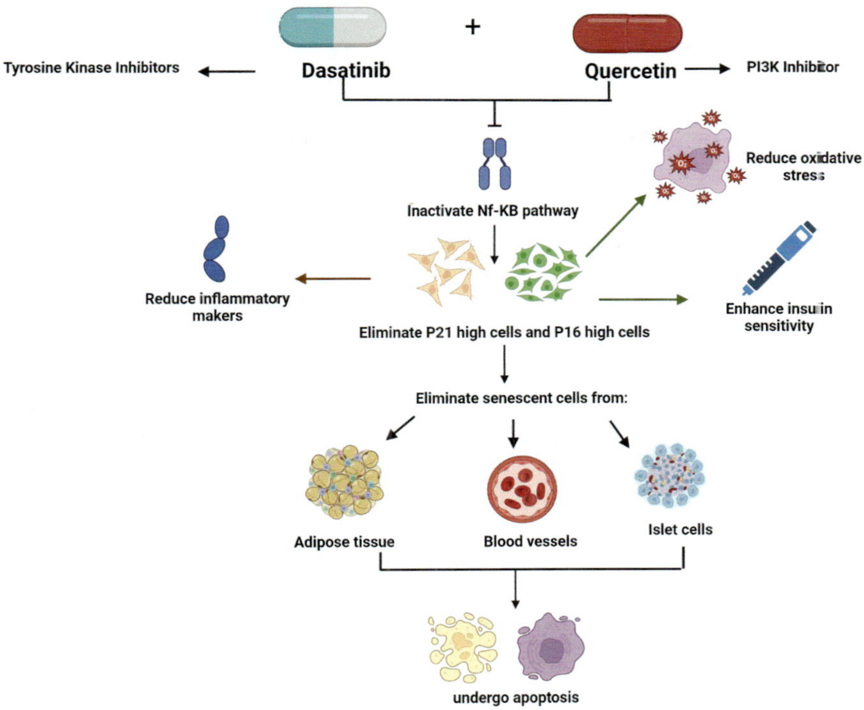

Figure 8.2 Mechanism of dasatinib and quercetin as senotherapeutics.

Quercetin is a natural flavonoid and a PI3K inhibitor. Numerous fruits, vegetables, and grains contain quercetin. A common use for it is as a dietary supplement. Quercetin has been proven to reduce inflammation and oxidative stress, which are crucial in the progression of diabetes. By blocking anti-apoptotic mechanisms, quercetin specifically targets senescent endothelium and mesenchymal cells (Kondoh and Hara 2022; Salaami et al. 2021).

A combination of dasatinib with quercetin was used clinically as the first senolytic in 2015. The combination of dasatinib with quercetin decreased the β-gal$^+$ dispersed islet cells. It even reduced blood glucose levels in an insulin-resistant model (Iwasaki, Abarca, and Aguayo-Mazzucato 2023). When quercetin and dasatinib are combined, the senolytic effect improves, which boosts the combination's effectiveness in reducing senescent cells in tissues affected by age-related illnesses, such as diabetes. Research has indicated that the co-administration of dasatinib and quercetin is better than the use of either drug alone in the eradication of senescent cells. Preclinical models and a few limited clinical trials have been used to explore this combination (H. Zhang et al. 2023). Dasatinib and quercetin therapy has the potential to enhance insulin sensitivity and management of type 2 DM, thus eliminating senescent cells specifically from adipose tissue and blood vessels.

Combining the two can help lessen the chronic inflammation linked to diabetes by reducing the pro-inflammatory discharges from senescent cells (Kim and Kim 2019). Kondoh et al. gave a diet with high fat to mice, thus causing obesity and diabetes. p21-high cells accumulated within 2 months. After 10 months, p16-high cells also accumulated. Senotherapy with dasatinib and quercetin inactivated the NF-kB pathway in p21-high cells and eliminated both p21-high cells and p16-high cells, thus resulting in reducing glucose intolerance and insulin sensitivity (Kondoh and Hara 2022). In diabetic individuals, dasatinib and quercetin therapy lower the complications such as retinopathy, nephropathy, and heart diseases. Clinical trials on a larger scale are required to verify the safety and effectiveness of dasatinib and quercetin, particularly for long-term usage in diabetic patients, despite the encouraging results of preclinical research (L. Zhang et al. 2023).

Dasatinib is a powerful medication intended to treat cancer; thus, it can have serious adverse effects such as immunosuppression, which should be carefully monitored when thinking about using it for other purposes. To reduce hazards and optimize benefits, research is still ongoing that determines the adequate dose regimens for the senolytic effects of dasatinib and quercetin, particularly in diabetes. Combining dasatinib and quercetin may target the fundamental causes of cellular senescence and aging in diabetes, thus providing a novel therapeutic approach for controlling the condition and its consequences (Chaib, Tchkonia, and Kirkland 2022).

8.4.2 Navitoclax

It is a senolytic agent targeted at ABT263. It is from a Bcl-2 inhibitor. It targets the Bcl-2, Bcl-xL, and Bcl-w proteins that are involved in controlling apoptosis. Navitoclax was first used as an anti-cancer medication (Choi et al. 2022). Navitoclax encourages cancer cells to undergo apoptosis by blocking these proteins. Senescent cells accumulate damage over time but frequently depend on anti-apoptotic proteins to prevent cell death. Due to the disruption of these proteins by navitoclax, senescent cells are more prone to apoptosis. Navitoclax significantly reduces the senescent cells in tissues by triggering apoptosis in cells that express high levels of Bcl-2 family proteins (Rubin de Celis and Bonner-Weir 2023). Navitoclax removes senescent cells from tissues that respond to insulin thereby potentially increasing insulin sensitivity. It reverses β-cell functioning and identity that was lost by β-cell senescence as well as reduces insulin resistance. Navitoclax is a small-molecule drug as a senolytic agent (Shakeri et al. 2018). It is primarily known for its role in targeting apoptotic pathways and making it a potent tool for selectively eliminating senescent cells that undergo deposition on aging and cause age-related diseases including DM as shown in Figure 8.3. Senescent cells thus contribute to persistent inflammation due to diabetes by secreting pro-inflammatory cytokines. By eliminating the cause of the inflammation, navitoclax may be able to lessen it (Atkinson et al. 2011). Navitoclax prevents or mitigates the effects of diabetes-related problems such as retinopathy, nephropathy, and atherosclerosis by specifically targeting senescent cells

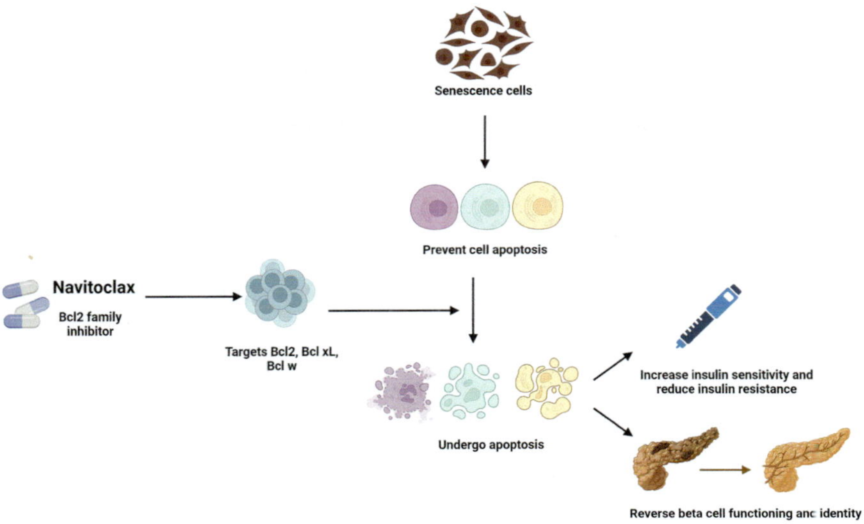

Figure 8.3 Mechanism of navitoclax as senotherapeutic.

in vascular tissues. Navitoclax has demonstrated efficacy in treating metabolic problems and aging-related health markers, as well as lowering the senescent cells of animal experiments (Power et al. 2023). The potency and safety of navitoclax as a senolytic drug have been the subject of a few early-stage clinical investigations. Aguayo-Mazzucato et al. conducted in vitro studies, animal studies, and clinical studies on navitoclax and showed reduced glucose levels compared to non-treated groups (Aguayo-Mazzucato et al. 2019).

Navitoclax acts on the Bcl-2 family of proteins, which can lead to serious adverse effects. One of these adverse effects is thrombocytopenia, or a decrease in platelet count, which raises the possibility of bleeding. This is a serious issue, particularly when it comes to long-term use or people with underlying medical concerns. It is critical to determine the ideal dosage that minimizes toxicity while maintaining efficacy in eradicating senescent cells (Cha, Aguayo-Mazzucato, and Thompson 2023). To lessen adverse effects, researchers are investigating intermittent dosing techniques. Although navitoclax shows promising effects, further research is necessary to comprehend how to use it in conjunction with other treatments and what the long-term effects will be. This is especially important for metabolic illnesses like diabetes. Navitoclax may be used in conjunction with other senolytics or anti-diabetic medications to maximize therapeutic benefits and reduction in side effects (Motlagh, Pipella, and Thompson 2024). To maximize its utility more studies are necessary to completely analyze the hazards and advantages of its indication in therapeutic settings such as for non-cancerous illnesses (Quarta and Demaria 2024).

8.4.3 Alvespimycin

Alvespimycin is also known as 17-DMAG and is primarily used as an anti-cancer agent. Alvespimycin is an HSP90 inhibitor. It is a heat shock protein 90 that is a highly express chaperone protein. It plays a major role in stabilizing and degrading many client proteins that help in cell proliferation, angiogenesis, and oncogenesis (L. Zhang et al. 2023). The inhibition of HSP90 can destabilize and lead to the degradation of several client proteins involved in cell growth, survival, and differentiation. Chaperone proteins like HSP90 help different client proteins to fold and operate accurately. Alvespimycin can degrade these client proteins by blocking HSP90, thus lowering the survival rate of tumor cells (Boccardi and Mecocci 2021). The disruption of HSP90 function can accumulate the misfolded proteins and therefore cause cellular stress responses and potentially lead to apoptosis as shown in Figure 8.4. Senescent cells depend on molecular chaperones such as HSP90 to survive and frequently show elevated stress responses. Alvespimycin may function as a senolytic drug by making senescent cells more susceptible to apoptosis by inhibition of HSP90. Proteases, growth factors, and pro-inflammatory cytokines are among the components of the SASP that contribute to tissue dysfunction and the advancement of age-related illnesses, including diabetes (Spinelli et al. 2023). Alvespimycin has the potential to lessen SASP and its negative consequences by focusing on the cellular stress pathways in senescent cells. Alvespimycin may enhance insulin sensitivity and metabolic health in diabetics by lessening the load of senescent cells and the inflammatory secretions they produce. Diabetes-related problems like atherosclerosis, nephropathy, and retinopathy may be avoided or made better by reducing SASP-related inflammation (Novoselova et al. 2023). Tesch et al. induced diabetes in mice using a low dose of streptozotocin; after 28 days the markers of senescence were elevated. Animals were treated with alvespimycin and reduced the markers of renal senescence. Further treatment was done with ASK1 inhibitor GS-444217 that reduced impairment of kidney function. Thus, senotherapeutics prevent tubulointerstitial fibrosis in diabetic nephropathy.

Alvespimycin can be hazardous and have off-target effects. This is significant for inhibiting HSP90 in normal cells that are dependent on chaperone functions to survive. Thus the therapeutic window is narrowed, necessitating cautious dosage and administration (Phillips et al. 2024). Alvespimycin has various adverse drug reactions in cancer clinical trials such as hepatotoxicity, gastrointestinal issues, and cardiovascular problems. The challenge of alvespimycin is finding a therapeutic dose that targets sick cells efficiently without seriously harming healthy cells. Thus to increase effectiveness and lessen negative effects, alvespimycin may be used in conjunction with other senotherapeutics or anti-diabetic medications (Narasimhan et al. 2021). More studies are required to fully analyze the impact of alvespimycin on senescent cells and its potential for the treatment of metabolic disorders like diabetes.

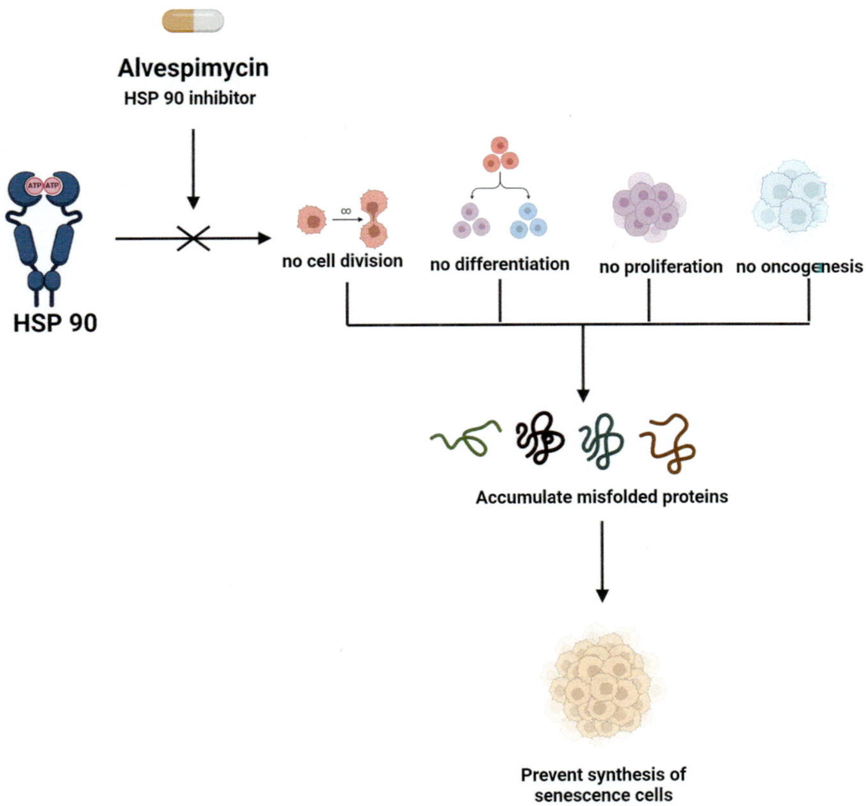

Figure 8.4 Mechanism of alvespimycin as senotherapeutic.

8.4.4 Metformin

Metformin is a drug often recommended for type 2 DM. It is also used to target senescent cells that proliferate with aging and are linked to several disorders associated with aging. Metformin mainly functions by increasing insulin sensitivity and decreasing the synthesis of glucose in the liver. Metformin has been studied for its possible advantages in aging and age-related disorders in addition to its main function (Kulkarni, Gubbi, and Barzilai 2020). Metformin has an impact on cellular metabolism and mitochondrial activity. It does this by activating AMP-activated protein kinase that has an impact on a number of cellular processes such as oxidative stress and inflammation, both of which are linked to aging and cellular senescence as shown in Figure 8.5 (Calabrò et al. 2024). Metformin lowers oxidative stress and inflammation, which are two major elements in aging that cause cellular senescence. According to certain research, metformin may increase longevity and postpone the onset of age-related illnesses. In people with diabetes,

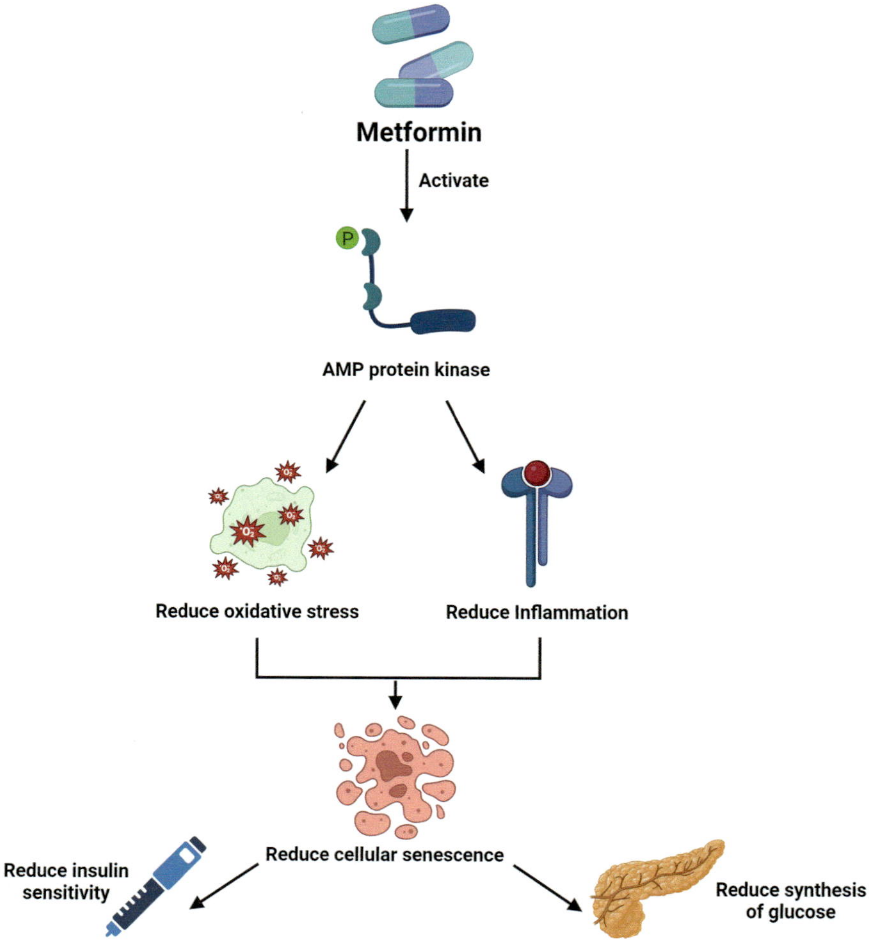

Figure 8.5 Mechanism of metformin as senotherapeutic.

it decreases risk of heart disease and cancer. The precise effects of metformin on senescent cells are still being studied. Metformin does not specifically target senescent cells, but it may have an indirect impact on the process due to its effects on inflammation and metabolism (Murakami, Inagaki, and Kondoh 2022). Further study is required to completely understand its potential advantages in this situation. Metformin lacks official recognition as a senotherapeutic medication because of its effects on cellular metabolism, inflammation, and oxidative stress, metformin has been shown to be helpful in the management of diabetes (Acar et al. 2021).

8.4.5 Canagliflozin

Canagliflozin is a sodium-glucose cotransporter 2 (SGLT2) inhibitor that primarily helps in managing type 2 DM by reducing glucose concentration. It works by preventing the reabsorption of glucose from the kidneys and back into the bloodstream leading to increased glucose excretion in the urine. This results in lower blood sugar levels and can have additional benefits beyond glycemic control. SGLT2 inhibitors block the SGLT2 protein in the kidneys that are responsible for reabsorbing glucose into the blood (Katsuumi et al. 2024). By inhibiting this protein, these medications promote glucose excretion into urine, thereby lowering blood sugar levels as shown in Figure 8.6. Other SGLT2 inhibitors include empagliflozin and dapagliflozin. SGLT2 inhibitors often lead to modest weight loss by glucose excretion in the urine. These medications reduce the severe adverse events in patients with type 2 DM (Stenlöf et al. 2013). Katsuumi et al. showed that canagliflozin reduced senescent cells. In an in-vivo study therapy with canagliflozin improved inflammation of adipose tissue and metabolic dysfunction, elevating the lifespan of mice by prevention of aging (Katsuumi et al. 2024). They can reduce the progression of diabetic complications such as nephropathy and kidney failure. SGLT2 inhibitors have been associated with improvements in metabolic health that can influence age-related processes. By reducing hyperglycemia, they help mitigate oxidative stress and inflammation caused by cellular senescence (Karagiannis, Bekiari, and Tsapas 2017). By improving cardiovascular and renal health, SGLT2 inhibitors may contribute to overall health and longevity, thus influence aging outcomes. While SGLT2 inhibitors are not classified as senotherapeutic agents, their impact on glucose metabolism, cardiovascular health, and renal function can indirectly influence aging process. They help manage conditions that

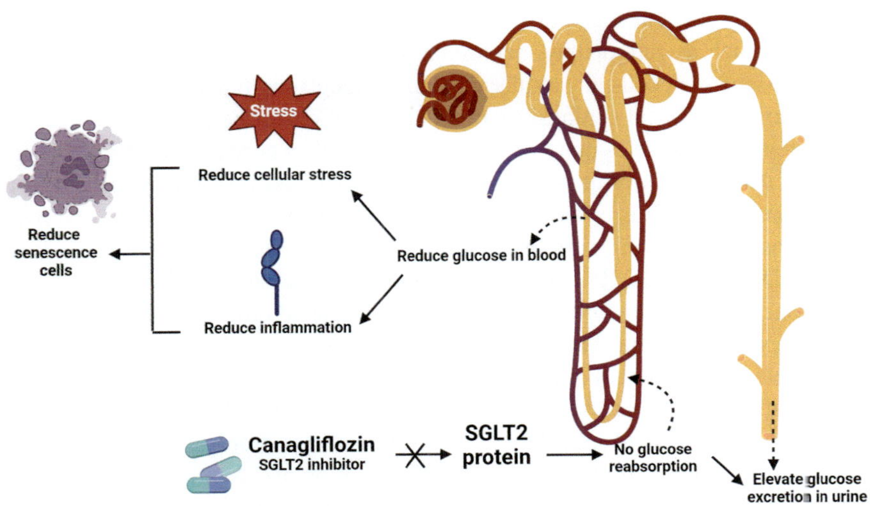

Figure 8.6 Mechanism of canagliflozin as senotherapeutic.

are prevalent in older adults and are associated with aging such as heart disease and kidney damage (Phillips et al. 2024). The primary use of SGLT2 inhibitors remains in managing T2DM and its complications. Their role as a senotherapeutic agent is not yet established in clinical practice. SGLT2 inhibitors are primarily used to manage type 2 DM but have additional benefits such as weight loss, cardiovascular protection, and renal health. Their potential role in senotherapy is an area of emerging interest, as their effects on metabolic health, inflammation, and oxidative stress could influence aging process and age-related diseases (Troise et al. 2024). Even though research on its potential as senotherapy is ongoing, future studies could demonstrate how it could support the health advantages of aging.

8.5 ROLE OF SENOTHERAPEUTICS IN DIABETIC COMPLICATIONS

Due to the senolytic properties and capacity to lower oxidative stress and inflammation, dasatinib and quercetin are potential therapy for DM. In diabetic individuals, dasatinib and quercetin therapy lowers consequences including retinopathy, nephropathy, and heart disease. Clinical trials on a larger scale are required to verify the safety and effectiveness of dasatinib and quercetin, particularly for long-term usage in diabetic patients, despite the encouraging results of preclinical research. To determine their roles in clinical practice, enhance treatment plans, and guarantee patient safety ongoing research is essential. They provide intriguing areas for more research because of their potential to enhance the outcomes for people with diabetes (L. Zhang et al. 2023). Navitoclax's capacity to target senescent cells and lower inflammation makes it a promising treatment option for controlling DM complications. Navitoclax prevents or mitigates the effects of diabetes-related problems such as retinopathy, nephropathy, and atherosclerosis by specifically targeting senescent cells in vascular tissues. Although additional study is required, particularly in clinical settings, its methods of action fit the pathophysiology of issues related to diabetes quite well. Further research is necessary to determine its efficacy, safety, and usefulness in the management of diabetes (Power et al. 2023). Alvespimycin's actions of HSP90 inhibition, reduction in inflammation, and possible senescent cell targeting make it a prospective therapeutic option for controlling DM problems. Its effects on cellular stress responses, inflammation, and senescence help to cure DM problems. Diabetes-related problems like atherosclerosis, nephropathy, and retinopathy may be avoided or made better by reducing SASP-related inflammation. Preclinical investigations are encouraging, but more investigation and clinical trials are necessary to determine adverse drug reactions, effectiveness, as well as usefulness in treating diabetes problems. Its potential to influence important pathways linked to inflammation and cellular stress makes it a promising option for managing diabetes in the future (Novoselova et al. 2023). When it comes to treating type 2 DM mellitus, canagliflozin is a great medication choice, especially for those who are at risk of cardiovascular and renal problems. Due to its many advantages, which include better glucose control, weight loss, cardiovascular protection, and renal protection, it is a crucial component of diabetes care plans. Further investigation will help to better understand its long-term effects and maximize its application in a variety of patient populations. In addition to lowering blood sugar, metformin is a vital component of type 2 DM treatment. For people at risk of problems from diabetes, its effects on weight control, cardiovascular health, renal protection, and possible anti-cancer qualities make it a beneficial treatment option. The advantages of metformin and its long-term effects on the health of people with diabetes are still being investigated (Katsumi et al. 2024).

8.6 CHALLENGES AND FUTURE PATHS OF SENOTHERAPEUTICS IN DIABETES MELLITUS

Senescent cells are involved in tissue repair and wound healing Creating senotherapeutics that can target senescent cells in particular tissues like vascular endothelial cells or pancreatic β-cells selectively while sparing other essential cell functions. Senotherapeutics are still being researched, and although they have a lot of promises, additional clinical trials are required to properly comprehend their function and efficacy in the treatment of diabetes. Senescent cells vary widely in their secretory patterns and functions, therefore exhibiting great heterogeneity (Power et al. 2023). Thus, it is challenging to find targets or uniform indicators for senescent cells in diabetes. Senescent cells have diverse functions within the body and getting rid of them entirely can have severe consequences. Senescent cells improves wound healing and tissue repair, both of which are essential for the control of diabetes (Cha, Aguayo-Mazzucato, and Thompson 2023). Hence, further research is required to determine the safety and effectiveness of senotherapeutics.

One of the challenges still present is getting senotherapeutic drugs to target tissues and sparing other organs. Senolytic medications must be delivered effectively to reach the right target tissues. In vivo studies have shown that senolytics provide short-term benefits but uncertainty on long-term implications in clinical use (Quarta and Demaria 2024). Extended use of senotherapeutics may result in unanticipated outcomes, particularly in conditions like diabetes which require long-term treatment (Spinelli et al. 2023). Senotherapeutics may have a greater therapeutic impact when combined with already available diabetes medications such as insulin sensitizers or anti-inflammatory medicines.

Senolytics and glucose-lowering drugs may work to improve insulin sensitivity and eliminate dangerous senescent cells. Targeting adipose tissue or senescent β-cells may enhance insulin production and decrease insulin resistance. To do this, tissue-specific marker research will be essential. Finding specific biomarkers for diabetic senescence is essential for monitoring the course of the condition and the effectiveness of treatment (Novoselova et al. 2023). SASP factors and p16INK4a expression are examples of biomarkers that may be used to track the effects of senotherapeutics in clinical settings. Senotherapeutics may be applied to people who are at risk to postpone the onset of diabetes. For example, early senescence-targeting medicines may be beneficial for those with obesity, metabolic syndrome, or a family history of diabetes. In order to precisely reverse or prevent senescence in diabetes, future research may concentrate on using genetic technologies such as CRISPR to modify genes implicated in cellular senescence processes (Phillips et al. 2024). Results may be enhanced by customizing senotherapeutics according to a patient's genetic profile, disease stage, or senescent cell burden. Using personalized techniques would help in determining whether senolytic or senomorphic medicines are best for the state of each patient. To determine the safety and potency of senotherapeutics in diabetes, more clinical studies are required. Senotherapeutics have enormous potential to treat diabetes, especially when it comes to targeting the cellular senescence–related mechanisms that underlie the condition (Katsuumi et al. 2024). Senotherapeutics for diabetes will probably combine customized medicine, combination treatments, and improvements in tissue-specific targeting in the future.

REFERENCES

Acar, Mustafa Burak, Şerife Ayaz-Güner, Zeynep Gunaydin, Musa Karakukcu, Gianfranco Peluso, Giovanni Di Bernardo, Servet Özcan, and Umberto Galderisi. 2021. "Proteomic and Biological Analysis of the Effects of Metformin Senomorphics on the Mesenchymal Stromal Cells." *Frontiers in Bioengineering and Biotechnology* 9 (October): 730813. https://doi.org/10.3389/FBIOE.2021.730813/BIBTEX.

Aguayo-Mazzucato, Cristina. 2020. "Functional Changes in Beta Cells during Ageing and Senescence." *Diabetologia* 63 (10): 2022–2029. https://doi.org/10.1007/S00125-020-05185-6/FIGURES/3.

Aguayo-Mazzucato, Cristina, Joshua Andle, Terrence B. Lee, Ayush Midha, Lindsay Talemal, Vaja Chipashvili, Jennifer Hollister-Lock, Jan van Deursen, Gordon Weir, and Susan Bonner-Weir. 2019. "Acceleration of β Cell Aging Determines Diabetes and Senolysis Improves Disease Outcomes." *Cell Metabolism* 30 (1): 129–142.e4. https://doi.org/10.1016/J.CMET.2019.05.006.

Atkinson, Mark A., Jeffrey A. Bluestone, George S. Eisenbarth, Matthias Hebrok, Kevan C. Herold, Domenico Accili, Massimo Pietropaolo, Peter R. Arvan, Matthias Von Herrath, Dorene S. Markel, and Christopher J. Rhodes. 2011. "How Does Type 1 Diabetes Develop?: The Notion of Homicide or β-Cell Suicide Revisited." *Diabetes* 60 (5): 1370–1379. https://doi.org/10.2337/DB10-1797.

Boccardi, Virginia, and Patrizia Mecocci. 2021. "Senotherapeutics: Targeting Senescent Cells for the Main Age-Related Diseases." *Mechanisms of Ageing and Development* 197 (July). https://doi.org/10.1016/J.MAD.2021.111526.

Calabrò, Anna, Giulia Accardi, Anna Aiello, Calogero Caruso, Damiano Galimberti, and Giuseppina Candore. 2024. "Senotherapeutics to Counteract Senescent Cells Are Prominent Topics in the Context of Anti-Ageing Strategies." *International Journal of Molecular Sciences* 25 (3). https://doi.org/10.3390/IJMS25031792.

Cha, Jeeyeon, Cristina Aguayo-Mazzucato, and Peter J. Thompson. 2023. "Pancreatic β-Cell Senescence in Diabetes: Mechanisms, Markers and Therapies." *Frontiers in Endocrinology* 14 (August): 1212716. https://doi.org/10.3389/FENDO.2023.1212716/BIBTEX.

Chaib, Selim, Tamar Tchkonia, and James L. Kirkland. 2022. "Cellular Senescence and Senolytics: The Path to the Clinic." *Nature Medicine* 28 (8): 1556–1568. https://doi.org/10.1038/S41591-022-01923-Y.

Chait, Alan, and Laura J. den Hartigh. 2020. "Adipose Tissue Distribution, Inflammation and Its Metabolic Consequences, Including Diabetes and Cardiovascular Disease." *Frontiers in Cardiovascular Medicine* 7 (February): 522637. https://doi.org/10.3389/FCVM.2020.00022/BIBTEX.

Choe, Sung Sik, Jin Young Huh, In Jae Hwang, Jong In Kim, and Jae Bum Kim. 2016. "Adipose Tissue Remodeling: Its Role in Energy Metabolism and Metabolic Disorders." *Frontiers in Endocrinology* 7 (April): 178543. https://doi.org/10.3389/FENDO.2016.00030/BIBTEX.

Choi, Ji Young, Samantha F. Yee, Tzvetelina Tchangalova, Guang Yang, and John P. Fisher. 2022. "Recent Advances in Senotherapeutics Delivery." *Tissue Engineering: Part B, Reviews* 28 (6): 1223–1234. https://doi.org/10.1089/TEN.TEB.2021.0212.

Eguchi, Kosei, and Ryozo Nagai. 2017. "Islet Inflammation in Type 2 Diabetes and Physiology." *The Journal of Clinical Investigation* 127 (1): 14. https://doi.org/10.1172/JCI88877.

Galicia-Garcia, Unai, Asier Benito-Vicente, Shifa Jebari, Asier Larrea-Sebal, Haziq Siddiqi, Kepa B. Uribe, Helena Ostolaza, and César Martín. 2020. "Pathophysiology of Type 2 Diabetes Mellitus." *International Journal of Molecular Sciences* 21 (17): 1–34. https://doi.org/10.3390/IJMS21176275.

Hossain, Md Jamal, Md Al-Mamun, and Md Rabiul Islam. 2024. "Diabetes Mellitus, the Fastest Growing Global Public Health Concern: Early Detection Should Be Focused." *Health Science Reports* 7 (3). https://doi.org/10.1002/HSR2.2004.

Iwasaki, Kanako, Cristian Abarca, and Cristina Aguayo-Mazzucato. 2023. "Regulation of Cellular Senescence in Type 2 Diabetes Mellitus: From Mechanisms to Clinical Applications." *Diabetes & Metabolism Journal* 47 (4): 441–453. https://doi.org/10.4093/DMJ.2022.0416.

Karagiannis, Thomas, Eleni Bekiari, and Apostolos Tsapas. 2017. "Canagliflozin in the Treatment of Type 2 Diabetes: An Evidence-Based Review of Its Place in Therapy." *Core Evidence* 12 (March): 1. https://doi.org/10.2147/CE.S109654.

Katsuumi, Goro, Ippei Shimizu, Masayoshi Suda, Yohko Yoshida, Takaaki Furihata, Yusuke Joki, Chieh Lun Hsiao, Liang Jiaqi, Shinya Fujiki, Manabu Abe, Masataka Sugimoto, Tomoyoshi Soga, and Tohru Minamino. 2024. "SGLT2 Inhibition Eliminates Senescent Cells and Alleviates Pathological Aging." *Nature Aging* 4 (7): 926–938. https://doi.org/10.1038/S43587-024-00642-Y.

Kim, Eok Cheon, and Jae Ryong Kim. 2019. "Senotherapeutics: Emerging Strategy for Healthy Aging and Age-Related Disease." *BMB Reports* 52 (1): 47–55. https://doi.org/10.5483/BMBREP.2019.52.1.293.

Kondoh, Hiroshi, and Eiji Hara. 2022. "Targeting P21 for Diabetes: Another Choice of Senotherapy." *Cell Metabolism* 34 (1): 5–7. https://doi.org/10.1016/j.cmet.2021.12.008.

Kruczkowska, Weronika, Julia Gałęziewska, Mateusz Kciuk, Adrianna Gielecińska, Elżbieta Płuciennik, Zbigniew Pasieka, Lin Yong Zhao, Yi Jin Yu, Damian Kołat, and Żaneta Kałuzińska-Kołat. 2024. "Senescent Adipocytes and Type 2 Diabetes—Current Knowledge and Perspective Concepts." *Biomolecular Concepts* 15 (1). https://doi.org/10.1515/BMC-2022-0046.

Kulkarni, Ameya S., Sriram Gubbi, and Nir Barzilai. 2020. "Benefits of Metformin in Attenuating the Hallmarks of Aging." *Cell Metabolism* 32 (1): 15–30. https://doi.org/10.1016/J.CMET.2020.04.001.

Li, Z, Tian M, Wang G, Cui X, Ma JE, Liu S, Shen B, Liu F, Wu K, Xiao X, and Zhu C. 2023. "Senotherapeutics: An emerging approach to the treatment of viral infectious diseases in the elderly." *Frontiers in Cellular and Infection Microbiology* 13: 1098712.

McHugh, Domhnall, and Jesús Gil. 2018. "Senescence and Aging: Causes, Consequences, and Therapeutic Avenues." *The Journal of Cell Biology* 217 (1): 65. https://doi.org/10.1083/JCB.201708092.

Motlagh, Roozbeh Akbari, Jasmine Pipella, and Peter J. Thompson. 2024. "Exploring Senescence as a Modifier of β Cell Extracellular Vesicles in Type 1 Diabetes." *Frontiers in Endocrinology* 15 (August): 1422279. https://doi.org/10.3389/FENDO.2024.1422279/BIBTEX.

Murakami, Takaaki, Nobuya Inagaki, and Hiroshi Kondoh. 2022. "Cellular Senescence in Diabetes Mellitus: Distinct Senotherapeutic Strategies for Adipose Tissue and Pancreatic β Cells." *Frontiers in Endocrinology* 13 (March). https://doi.org/10.3389/FENDO.2022.869414.

Narasimhan, Akilavalli, Rafael R. Flores, Paul D. Robbins, and Laura J. Niedernhofer. 2021. "Role of Cellular Senescence in Type II Diabetes." *Endocrinology* 162 (10): 1–12. https://doi.org/10.1210/endocr/bqab136.

Novoselova, Elena G., Sergey M. Lunin, Maxim O. Khrenov, Olga V. Glushkova, Tatiana V. Novoselova, and Svetlana B. Parfenyuk. 2023. "The Possible Role of B-Cell Senescence in the Development of Type 2 Diabetes Mellitus." *Cellular Physiology and Biochemistry: International Journal of Experimental Cellular Physiology, Biochemistry, and Pharmacology* 57 (1): 34–48. https://doi.org/10.33594/000000606.

Palmer, Allyson K., Birgit Gustafson, James L. Kirkland, and Ulf Smith. 2019. "Cellular Senescence: At the Nexus between Ageing and Diabetes." *Diabetologia* 62 (10): 1835–1841. https://doi.org/10.1007/S00125-019-4934-X.

Palmer, Allyson K., Tamara Tchkonia, Nathan K. LeBrasseur, Eduardo N. Chini, Ming Xu, and James L. Kirkland. 2015. "Cellular Senescence in Type 2 Diabetes: A Therapeutic Opportunity." *Diabetes* 64 (7): 2289–2298. https://doi.org/10.2337/DB14-1820.

Phillips, Paige Charlotte Alison, Mafalda de Sousa Loreto Aresta Branco, Chelsy Louise Cliff, Joanna Kate Ward, Paul Edward Squires, and Claire Elizabeth Hills. 2024. "Targeting Senescence to Prevent Diabetic Kidney Disease: Exploring Molecular Mechanisms and Potential Therapeutic Targets for Disease Management." *Diabetic Medicine: A Journal of the British Diabetic Association*. https://doi.org/10.1111/DME.15408.

Power, Helen, Peter Valtchev, Fariba Dehghani, and Aaron Schindeler. 2023. "Strategies for Senolytic Drug Discovery." *Aging Cell* 22 (10). https://doi.org/10.1111/ACEL.13948.

Quarta, Marco, and Marco Demaria. 2024. "On the Past, Present and Future of Senotherapeutics." *NPJ Aging* 10 (1). https://doi.org/10.1038/S41514-024-00139-3.

Roger, L, Tomas F, and Gire V. 2021. "Mechanisms and Regulation of Cellular Senescence." *Int J Mol Sci.* 22 (23): 13173. https://doi.org/10.3390/ijms222313173. PMID: 34884978; PMCID: PMC8658264.

Rubin de Celis, Maria F., and Susan Bonner-Weir. 2023. "Reversing and Modulating Cellular Senescence in Beta Cells, a New Field of Opportunities to Treat Diabetes." *Frontiers in Endocrinology* 14. https://doi.org/10.3389/FENDO.2023.1217729.

Salaami, Omid, Chia Ling Kuo, Matthew T. Drake, George A. Kuchel, James L. Kirkland, and Robert J. Pignolo. 2021. "Antidiabetic Effects of the Senolytic Agent Dasatinib." *Mayo Clinic Proceedings* 96 (12): 3021–3029. https://doi.org/10.1016/J.MAYOCP.2021.06.025.

Shakeri, Hadis, Katrien Lemmens, Andreas B. Gevaert, Guido R.Y. De Meyer, and Vincent F.M. Segers. 2018. "Cellular Senescence Links Aging and Diabetes in Cardiovascular Disease." *American Journal of Physiology. Heart and Circulatory Physiology* 315 (3): H448–H462. https://doi.org/10.1152/AJPHEART.00287.2018.

Spinelli, Rosa, Ritesh Kumar Baboota, Silvia Gogg, Francesco Beguinot, Matthias Blüher, Annika Nerstedt, and Ulf Smith. 2023. "Increased Cell Senescence in Human Metabolic Disorders." *The Journal of Clinical Investigation* 133 (12). https://doi.org/10.1172/JCI169922.

Stenlöf, K., W.T. Cefalu, K.A. Kim, M. Alba, K. Usiskin, C. Tong, W. Canovatchel, and G. Meininger. 2013. "Efficacy and Safety of Canagliflozin Monotherapy in Subjects with Type 2 Diabetes Mellitus Inadequately Controlled with Diet and Exercise." *Diabetes, Obesity & Metabolism* 15 (4): 372–382. https://doi.org/10.1111/DOM.12054.

Troise, Dario, Silvia Mercuri, Barbara Infante, Vincenzo Losappio, Luciana Cirolla, Giuseppe Stefano Netti, Elena Ranieri, and Giovanni Stallone. 2024. "MTOR and SGLT-2 Inhibitors: Their Synergistic Effect on Age-Related Processes." *International Journal of Molecular Sciences* 25 (16). https://doi.org/10.3390/IJMS25168676.

Zhang, Huantong, Han Zhou, Xin Shen, Xingchen Lin, Yuke Zhang, Yiyi Sun, Yi Zhou, Lei Zhang, and Dayong Zhang. 2023. "The Role of Cellular Senescence in Metabolic Diseases and the Potential for Senotherapeutic Interventions." *Frontiers in Cell and Developmental Biology* 11. https://doi.org/10.3389/FCELL.2023.1276707/FULL.

Zhang, Lei, Louise E. Pitcher, Vaishali Prahalad, Laura J. Niedernhofer, and Paul D. Robbins. 2023. "Targeting Cellular Senescence with Senotherapeutics: Senolytics and Senomorphics." *The FEBS Journal* 290 (5): 1362–1383. https://doi.org/10.1111/FEBS.16350.

Chapter 9

Bringing Senotherapeutics from Research to Patient Care

Status and Challenges

Razia Khanam

9.1 INTRODUCTION

The initial discovery of senolytic drugs focused on targeting antiapoptotic pathways in senescent cells, while more recent senotherapeutics have been identified through specific targeting of senescent cell markers. The ongoing failure of existing therapies and/or therapeutic ineffectiveness drives the persistent demand for better drugs with novel targets. While pharmaceutical industries invest billions in drug development, scientists also work tirelessly to identify novel targets of drug action. Targeting cellular senescence to reverse aging or treat neurological disorders, cancer, diabetes, and other conditions is a recent medical challenge. If proven effective, it has the potential to revolutionize the entire paradigm of disease treatment and management. Studies done so far cannot deny the crucial role of cellular senescence in human health, in principle. Its precise role in tissue repair, wound healing and tumor suppressive mechanisms by halting the proliferation of damaged cells have proved to be highly beneficial. However, the detrimental effects, like accumulation of senescent cells linked to aging and age-related diseases due to chronic inflammation and tissue dysfunction driven by the senescence-associated secretory phenotype (SASP), cannot be overlooked (Yoon & Han 2024; Quarta & Demaria 2024).

Based on the different subsets of senescent cells and their varied contribution in the process of tissue repair and regeneration, the existence of phenotypic diversity has come into the limelight. For instance, while expressing senescence markers, cells like neurons and adipocytes maintain partial functionality, but macrophages do not. Consequently, the development of novel agents that selectively target specific senescent cell populations has become a critical priority, leading to the ongoing advancement of second-generation senotherapeutics. While first-generation senolytics primarily aim to eliminate persistent senescent cells or suppress the secretion of SASP factors, second-generation approaches-such as senoblockers and senoreversers-are designed to prevent the onset of cellular senescence or reverse it, respectively.

DOI: 10.1201/9781003493969-9

Figure 9.1 shows an overview of first- and second-generation senotherapeutic drugs. The first-generation drugs have reached the clinical trials, whereas second-generation drugs are in the development stage (Quarta & Demaria 2024).

The field of senotherapeutics is currently experiencing rapid growth, with a significant number of clinical trials underway. Table 9.1 shows the clinical trials status of senolytic drugs and their key outcomes, whereas Table 9.2 depicts the status of clinical trials of senomorphic agents. Table 9.3 demonstrates few examples of senotherapeutics in clinical trials for specific age-related diseases

The present data shows that senotherapeutics have moved from promising preclinical models to active human clinical trials. While early results show potential for improving age-related conditions and eliminating senescent cells, the field is still in its early to middle stages, with ongoing trials seeking to establish long-term safety, efficacy, and optimal application for a wide range of diseases. To further establish these drugs in clinical settings, there is an utmost requirement of ambitious initiatives like:

- Identifying specific biomarkers that can accurately detect and monitor in-vivo senescent cells and assess their efficacy in various treatments.
- Understanding senescence heterogeneity to explore how senescence varies across different cell types and conditions.
- Developing targeted therapies to create interventions that can modulate senescence pathways with minimal adverse or toxic effects.
- Integrating various disciplines like genetics, molecular biology, and clinical research to translate the present findings into therapeutic strategies to improve health, reverse aging and other related disorders.
- Collaborating multi-centric advanced single-cell technologies for understanding the dynamic nature of senescence.
- Increasing governmental, non-profit, and private investments to accelerate research and clinical translation.

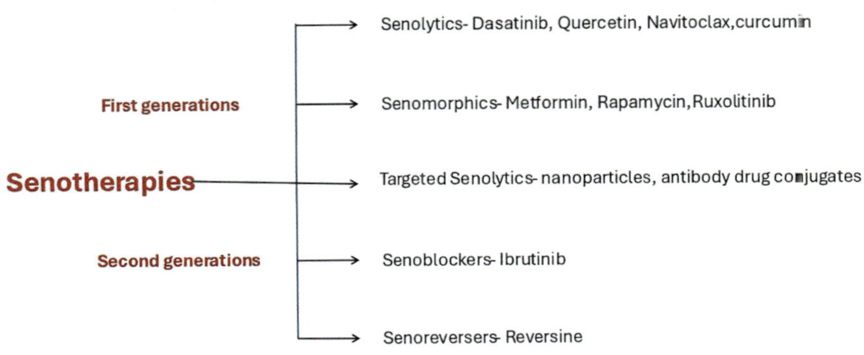

Figure 9.1 Overview of first and second generations senotherapeutic drugs.

Table 9.1 Prominent Senolytic Drugs in Preclinical and Clinical Studies

Drug Name	*Mechanism of Action*	*Preclinical Outcomes*	*Clinical Trial Status*	*Key Clinical Outcomes*	*References*
Dasatinib + quercetin (D+Q)	Tyrosine kinase inhibitor + BCL-2/PI3K/AKT inhibitor	Ameliorated age-related symptoms in mice; improved function in models of various age-related diseases	Phase 2 (IPF, AD, frailty, CKD, etc.)	Improved physical function in IPF; significantly decreases senescent cell burden in humans; CNS penetrance of dasatinib in AD	Gonzales et al. (2022); Hickson et al. (2019)
Navitoclax (low dose) ± venetoclax	BCL-2 family inhibitor	Eliminated senescent cardiomyocytes in mice; attenuated cardiac remodeling after injury	Phase 2/3 (various cancers)	Well tolerated, promising efficacy in patients with relapsed/refractory acute lymphoblastic leukemia or lymphoblastic lymphoma	Pullarkat et al. (2021)
Fisetin	BCL-xL, HIF-1α, PI3K inhibitor	Reduced senescence markers and extended lifespan in mice	Phase 2 (breast cancer survivors, frailty, COVID-19)	–	Farsad-Naeimi et al. (2018); Guo et al. (2019); Verdoorn et al. (2021); Wissler Gerdes et al. (2021)

Table 9.2 Prominent Senomorphic Drugs in Preclinical and Clinical Studies

Drug Name	*Mechanism of Action*	*Preclinical Outcomes*	*Clinical Trial Status*	*Key Clinical Outcomes*	*References*
Rutin	Interferes with ATM-HIF1α and ATM-TRAF6	Dampened SASP expression in senescent cells	Preclinical	–	Liu et al. (2024)
Ruxolitinib	JAK2/STAT3 inhibitor	Mitigated cardiomyocyte senescence in septic cardiomyopathy	Approved (myeloproliferative diseases)	Comparable efficacy to senolytics in preclinical SCM model	Verstovsek et al. (2017)
Resveratrol	Antioxidant, SIRT1 activator	Neuroprotective effects in AD models	Phase 2 (AD)	Reduced oxidative stress; potential delay in cognitive impairment	Liu et al. (2025)
Rapamycin	mTOR inhibitor	Prevented cognitive deficits and reduced AD pathology in mouse models	Phase 2a (AD)	–	Svensson et al. (2024)
Metformin	AMPK agonist, mTOR inhibitor	Extended lifespan in animal models; reduced age-related diseases in observational human studies	Approved (type 2 diabetes)	Potential reduction in cardiovascular disease and cancer incidence	Amin et al. (2019)

Table 9.3 Examples of Senotherapeutics in Clinical Trials for Specific Age-Related Diseases

Disease	*Senotherapeutic Agent(s)*	*Clinical Trial Phase*	*NCT Number (if available)*	*Key Objectives/Outcomes*	*References*
Diabetic macular edema	UBX1325	Phase 2B	–	Evaluate efficacy and safety	Klier et al. (2025)
Alzheimer's disease	Dasatinib + quercetin	Phase 2	NCT04685590	Evaluate safety, tolerability, and efficacy; assess CNS penetrance	Guerrero et al. (2021)
Breast cancer survivors (frailty)	Fisetin	Phase 2	NCT05595499,	Improve physical function; prevent frailty	ClinicalTrials.gov
Triple-negative breast cancer	Dasatinib + quercetin + chemotherapy	Phase 2	–	Evaluate efficacy and safety in chemo-resistant patients	Lewińska et al. (2022)

There is also the scope of more interventions like:

- *Microbiome and microbiota role in senescence*: The gut microbiota influences cellular senescence and skin disruption through the gut-skin axis and secretion of microbial metabolites. Metabolomics can be used to identify and quantify metabolites involved in senescence. Probiotics, prebiotics, and postbiotics may come up as effective alternatives to delay senescence, considering the relationship between microbiome and healthy aging. For this approach to be rationalized, the identification of specific microbial signatures or metabolites as biomarkers for biological age and senescence burden is required. Combination strategies using senotherapeutics and microbiota-senescence axis modulators for synergistic anti-aging effects can also revolutionize the approach to longevity and age-related diseases (Boyajian et al. 2021; Sharma & Padwad 2020).
- *Integration with senotherapeutics with gerotherapeutics*: Gerotherapeutics are known to modulate the molecular and cellular hallmarks of aging, shifting the medical focus from treating individual diseases to addressing the root processes of aging itself. The primary goal is to extend health span, not merely lifespan, representing a transformative shift in medical paradigms from a disease-centered model to an aging-centered approach. Notably, recent research highlights fisetin as a promising senotherapeutic agent with both geroprotective and senolytic properties, offering a compelling foundation for the development of next-generation therapeutics (Spiegel 2025).
- The integration of artificial intelligence (AI) into the clinical development of senotherapeutics at every stage has the potential to revolutionize drug discovery and accelerate therapeutic advancement. By streamlining target identification, optimizing compound screening, and enabling predictive modeling of treatment outcomes, AI integration can significantly enhance the efficiency and precision of senotherapeutic drug development.

To summarize, the senotherapeutics (senolytics, senomorphics, senoreversers etc.) target removing the harmful senescent cells, reducing chronic inflammation, suppressing SASP, improving the surrounding environment, exerting multi-system effects, acting on aging hallmarks, and so on. Overall, all these approaches show that senotherapeutics offer a holistic approach towards disease management, thereby making them a foundational, preventive, and integrative therapeutic strategy. In conclusion, the clinical translation of senescence-targeting therapies is still in its early stages, however the underlying conceptual and technological foundations are advancing rapidly. Senolytics and senomorphics hold the potential not only to revolutionize the management of chronic, age-related diseases but also to transform the healthcare model-from reactive disease treatment to proactive health preservation-ushering in a new era in the science of aging and regenerative medicine.

REFERENCES

Amin S, Lux A, O'Callaghan F. 2019. "The journey of metformin from glycaemic control to mTOR inhibition and the suppression of tumour growth." *Br J Clin Pharmacol* 85 (1): 37–46. https://doi.org/10.1111/bcp.13780.

Boyajian JL, Ghebretatios M, Schaly S, Islam P, Prakash S. 2021. "Microbiome and human aging: Probiotic and prebiotic potentials in longevity, skin health and cellular senescence." *Nutrients* 13 (12): 4550. https://doi.org/10.3390/nu13124550.

Farsad-Naeimi A, Alizadeh M, Esfahani A, Darvish Aminabad E. 2018. "Effect of fisetin supplementation on inflammatory factors and matrix metalloproteinase enzymes in colorectal cancer patients." *Food Funct* 9 (4): 2025–2031. https://doi.org/10.1039/c7fo01898c.

Gonzales MM, Garbarino VR, Marques Zilli E, Petersen RC, Kirkland JL, Tchkonia T, et al. 2022. "Senolytic therapy to modulate the progression of Alzheimer's disease (SToMP-AD): A pilot clinical trial." *J Prev Alzheimers Dis* 9 (1): 22–29. https://doi.org/10.14283/jpad.2021.62.

Guerrero A, De Strooper B, Arancibia-Cárcamo IL. 2021. "Cellular senescence at the crossroads of inflammation and Alzheimer's disease." *Trends Neurosci* 44 (9): 714–727. https://doi.org/10.1016/j.tins.2021.06.007.

Guo G, Zhang W, Dang M, Yan M, Chen Z. 2019. "Fisetin induces apoptosis in breast cancer MDA-MB-453 cells through degradation of HER2/neu and via the PI3K/AKT pathway." *J Biochem Mol Toxicol* 33 (4): e22268. https://doi.org/10.1002/jbt.22268.

Hickson LJ, Langhi Prata LGP, Bobart SA, Evans TK, Giorgadze N, Hashmi SK, et al. 2019. "Senolytics decrease senescent cells in humans: Preliminary report from a clinical trial of dasatinib plus quercetin in individuals with diabetic kidney disease." *EBioMedicine* 47: 446–456. https://doi.org/10.1016/j.ebiom.2019.08.069.

Klier S, Dananberg J, Masaki L, Bhisitkul RB, Khanani AM, Maturi R, et al. 2025. "Safety and efficacy of senolytic UBX1325 in diabetic macular edema." *NEJM Evid* 4 (5): EVIDoa2400009. https://doi.org/10.1056/EVIDoa2400009.

Lewińska A, Przybylski P, Adamczyk-Grochala J, Błoniarz D, Litwinienko G, Wnuk M. 2022. "Senolysis-based elimination of chemotherapy-induced senescent breast cancer cells by quercetin derivative with blocked hydroxy groups." *Cancers (Basel)* 14 (3): 605. https://doi.org/10.3390/cancers14030605.

Liu H, Xu Q, Wufuer H, Li Z, Sun R, Jiang Z, et al. 2024. "Rutin is a potent senomorphic agent to target senescent cells and can improve chemotherapeutic efficacy." *Aging Cell* 23 (1): e13921. https://doi.org/10.1111/acel.13921.

Liu X, Baxley S, Hebron M, Turner RS, Moussa C. 2025. "Resveratrol attenuates CSF markers of neurodegeneration and neuroinflammation in individuals with Alzheimer's disease." *Int J Mol Sci* 26 (11): 5044. https://doi.org/10.3390/ijms26115044.

Pullarkat VA, Lacayo NJ, Jabbour E, Rubnitz JE, Bajel A, Laetsch TW, et al. 2021. "Venetoclax and Navitoclax in combination with chemotherapy in patients with relapsed or refractory acute lymphoblastic leukemia and lymphoblastic lymphoma." *Cancer Discov* 11 (6): 1440–1453. https://doi.org/10.1158/2159-8290.CD-20-1465.

Quarta M, Demaria M. 2024. "On the past, present and future of senotherapeutics." *NPJ Aging* 10 (1): 11. https://doi.org/10.1038/s41514-024-00139-3.

Sharma R, Padwad Y. 2020. "Probiotic bacteria as modulators of cellular senescence: Emerging concepts and opportunities." *Gut Microbes* 11 (3): 335–349. https://doi.org/10.1080/19490976.2019.1697148.

Spiegel M. 2025. "Fisetin as a blueprint for senotherapeutic agents—elucidating gero-protective and senolytic properties with molecular modeling." *Chemistry* 31 (16): e202403755. https://doi.org/10.1002/chem.202403755.

ClinicalTrials.gov. 2025. *Fisetin to Improve Physical Function in Stage I–III Breast Cancer Survivors.* NCT05595499 [cited 2025 Nov 25]. Available from: ClinicalTrials.gov

Svensson JE, Bolin M, Thor D, Williams PA, Brautaset R, Carlsson M, et al. 2024. "Evaluating the effect of rapamycin treatment in Alzheimer's disease and aging using in vivo imaging: The ERAP phase IIa clinical study protocol." *BMC Neurol* 24 (1): 111. https://doi.org/10.1186/s12883-024-03596-1.

Verdoorn BP, Evans TK, Hanson GJ, Zhu Y, Langhi Prata LGP, Pignolo RJ, et al. 2021. "Fisetin for COVID-19 in skilled nursing facilities: Senolytic trials in the COVID era." *J Am Geriatr Soc* 69 (11): 3023–3033. https://doi.org/10.1111/jgs.17416.

Verstovsek S, Gotlib J, Mesa RA, Vannucchi AM, Kiladjian JJ, Cervantes F, et al. 2017. "Long-term survival in patients treated with ruxolitinib for myelofibrosis: COMFORT-I and -II pooled analyses." *J Hematol Oncol* 10 (1): 156. https://doi.org/10.1186/s13045-017-0527-7.

Wissler Gerdes EO, Misra A, Netto JME, Tchkonia T, Kirkland JL. 2021. "Strategies for late phase preclinical and early clinical trials of senolytics." *Mech Ageing Dev* 200: 111591. https://doi.org/10.1016/j.mad.2021.111591.

Yoon JH, Han HJ. 2024. "Senotherapeutics: Different approaches of discovery and development." *Mol Cells* 47 (1): 100002. https://doi.org/10.1016/j.mocell.2023.10.001.

Index

Note: Page locators in **bold** indicate a table and page locators in *italics* indicate a figure